# TREATING INTERNALIZING DISORDERS IN CHILDREN AND ADOLESCENTS

# Treating Internalizing Disorders in Children and Adolescents

*Core Techniques and Strategies*

Douglas W. Nangle, David J. Hansen,
Rachel L. Grover, Julie Newman Kingery,
Cynthia Suveg, and Contributors

THE GUILFORD PRESS
New York   London

*To our loving and supportive families, and to the
children and families who have been our clients
and enlightened us as clinicians*

Copyright © 2016 The Guilford Press
A Division of Guilford Publications, Inc.
370 Seventh Avenue, Suite 1200, New York, NY 10001
www.guilford.com

Printed in the United States of America

This book is printed on acid-free paper.

Last digit is print number:   9   8   7   6   5   4   3   2   1

The authors have checked with sources believed to be reliable in their efforts to
provide information that is complete and generally in accord with the standards
of practice that are accepted at the time of publication. However, in view of the
possibility of human error or changes in behavioral, mental health, or medical
sciences, neither the authors, nor the editor and publisher, nor any other party who
has been involved in the preparation or publication of this work warrants that the
information contained herein is in every respect accurate or complete, and they are
not responsible for any errors or omissions or the results obtained from the use of
such information. Readers are encouraged to confirm the information contained in
this book with other sources.

Library of Congress Cataloging-in-Publication Data is available from the publisher.

ISBN 978-1-4625-2626-0

# About the Authors

**Douglas W. Nangle, PhD,** is Professor and Director of the Doctoral Program in Clinical Psychology at the University of Maine. He has published extensively in the areas of social skills assessment and treatment, child and adolescent peer relations, and cognitive-behavioral treatments. An award-winning teacher and mentor, he has advised, taught, and provided clinical supervision for doctoral students for more than 20 years.

**David J. Hansen, PhD,** is Professor of Psychology, Director of the Clinical Psychology Training Program, and Director of the Center for Brain, Biology and Behavior at the University of Nebraska–Lincoln. His primary research area is child maltreatment (sexual abuse, physical abuse, and neglect), including assessment and intervention with victims and families, and the consequences and prevention of maltreatment.

**Rachel L. Grover, PhD,** is Associate Professor of Psychology at Loyola University Maryland, where she teaches undergraduate and graduate courses in child development, research methods, and child therapy. She conducts research on child anxiety as well as social competence in the teen and emerging adulthood years.

**Julie Newman Kingery, PhD,** is Associate Professor of Psychology at Hobart and William Smith Colleges in Geneva, New York. Her research examines the role of peer relationships as predictors of psychological and academic adjustment, particularly across the middle school transition, as well as factors related to the etiology and maintenance of anxiety in youth. She also has a particular interest in the developmentally sensitive implementation of cognitive-behavioral therapy with children and adolescents.

**Cynthia Suveg, PhD,** is Associate Professor of Psychology and Associate Director of Clinical Training in the Clinical Doctoral Program at the University of Georgia. Her research broadly examines the role of emotion-regulation processes in child adjustment.

# Contributors

**Matthew W. Kirkhart, PhD,** is Associate Professor and Chair of the Department of Psychology at Loyola University Maryland. His current research focuses on the cognitive processes involved with second-language acquisition and the identification of psychological factors associated with successful adaptation to chronic medical conditions.

**Amber A. Martinson, PhD,** is a medical psychologist at the VA Salt Lake City Health Care System, U.S. Department of Veterans Affairs. Her research interests include biological correlates of stress, sexual trauma, and chronic pain. Her clinical focus is on veterans with comorbid mental and medical conditions, including chronic pain, dementia, and life-limiting illness.

**Diana Morelen, PhD,** is a postdoctoral fellow in Clinical Child Psychology at the University of Michigan Department of Psychiatry. Her research focuses on the origins of children's emotion-related competencies and the role of these competencies in children's mental health. Dr. Morelen is interested in familial and environmental processes that influence and shape children's development of emotion regulatory processes, how emotion development occurs within diverse contexts, and how emotional processes help explain the intergenerational transmission of risk from parental to child psychopathology.

**Matthew P. Mychailyszyn, PhD,** is Assistant Professor of Psychology at Towson University. He is a licensed psychologist who conducts his clinical work at Mt. Washington Pediatric Hospital in Baltimore. Dr. Mychailyszyn's clinical and research interests focus on issues with pediatric feeding disorders as well as cognitive-behavioral therapy and parent training to address internalizing disorders and disruptive behaviors in youth.

**Jason M. Prenoveau, PhD,** is a licensed clinical psychologist and Associate Professor of Psychology at Loyola University Maryland. His research focuses on the etiology, phenomenology, and treatment of disorders of anxiety and fear.

**Jennifer Sauvé, PhD,** is a postdoctoral fellow in Child and Family Psychology at the University of Southern California University Center for Excellence in Developmental Disabilities/Children's Hospital Los Angeles. Her major interests include social relationships, anxiety, and adjustment among children and adolescents.

**Alayna Schreier, MA,** is a doctoral candidate in Clinical Psychology at the University of Nebraska–Lincoln. Her research interests include prevention and intervention for at-risk and maltreating families, early childhood intervention programs, and policy related to child welfare.

**Kristel Thomassin, PhD,** is Assistant Professor in the School of Psychology at the University of Ottawa. Her research focuses on children's emotional development, including the ways in which the family system contributes to children's development of adaptive emotion skills and the role of these emotion skills in child psychopathology. Dr. Thomassin seeks to translate this knowledge to the clinical care context as a means of gaining insight into how treatment approaches might be adapted to maximize therapeutic outcomes for youth.

**Tiffany West, PhD,** is Assistant Professor at the University of Arkansas for Medical Sciences and the Arkansas Children's Hospital. Her research and clinical interests are in the field of childhood traumatic stress and disruptive behavior disorders.

**Monica R. Whitehead, MS,** is a doctoral candidate in Clinical Psychology at the University of Georgia. Her research interests include social and emotional functioning of anxious youth and examining factors related to the therapeutic alliance and treatment outcome.

# Contents

# 1

## Introduction

It was not hard to find the inspiration for writing this book. Across our many years of collective practice, teaching, and supervision experience, we continually faced a similar frustration stemming from attempts to answer one simple question: Where could a student, instructor, or practitioner find comprehensive coverage of the underlying theoretical rationale and the "nuts and bolts" of the therapeutic techniques comprising the various evidence-based treatments? Not in journal articles, which offer very few, if any, specifics on the evaluated treatments. Book chapters offer more details than journal articles, but they tend to be organized by the specific disorder. Coverage of the etiology, assessment, and summaries of several different treatment approaches leaves insufficient room for the fine points on the underlying procedures and techniques of various treatments. Next in line are the treatment manuals. Although these offer far more practical information than articles and chapters, they also tend to have significant gaps in coverage and include very little on the conceptual underpinnings of the treatment strategies. Manuals most often describe multicomponent treatment packages, and the level of detail included for each component varies widely. For this reason, it is often necessary to consult a few different sources and "piece together" the information needed for implementation. And even then, there is no guarantee that such patchworking attempts will fill all of the gaps.

To help meet these needs, we took a much different approach in the development of this book, which is organized by the core elements of evidence-based treatments (EBTs) for internalizing disorders in children and adolescents. For example, EBTs for depression in youth consist of combinations of more basic elements, such as psychoeducation, relaxation training, problem solving, activity scheduling, cognitive skills, social skills training, and self-monitoring (Chorpita, Daleiden, & Weisz, 2005). Focusing on these basic or core elements offered important advantages over the more commonly encountered "treatment-by-disorder" approach. Devoting entire chapters to each element allowed for more in-depth coverage that includes the theoretical rationale behind each treatment strategy as well as "step-by-step" implementation suggestions. The included elements are the building blocks of the multicomponent EBTs. Once learned, they can facilitate manual use and be more flexibly applied to treat a wide range of presenting concerns.

Based upon growing discontent with some of the byproducts of the EBT movement, others have been touting the benefits of such "deconstruction" efforts as well (e.g., Chorpita & Daleiden, 2009; Garland et al., 2014). Before describing these efforts in more detail, a brief review of the EBT movement and some of the challenges encountered along the way is needed to provide a broader context for the core elements approach used for this book.

## THE MOVEMENT TOWARD EBTs AND SOME UNINTENDED CONSEQUENCES

Since Eysenck (1952) first asserted that psychotherapy was no more effective than the passage of time, several meta-analytic reviews have refuted that claim with child and adolescent samples (e.g., Casey & Berman, 1985; Weiss & Weisz, 1995; Weisz, Weiss, Alicke, & Klotz, 1987; Weisz, Weiss, Han, Granger, & Morton, 1995). On average, treated children scored better than about 76% of control group children across a variety of outcome measures (Casey & Berman, 1985). Further, it appears that not all treatments are equal in their effectiveness. Three meta-analyses have found that behavioral interventions result in larger effect sizes than nonbehavioral interventions (Casey & Berman, 1985; Weiss & Weisz, 1995; Weisz et al., 1987).

With the overall efficacy of child and adolescent treatments established, the field moved toward identifying the most effective treatments for particular disorders, a trend embodied by the empirically supported treatment (EST) movement (Chambless & Hollon, 1998; Task Force on Promotion and Dissemination of Psychological Procedures, 1995). The original EST list included only three "well-established" treatments and one "probably efficacious" treatment for children and adolescents, but the list was expanded in a subsequent task force review (Lonigan, Elbert, & Bennett Johnson, 1998). These efforts helped to build consensus on a standard set of guidelines for evaluating treatments and have had a transformative impact on the field. Nevertheless, the movement has also had some unintended consequences and its fair share of critics. A thorough review of these consequences and critiques is beyond the scope of this introduction, but some are particularly noteworthy in forming a rationale for our core element approach.

Many of the criticisms have targeted the "manualization" of psychotherapy, a byproduct of the EST movement. One of the criteria for meeting either "well-established" or "probably efficacious" status is the use of a treatment manual (Task Force on Promotion and Dissemination of Psychological Procedures, 1995). Manuals have played a critical role in the evaluation and dissemination of ESTs and often offer practical "how-to" information on treatment implementation. By operationalizing a treatment, manuals also promote adherence and reduce variability across clinicians (Ollendick, King, & Chorpita, 2006). At the same time, however, manuals have been criticized for limiting clinical innovation, ignoring the role of common factors (i.e., things all therapies have in common), promoting adherence to a single theoretical perspective, overemphasizing particular techniques, relying on diagnosis to match children to treatment, and disregarding the need to flexibly adapt treatment to meet the needs to individual clients (Herschell, McNeil, & McNeil, 2004).

Relying on diagnosis to match children to treatments has led to some significant concerns. A treatment-by-disorder approach does not reflect the complexity of the cases actually seen in practice, in which comorbidity is the norm (Angold, Costello, & Erklani, 1999). Another problem is that many disorders and clinical problem areas lack an established EST. Efforts to close this gap have uncovered further concerns. More than a decade ago, Kazdin (2000) estimated that there were some 500 documented treatments for youth, more than 35 of which met the two most stringent effectiveness standards (Chambless & Ollendick, 2001). For practitioners, the task of determining which treatment to use in a particular case has become increasingly complex, not to mention the challenge of attaining and maintaining sufficient levels of competence to carry them out. For researchers, time and resource limitations render the task of submitting the 500 documented treatments to controlled evaluation impossible to carry out.

For our purposes, the fact that manuals have seemingly come to *define* rather than exemplify treatment is one of the more significant problems (Westen & Weinberger, 2005). Specific treatment protocols are now often emphasized over the theoretically based treatment components (Chorpita et al., 2005). For example, cognitive-behavioral therapy (CBT) is a "probably efficacious" treatment for anxiety in youth (Silverman, Pina, & Viswesvaran, 2008). This treatment is exposure-based with psychoeducation, cognitive restructuring, relaxation, and contingency management components. Although there are many ways to operationalize this package, the Coping Cat manual (Kendall & Hedtke, 2006), by virtue of its established evidence base (e.g., Kendall et al., 1997; Kendall, Hudson, Gosch, Flannery-Schroeder, & Suveg, 2008), has come to be considered a "blueprint" of sorts. This is an interesting example because exposure is a key element that holds a prominent place in the history of behavior therapy. Like other elements, it has its own rich conceptual and empirical base (e.g., Nakamura, Pestle, & Chorpita, 2009; Peris et al., 2015; Seligman & Ollendick, 2011). The Coping Cat manual outlines just one of many possible ways to implement exposure. As aptly stated by Roth and Pilling (2008), a manual ends up specifying both "wheat and chaff" in that the overall package has demonstrated effectiveness but there is little "empirical basis for sifting effective from potentially ineffective strategies" (p. 131). Whether the steps laid out in the Coping Cat manual are the best ways to do exposure—or what combination, what order, and what "dose" of the constituent components are best—are not known. Another issue is that those regularly relying on such a protocol for guidance in conducting exposure (and other components) run the risk of losing touch with the treatment's historical, theoretical, and empirical foundations.

Concerns with the EST approach and more general trends in health care policy helped usher in the evidence-based practice of psychology (EBPP) movement, the latest iteration in this move toward improving the translation of psychological science into clinical practice (American Psychological Association, 2006). EBPP is considered to be a more comprehensive approach than EST. The EST approach starts with a treatment and whether it is effective for a certain disorder, whereas the EBPP approach starts with a patient and whether there is research evidence that will assist in achieving the best outcome. As such, EBPP encompasses consideration of the best available research evidence, clinical expertise, and patient characteristics. This new approach, however, does not address all of the concerns with EST outlined above and, in fact, can actually serve to amplify them. For example, the question of what treatment works for a given disorder now becomes what treatment works for a disorder when delivered by whom and for a child with what characteristics. Sensitivity to these factors can complicate clinical decision making and require increased judgment and flexibility in the application of treatments (American Psychological Association, 2006).

## A COMMON ELEMENTS APPROACH

To address some of the issues related to reliance on manuals and the need for increased flexibility in developing treatments, some have called for the "deconstruction" of evidence-based treatment packages to identify common elements that cut across protocols for a variety of disorders and clinical problem areas (e.g., Chorpita & Daleiden, 2009; Chorpita et al., 2005; Garland et al., 2014; Garland, Hawley, Brookman-Frazee, & Hurlburt, 2008). Chorpita and colleagues led the way in these efforts with the introduction of their distillation and matching model (DMM; Chorpita et al., 2005). In the distillation portion of the model, the authors propose that treatment protocols be viewed as composites of individual strategies, techniques, or components (i.e., practice elements) rather than single units of analysis. Examples of practice elements are activity scheduling, cognitive strategies and coping skills, parent praise, problem solving, self-monitoring, and time-out. Matching refers to a method for summarizing client, setting, or other study characteristics (such as diagnosis, age, gender, and ethnicity) that might be relevant when choosing a treatment. Applying the model, evidence-based treatment protocols could be coded in terms of their practice elements and the data analyzed to determine what practice elements are associated with successful treatments by diagnosis, age, gender, or ethnicity.

In an application of the DMM, Chorpita and Daleiden (2009) coded 615 treatment protocols derived from 322 randomized clinical trials with children and adolescents. Only "winning" treatments (i.e., those demonstrating effectiveness when compared to another active treatment or control group) were included in the analyses. The content of these protocols was then coded in terms of the presence or absence of 61 practice elements (14 removed, owing to low base rates). Matching variables, including age, gender, ethnicity, and problem area, were also coded. Using a complex data reduction approach, the authors identified meaningful patterns in the frequency of practice elements by matching the variables. For example, the most common practice elements for anxiety were exposure, relaxation, cognitive strategies, modeling, and psychoeducational–child. For depressed mood, the most common practice elements were cognitive strategies, psychoeducation with the child, maintenance and relapse prevention, activity scheduling, problem solving, and self-monitoring. These patterns did not differ by age or gender, but they did vary somewhat by ethnicity. For example, depression treatments targeting African American participants used a more restricted set of practices, including cognitive strategies, communication skills, and more frequent use of family therapy, whereas those targeting Hispanic youth had a higher frequency of psychoeducation with the parent and parent coping strategies and did not include goal setting and self-reward/self-praise.

This common element approach can be applied in a number of ways and offers advantages over more typical methods for selecting treatments (Chorpita et al., 2005). In selecting a treatment, a clinician could examine the practice element profiles (e.g., practice elements associated with successful treatments by problem area, age, gender, or ethnicity) to determine a best match for a child's problems and characteristics. Once selected, the clinician could choose a manual with content that best matches the resulting profile. For cases in which there is no established manual, the information could be used to identify the closest match based on the entire literature. In cases in which there are multiple manuals with empirical support, the resulting profile could provide a set of the most reliably tested practice elements for comparison purposes.

Another application would enhance flexibility by facilitating the "modular" reassembly of the practice elements to match specific targets. For example, in his modularized treatment for children with anxiety disorders, Chorpita (2006) describes a core treatment plan (i.e., psychoeducation, exposure tasks, and maintenance/relapse prevention) that can be supplemented as needed for a particular child, with one or more modules addressing disruptive behavior (e.g., timeout), parent behaviors that interfere with progress (e.g., active ignoring), depression (e.g., cognitive restructuring), poor motivation (e.g., praise and rewards), and social skills deficits (e.g., social skills training). In a recent controlled investigation, this type of modular design outperformed standard manual treatment and usual care conditions in the treatment of depression, anxiety, and conduct problems in youth (Weisz et al., 2012).

From our perspective, when it comes to implementation, an important limitation of the common elements approach is the continued reliance on manuals for guidance. As suggested by Garland and colleagues (2008), the identification and definition of common core elements can provide a useful language for clinicians. With time, the current focus on protocols may shift to more of a focus on the elements on which they are based. Intensive training and supervision could target common core techniques (e.g., exposure, relaxation, modeling, problem solving, cognitive restructuring) using effective methods to shape therapist behavior (e.g., behavioral rehearsal with feedback, video modeling, discussion of cases, printed materials and skills checklists, ongoing supervision). As the authors note, this type of training could improve the basic competencies of therapists and serve as a foundation for the implementation of particular treatment protocols with specific populations (Garland et al., 2008). Such training would not substitute for, but rather facilitate, the use of manuals.

## OVERVIEW OF THE BOOK

We liked the suggestion of Garland and colleagues (2008) that the common elements approach be used as a springboard for training, but were also painfully aware of the current lack of resources needed to make that happen. Thoughts, discussion, and idea sharing leading to this book predated the landmark publications of Chorpita and his colleagues (e.g., Chorpita & Daleiden, 2009; Chorpita et al., 2005). Instead, we were driven by practical training needs and what we saw as a gaping hole in the literature, one that we were constantly reminded of in our teaching and supervision duties. Below, we illustrate these needs using an example and then describe how we help address them in this book.

The typical scenario we faced was this: A graduate student comes in for clinical supervision, describes her assessment results, and asks for guidance on a suitable treatment. For illustration purposes, let's say that the case involves a 10-year-old girl with a diagnosis of major depressive disorder. The student is told to first scan the primary treatment literature and to consult the EBT list. After reading an excellent review by David-Ferdon and Kaslow (2008) and consulting the EBT list, she learns that group-based CBT is one potential treatment. As directed, she also delves into the primary literature and reviews some studies supporting the efficacy of this treatment (e.g., Stark, Reynolds, & Kaslow, 1987). When she becomes frustrated by the lack of detail in descriptions of what is actually done in this type of treatment, she is pointed to some book resources that provide further description (e.g., Kendall, 2012; Mash & Barkley, 2006; Weisz & Kazdin, 2010). After reviewing those, she returns and asks, "Yes, but what would I actually do in a session?" A representative manual is suggested (e.g., Stark et al., 2007). Recognizing the fact that she will need to adapt this group treatment for her individual case, she is at least pleased with the structure provided by the manual.

All is going well until she returns for supervision, noting that the manual instructed her to "model" giving more meaningful compliments to others and admitting that, although the manual gives a number of such instructions, she really has never been taught about modeling as an intervention technique. She asks for some helpful resources, and the supervisor is taken a bit off-guard. One solution may be to check other manuals for guidance, but although most mention modeling, none seems to actually describe how to do it. Another option is to scan the office bookshelves, but this too comes up empty in terms of practical "how-to" advice. Finally, it is to the web, where a long time searching and sifting leads to one or two resources from either the education or applied behavior analysis field (e.g., *www.txautism.net/uploads/target/VideoModeling.pdf*). Surely, there must be something! Modeling is such an established intervention technique (see Southam-Gerow & Chorpita, 2006, for a review). Beyond practical implementation suggestions, it would also be nice to be able to connect the student with modeling's substantial historical and theoretical bases (e.g., Bandura & Walters, 1963), but it is similarly difficult to find a summative resource for that purpose.

## Identifying the Core Elements

The first step in the process of formulating this book was to select the core elements. Because we were targeting internalizing disorders more generally, one of the complicating factors in this process was judging the relative ranking of elements essential in the treatment of some disorders but not others (e.g., exposure, activity scheduling). In the initial step of this process, the first three authors independently generated rank-ordered lists of the top 15 core elements found in the EBTs (i.e., well established or probably efficacious) for anxiety and mood disorders. Second, using the DMM (Distillation and Matching Model) analyses of Chorpita and Daleiden (2009), these same authors each developed a set of decision rules to generate a list of the most commonly occurring practice elements for internalizing syndromes.

An example of one set was (1) scan the Chorpita and Daleiden (2009) lists for anxiety and mood disorders, (2) identify a proportion (e.g., .50 would indicate that 50% of EBTs for a problem area used the practice element) cutoff point, (3) rank-order the resulting elements for anxiety and then mood disorders based on the proportions, (4) for overlapping elements (anxiety, mood) multiply the relative ranking and prioritize lowest products, and (5) consider the relative rankings of nonoverlapping elements. Finally, we surveyed 30 leading clinical child psychologists, many of whom were manual developers themselves. They were asked to rate how important each of 16 different elements was in the treatment of internalizing disorders and to add to the list if necessary.

This process resulted in agreement on the following core elements for this book: exposure tasks, cognitive strategies, problem-solving training, modeling, relaxation training, psychoeducation, social skills training, praise and rewards, activity scheduling, self-monitoring, goal setting, homework, and maintenance and relapse prevention.

## Chapter Content

Essential to our purpose was the devotion of an entire chapter to each included core element. This allowed for the type of detailed coverage not found in existing resources. Given an authored book, we were able to use a standardized chapter format, an instructional advantage over the more variable formats found in edited books. On a related note, the edited volumes tend to be organized by specific disorder and often are authored by the same small pool of experts, resulting in a fairly similar coverage across resources.

Each chapter follows this outline:

- Background of the Element
  - Brief History
  - Theory Base
  - Evidence Base
- The Element in Practice
  - "Core of the Core" Element
  - Developmental Adaptations
  - Diversity Considerations
- Conclusions
- The Element in Representative EBT Manuals
- Task Analysis of the Element
- Illustrative Case Example

The first half of each chapter covers the background of the element. This starts with a brief history, tracing back to the key points in the development of the element. Next, the theoretical basis underlying the use of the element is described. Importantly, this theory base coverage is *directly* linked to the element's application in the treatment of internalizing distress. Background coverage ends with a summary of the element's evidence base—as a stand-alone treatment, if applicable, and as part of a multicomponent intervention package. As part of this section, a table summarizing the element's inclusion in representative EBT manuals for internalizing disorders is included.

With the "bases" covered, the second half of each chapter turns to practical "how-to" information needed to apply the element. A hallmark feature of this section is the "core of the core" element section and its accompanying task analysis. Step-by-step guidance on implementation from beginning to end is provided in clear, easy-to-follow language. This is followed by suggestions for how to adapt the element for different developmental levels and to youth from diverse backgrounds. Each chapter closes with an illustrative case example.

## How to Use This Book

We envision this book being used to fill the niche previously described. As such, it is not considered a stand-alone source sufficient to guide treatment. This book provides comprehensive coverage of the core elements associated with the EBTs for internalizing disorders in youth, but it does not address all of the limitations of the common elements approach (Chorpita, Becker, & Daleiden, 2007; Garland et al., 2008). For instance, just because the identified core elements more frequently appear in EBTs does not mean that they are necessary or sufficient for exacting clinical change. Further, although combinations of certain elements are described, the book provides very little guidance on sequencing, coordination, intensity, and duration of the elements. Manuals can be very helpful in this regard, but, as discussed previously, they come with their own set of limitations. Finally, by drawing attention to the techniques and procedures used in EBTs, we do not want to leave the impression that other contextual factors, such as therapeutic alliance, are any less important. We assume that trainees and practitioners using this book will be developing and/or will have the requisite process competencies that ground all therapeutic endeavors.

With these caveats in mind, a solid grounding in the common core elements could help to facilitate the use of manuals for specific protocols targeting particular problem areas (Garland et al., 2008). This type of foundational training is often not done and would seem to be a much more efficient way to prepare future EBT practitioners. In addition to trainees who are learning the elements for the first time, more seasoned practitioners wanting a refresher on the basics will also find the book to be very useful, as will clinicians and researchers attempting to more flexibly apply individual elements or identify new element combinations for addressing particular problem areas. Collectively, it is our hope that the book will be helpful to educators, trainees, and practitioners interested in the conceptual underpinnings and practical considerations of evidence-based practices for youth with internalizing disorders.

# 2

## Exposure Tasks

### BACKGROUND OF THE ELEMENT

At the most basic level, exposure tasks involve intentional contact with a feared, yet safe, stimulus, and they are a core element of treatment programs for anxiety, trauma-based, and obsessive–compulsive disorders in youth (Freeman et al., 2014; Silverman, Ortiz, et al., 2008; Silverman, Pina, et al., 2008). Exposure tasks can take many forms, depending on the nature of the fear itself and the developmental level of the child as well as practical implementation issues. For instance, a therapist might assist a child who has a fear of speaking in class to overcome this fear by speaking in similar, but less-anxiety-provoking, situations (e.g., in front of the therapist, with familiar peers in a small group) until he or she is comfortable speaking in school. Other fears, such as worry about a parent dying, will necessarily be imaginal in nature. Regardless of the particular form, exposure tasks have a strong conceptual and empirical foundation (Jones, 1924; Nakamura et al., 2009; Peris et al., 2015), and this chapter begins with a brief review of this rich literature and the empirical base for the use of exposure tasks. The remainder of the chapter is practical, focusing on implementation of this strategy, with attention to developmental and diversity considerations. An illustrative case example of the use of exposure tasks in the treatment of a 9-year-old Hispanic boy with separation anxiety disorder is also included at the end.

## Brief History

The history of exposure tasks can be traced back to the beginnings of behaviorism. In 1924, Jones published the classic report "A Laboratory Study of Fear: The Case of Peter" as a follow-up to Watson's (1921) study on the acquisition of fears. Using an 11-month-old boy, Watson showed that fears could be conditioned and that the fears could generalize to other similar stimuli without further conditioning. Jones wondered whether fears could be "unconditioned" and, if so, whether the "unconditioning" would generalize to similar stimuli. Working with Peter, almost a 3-year-old, Jones observed that he initially showed great fear in response to a white rabbit and similar objects (e.g., a rat, a fur coat)—fear so intense that in the presence of the rabbit Peter screamed and threw himself on the floor. Over the course of a few months, the rabbit was gradually introduced to Peter, first in a cage 12 feet away from the child, until finally Peter was able to interact with the rabbit, permitting it eventually to nibble at his fingers. Jones's (1924) very careful documentation of Peter's "degrees of tolerance" (p. 465) not only provided evidence that exposures work but also generated hypotheses about the mechanisms of the effect. For instance, Jones noted particularly successful encounters with the rabbit whenever it was presented while Peter was eating candy or when in the presence of a "brave" friend or favorite adult. Modeling also appeared to enhance the child's fear reduction, as willing attempts to approach the rabbit often followed observation of a peer interacting positively with the animal. Such early observations paved the way for the development of theories relating to exposure tasks, including counterconditioning and increases in self-efficacy, among others.

Despite Jones's early demonstrations, it was only decades later, during the 1950s and 1960s, that exposure tasks were finally considered seriously as methods of treating fears. The cultural climate of the time strongly opposed the rise of behavioral techniques in favor of psychodynamic approaches (Bandura, 2004). Mainstream therapists minimized the progress attributable to exposure treatments by noting that such strategies treated only the symptoms, not the underlying cause, of the problems. In contrast, proponents of behavior therapy argued that psychodynamic therapists attempted to block the use of behavioral strategies in part because they likely derived some personal satisfaction as well as greater sense of power from the admiration they often received from their patients (Wolpe, 1958). Behavior therapists, rather than holding positions of power, attempted to empower patients to effect change on their own; in fact, the use of behavioral strategies, including exposure tasks, could be completed by the patient relatively independently.

Despite initial resistance, the lack of empirical support for psychodynamic approaches, in combination with the accumulating evidence for the use of exposure tasks (Lazarus & Rachman, 1957; Wolpe, 1958) and other behavioral strategies, provided fertile ground for a paradigm shift in the conceptualization and treatment of psychological problems broadly and anxiety specifically (Bandura, 1961). Since the early use of exposure tasks, literally thousands of books and empirical articles have been published on this core treatment element. Not only are exposure tasks now considered an acceptable treatment approach, they are an *expected* element of treatment programs for anxiety and related disorders.

## Theory Base

Theoretical debates regarding how exposure tasks work are ongoing since Jones's now classic 1924 study documenting their effectiveness. In fact, years of subsequent research suggest that there may be multiple ways that exposure tasks reduce anxiety and that the mechanisms may vary by the situation, the task, person, and even within an individual. This section covers some of the primary ways that exposure tasks may effect positive change, including counterconditioning, changes in self-efficacy, and cognitive and emotion processing. Having a solid grasp of the principles upon which exposure tasks are based will greatly facilitate the implementation of this core treatment element.

Counterconditioning is one of the earliest theories of exposure tasks, first demonstrated by Jones (1924). Counterconditioning involves teaching (i.e., conditioning) a new response to a feared stimulus by pairing it with a pleasant or desired stimulus. In so doing, the individual comes to associate the once feared stimulus with something pleasant, thereby inducing either a neutral or positive emotional reaction in place of the fear response. For example, in Jones' study, she had Peter sit in a high chair eating a desirable food. Each day, the rabbit was presented a bit closer to the child while he ate the food; over a period of time the child's fear response was replaced by a more positive response to the rabbit. Jones further observed that the child's fear of the rabbit also diminished when in the presence of a favorite adult, again showing that a strong fear response could be eliminated when the feared object was paired with pleasant stimuli.

Systematic desensitization, which built upon the principles described by early behaviorists (e.g., Jones, 1924; Pavlov, 1927; Watson, 1924), was formally introduced by Wolpe in 1958 and involved counter-conditioning. Using progressive muscle relaxation as the anxiety-inhibiting response, Wolpe developed systematic desensitization, whereby individuals are first induced into a state of relaxation and then exposed to anxiety-provoking situations of increasing intensity until the individual no longer experiences an anxious response in the presence of the feared stimulus. Wolpe contended that inducing a physiological state incompatible with anxiety while in the presence of an anxiety-provoking stimulus could significantly reduce fear. In other words, one could not be anxious if in a relaxed state (i.e., response inhibition). Importantly, Wolpe believed that exposure to feared situations should occur gradually and that much care should be taken when constructing the exposure hierarchy.

In contrast to Wolpe, who believed that systematic gradual exposure was key, Marks (1987) suggested that flooding could also be effective in reducing the fear response, thus challenging one of the key principles of Wolpe's theory. In flooding, the individual is exposed immediately rather than gradually to the feared situation. Though relaxation or other coping strategies can also be employed during flooding, Marks noted that fear reduction *will* occur as long as the individual does not escape or avoid the feared stimulus. This notion that successful treatment of anxiety must include exposure tasks in some form, and preclude engagement in avoidant behaviors, is consistent with Mowrer's (1947) two-factor model of avoidance learning.

Mowrer (1947) proposed that fears develop through classical conditioning principles whereby a neutral stimulus is paired with a feared stimulus. The fear response prompts the individual to avoid the stimulus or escape when in its presence. Fear is then maintained via operant learning processes in which avoidance of the feared stimulus reduces the negative emotions that one experiences and thus serves as a negative reinforcer of the avoidance. Theoretically, to disrupt this learning process, an individual must not experience a reduction in negative arousal as a result of avoidance, but instead should experience a reduction in the anxious response in the presence of the stimulus. For instance, a child may have learned to fear speaking up in class because a classmate laughed at him (or her) each time he asked the teacher a question. The child has learned to avoid speaking up in class to reduce his negative arousal. However, suppose that the classroom situation has changed and the child is no longer able to avoid speaking up in class. Over time, after speaking several times in class with success, the child realizes that he no longer experiences high anxiety while talking. Extinction has occurred in this example because the child's learned feared response significantly diminished as a result of speaking up in class. Fears that are not learned can also be reduced as a result of repeated exposure, and in this case the fear reduction is termed habituation (for a nuanced discussion of the relations between extinction and habituation, see McSweeney & Swindell, 2002).

Although gradual exposure may not be necessary to effect change, this procedure may be more palatable to extremely fearful individuals who are reluctant to engage in exposure tasks. Engagement in mildly anxiety-provoking tasks before highly anxiety-inducing tasks may help to gradually build confidence in the ability to successfully manage fear. In fact, Bandura's (1977b) theory suggests that engagement in exposure tasks is effective in reducing anxiety because it helps to build a sense of self-efficacy. In particular, Bandura emphasized the differences between response–outcome and efficacy expectations. Whereas the former refers to the belief that a particular behavior will lead to some outcome, the latter is the belief that one can carry out the behavior needed to achieve a desirable outcome. Popular treatment programs for anxiety in youth often structure treatment so that the first half focuses on skills building and the second half on skills practice. Structuring treatment in this way may in fact have the result of enhancing coping skills and building self-efficacy to enable youth to engage successfully in exposure tasks in the latter part of treatment. Empirical research supports this notion. Following participation in a CBT program, 6- to 14-year-old children were asked how much they would be able to help themselves feel more comfortable in three anxiety-provoking situations that were specific to the child. Youth showed significant gains in coping efficacy from pre- to posttreatment and additional gains from posttreatment to the 1-year follow-up (Kendall et al., 2008). A later study conducted with nearly 500 youth ages 7–17 years showed that changes in coping self-efficacy mediated treatment gains (Kendall et al., 2016). Other research has likewise supported an increase in coping efficacy as a mediator of change (Prins & Ollendick, 2003).

The notion of modifying associations between a stimulus and a fear reaction to reduce fear is consistent with cognitive-mediation and emotion-processing models (e.g., Beck, Emery, & Greenberg, 1985; Foa & Kozak, 1986). In particular, several researchers suggest that therapy change occurs through the modification of emotion schemas (Leventhal, 1984) or cognitive-affective schemas (Safran & Greenberg, 1991).

Regardless of the particular terminology used, the general idea is that when an emotion is experienced a corresponding schema for that emotion is activated. The schema includes information about the emotion (including the situation itself) and the action tendencies that are associated with the emotion (L. F. Barrett, 1998). For instance, the general action tendency associated with fear is escape, whereas the action tendency associated with interest is approach. In people with anxiety disorders, emotion schemas may be distorted, and that, in turn, may lead to maladaptive responding. To modify the distorted schema, the schema must be activated through some sort of exposure, and information incompatible with the schema must be presented for new memories to form. Foa and Kozak (1986) refer to this as "emotional processing" and suggest that exposures are effective because they provide an opportunity for accurate information to be integrated into the fear structure. Through exposures, new and more accurate associations are formed, and fear is reduced. Research is needed to examine the ways in which exposures might exert their effects via cognitive or emotional structures, and empirical support is mixed regarding whether changes in anxious self-talk mediate treatment outcome (e.g., Kendall et al., 2015; Prins & Ollendick, 2003).

Collectively, numerous theories for the effectiveness of exposure tasks have been posited, though many are lacking in empirical support. Though the issue of *how* exposure tasks exert their positive effects is still widely debated, there is little question that they *do* work. The evidence base for the use of exposure tasks is strong; this next section reviews empirical evidence for the inclusion of exposure tasks as a core element of treatment programs for youth with anxiety, trauma-based, and obsessive–compulsive disorders.

## Evidence Base

Chorpita and Daleiden (2009) conducted a review of common elements in treatment programs for youth and found that the vast majority of psychosocial treatments for anxiety in youth included exposure tasks. Undoubtedly, a plethora of data supports the use of exposure-based CBT programs for child anxiety, with positive outcomes documented up to 19 years posttreatment (Benjamin, Harrison, Settipani, Brodman, & Kendall, 2013; for a review, see Seligman & Ollendick, 2011, and Table 2.1). Most recently, the largest randomized controlled trial included nearly 500 youth between the ages of 7 and 17 years with a primary anxiety disorder. Results showed that a combination of exposure-based CBT

**TABLE 2.1. The Exposure Tasks Element in Representative EBT Manuals**

| | |
|---|---|
| *Coping Cat* (Kendall & Hedtke, 2006) | • The use of exposure tasks is explicitly incorporated. The fear hierarchy is constructed within the first few sessions and modified accordingly throughout treatment until exposure tasks begin. A gradual approach is used, with "easy" exposure tasks lower on the hierarchy, followed by increasingly difficult tasks. |
| *C.A.T. Project* (Kendall, Choudhury, Hudson, & Webb, 2002) | • As in Coping Cat, exposure tasks are explicitly used throughout the treatment program, once coping skills have been taught. |
| *Family-Based Treatment for Young Children with OCD* (Freeman & Garcia, 2009) | • The use of exposure and response prevention is explicitly incorporated following several sessions of parent and child education. Therapists specifically model the use of exposure and response prevention and teach the parents how to scaffold. |
| *OCD in Children and Adolescents* (March & Mulle, 1998) | • After learning a variety of coping skills, the youth are taught to "talk back to OCD" by resisting urges to engage in obsessions and compulsions. The youth are exposed to a variety of situations that typically elicit urges to engage in rituals and are taught to "boss them back" through resistance. |
| *CBT of Childhood OCD: It's Only a False Alarm* (Piacentini, Langley, & Roblek, 2007) | • Therapists assist the youth in creating an exposure hierarchy during the first few sessions of treatment, and exposure and response prevention begin in the following session.<br>• The children provide "thermometer ratings" to facilitate accurate reporting of anxiety ratings. |
| *CBT for Social Phobia: Stand Up, Speak Out* (Albano & DiBartolo, 2007) | • The youth are initially taught a variety of coping skills as well as social skills and assertiveness training. Then, they explicitly engage in a variety of social-focused exposure tasks. |
| *When Children Refuse School: A CBT Approach* (Kearney & Albano, 2007): Chapters 4 and 5 on internalizing symptoms | • Exposure tasks begin very early in the treatment process. Imaginal exposures are used first, followed by *in vivo* exposure tasks. The caregivers are encouraged to coordinate exposure tasks with school personnel, and therapists help to troubleshoot issues as needed. |
| *Treating Trauma and Traumatic Grief in Children and Adolescents* (Cohen, Mannarino, & Deblinger, 2006) | • Exposure is an explicit component of this treatment program. The youth create a "trauma narrative" that serves as a gradual exposure and helps the youth to process the experience.<br>• The youth may also engage in *in vivo* exposure tasks when they develop generalized avoidant fears. For instance, if a child is fearful of attending a new school as a result of being abused by a teacher at a previous school, then *in vivo* exposure is used. |

*Note.* Some book titles are shortened to conserve space. See the References at the back of the book for full titles.

and sertraline resulted in the greatest improvements, with commensurate outcomes for the CBT and sertraline-only conditions (Walkup et al., 2008). CBT is now considered a "well-established" treatment for child anxiety (Chambless & Hollon, 1998).

Although exposure tasks are most often embedded within multicomponent CBT programs that include a variety of other components (e.g., psychoeducation, problem-solving training, cognitive restructuring), research has attempted to isolate their unique effects on treatment outcome. For example, Kendall et al. (1997) treated 9- to 14-year-old youth with primary anxiety disorders with CBT and compared outcomes to those of a waitlist condition. The first half of treatment focused on psychoeducation and teaching skills to manage anxiety, whereas the latter part consisted of exposure tasks. CBT showed clinically significant gains over the waitlist condition across several measures, and the effects were maintained at a 1-year follow-up. Additional analyses used pre-, mid-, and posttreatment data to compare positive treatment change during the first (i.e., education) and second (i.e., exposure-based) portions of treatment. Results showed that treatment change occurred only during the second portion of treatment, which included the use of exposure tasks. It could be that the exposure portion of treatment was the active ingredient of the treatment; alternatively, it could be that the skills learned in the first half of treatment helped the child to successfully implement the exposure tasks, and thus all components contributed to positive change. Because the study was not designed specifically to identify the active ingredients of the treatment component, firm conclusions cannot be drawn.

A study by Nakamura et al. (2009), however, used an interaction element multiple-baseline design to specifically isolate treatment effects. Changes in anxiety levels, cognitive errors, and treatment outcomes as a function of exposure and/or cognitive/coping skills were examined in four youth with a primary anxiety disorder. The particular research design allowed for the examination of these treatment outcomes based on the addition or subtraction of exposure or cognitive/coping skills following a baseline period. Though results indicated that cognitive education might be helpful in triggering positive change for some children, the most consistent positive results were found for the use of exposure tasks. In particular, following the education component of treatment, positive change occurred only when exposure was implemented. Child-reported cognitive errors also decreased only when exposure tasks were used. Taken together, findings for child report outcomes were fairly consistent, suggesting that exposure tasks were necessary for positive treatment change. It is important to note, however, that at least one other study has found a steep decline in anxiety early in CBT, prior to the start of treatment (Chu, Skriner, & Zandberg, 2013), suggesting the need for additional research on the active ingredients of therapeutic change.

A recent study by Peris et al. (2015) provides perhaps the most convincing evidence to date for the effectiveness of exposure tasks in treating anxiety disorders in youth. Using a sample of nearly 500 youth ages 7–17 years, trajectories of anxiety symptoms were examined following the introduction of relaxation training, cognitive restructuring, and exposure tasks. For comparison, trajectories of anxiety symptoms in a combination (CBT + medication), medication, and medication placebo condition were also included. Results indicated that treatment progress accelerated only following the introduction of cognitive restructuring and exposure tasks but not following the introduction of relaxation training. Importantly, the positive effects of exposure tasks on symptom severity and global impairment remained even after accounting for the effects of prior techniques. Younger children showed steeper rates of improvement following exposure tasks in comparison to adolescents, as did children in the combination (CBT + sertraline condition) compared to the CBT-only condition. Though the introduction of exposure tasks and cognitive restructuring were followed by accelerated rates of improvement, improvements were not specific to the domain that the strategies were intended to address (e.g., exposure tasks targeting avoidance behavior, cognitive restructuring targeting anxious self-talk).

Other research likewise suggests the superiority of exposure-based strategies versus relaxation in the treatment of obsessive–compulsive disorder (OCD; Freeman et al., 2008). Exposure-based treatment for OCD includes an exposure component, which involves having the child come into contact with the situations that trigger his or her obsessions, and a response prevention component that involves resisting the urge to perform a ritual. Much data support the use of exposure and response prevention for youth with OCD of all ages and within the context of both efficacy and effectiveness work (Abramowitz, Whiteside, & Deacon, 2005; Freeman, Sapyta, et al., 2014; Torp et al., 2015).

Research has also documented the effectiveness of intensive, exposure-based one-session treatment (OST) for the alleviation of specific phobias in youth (Muris, Merckelbach, Holdrinet, & Sijsenaar, 1998; Öst, Svensson, Hellström, & Lindwall, 2001). Most recently, Ollendick et al. (2009) compared OST, an education support treatment, and a waitlist control using a randomized design for the treatment of specific phobias in youth ages 7–16 years. The OST condition was based on the notion that fears and avoidance are maintained through the child's belief in a catastrophic outcome upon interaction with the feared stimulus. During OST, children were gradually exposed over a period of approximately 3 hours to variations of the feared stimulus and were encouraged to make new conclusions about the stimulus following each exposure. In this way, information incompatible with the preexisting beliefs about the stimulus was reinforced. Results showed a significant benefit of OST over the other two conditions on measures of impairment, the percentage of children diagnosis-free at both post-treatment and 6-month follow-up, and overall amount of clinical significant improvement. Based upon child and parent report, treatment satisfaction was also higher for the OST (as compared to the education) condition.

In contrast to the exposure-based one-session treatment of specific phobias, the treatment of trauma in children and adolescents using exposure-based strategies typically lasts several months. Nonetheless, much empirical support now exists for the use of such strategies in youth who have experienced trauma (Cohen, Deblinger, Mannarino, & Steer, 2004, 2006). Most recently, Foa, McLean, Capaldi, and Rosenfield (2013) demonstrated the effectiveness of prolonged exposure therapy with girls between the ages of 13 and 18 years who sought treatment at a rape crisis center, in comparison to a supportive counseling condition. Results indicated greater reductions in posttraumatic stress disorder (PTSD) symptoms, secondary outcomes (e.g., depression symptoms), and global functioning. Gains were maintained at the 1-year follow-up, suggesting long-term positive outcomes of prolonged exposure therapy. The evidence base for prolonged exposure therapy in treating other traumas in youth, and with youth of various developmental levels, remains to be examined.

Several studies have examined characteristics of exposure tasks that may moderate their effectiveness. For instance, though both imaginal and *in vivo* exposure tasks are frequently used, early research examining the effectiveness of this technique suggests that live may be more powerful than imaginal methods (Bandura, 1969; Marks, 1987; Ultee, Griffioen, & Schellekens, 1982). Despite these findings, imaginal exposures are often used when first beginning exposure tasks with children and when fears and anxieties are more abstract (Kendall, Robin, et al., 2005). Other research has examined children's behavior during exposure tasks and relations to outcome (Hedtke, Kendall, &

Tiwari, 2009). In a sample of 87 children ages 7–13 years with anxiety disorders, Hedtke et al. (2009) found that the use of safety-seeking behaviors (i.e., behaviors that function to increase a sense of safety in the presence of perceived threat and thus serve or can serve as a means of avoidance) during exposure tasks related to poorer treatment outcome on several measures. The only exposure characteristic that related to treatment outcome was the number of exposure tasks carried out, with a greater number of tasks associated with poorer outcome. This finding was in contrast to previous work that found a greater number of exposures related to better treatment outcome (Vande Voort, Svecova, Brown Jacobsen, & Whiteside, 2010). Fewer exposure tasks might have given the therapists more time to prepare for and process each exposure task, which may be more important for treatment outcomes than the number of tasks (Hedtke et al., 2009), and a later study allowed for a test of this hypothesis. Tiwari, Kendall, Hoff, Harrison, and Fizur (2013) examined the preparation for exposure tasks and the postprocessing of the task in relation to outcomes in a sample of 61 7- to 14-year-old youth with an anxiety disorder. Exposure task preparation was not related to the outcome, but postexposure processing was. Further analyses indicated that treatment responders were more likely to have been rewarded for completing the exposure task and were more likely to have been assigned an exposure task for homework than were treatment nonresponders. The authors speculated that processing of the exposure may have enabled the youth to challenge the maladaptive schemas associated with their feared stimulus. The processing of the exposure may have also enabled the youth to reflect on their coping efforts, gain a sense of control over the feared situations, and then build their self-efficacy. Finally, Gryczkowski et al. (2013) showed that earlier implementation of exposure tasks in the context of treatment programs that are shorter than typical manual-based CBT programs is associated with positive treatment outcomes.

Collectively, there is much empirical support for the use of exposure tasks in treating anxiety in youth. One might wonder, however, whether exposure tasks might negatively affect the therapeutic relationship, which has been related to treatment outcomes with highly anxious youth (Creed & Kendall, 2005; McLeod & Weisz, 2005). Kendall et al. (2009) examined this question and found that, across reporters, alliance showed an initial positive steep growth, followed by a reduced rate of growth, over the course of treatment for both the exposure-based treatment and the education/support condition. Importantly, the exposure-based treatment outperformed the education/support condition in diagnostic outcomes. Thus, exposure tasks are the treatment of choice for anxiety in youth and are unrelated to the therapeutic alliance.

## THE ELEMENT IN PRACTICE

The remainder of this chapter is practical, focusing on the implementation of exposure tasks. Issues of diversity and development when conducting exposure tasks are considered. The task analysis in Box 2.1 summarizes key steps involved in conducting an exposure task, and the case summary in Box 2.2 (at the end of the chapter) provides an illustrative example of the use of this core element.

### "Core of the Core" Element

A strong therapeutic alliance will provide a solid foundation for the introduction of exposure tasks. Assuming that a strong therapeutic alliance is already in place, there is no reason to worry that the implementation of exposure tasks will damage the relationship (Hedtke et al., 2009; Kendall, Robin, et al., 2005). Nonetheless, the therapist should be mindful that asking youth to face their fears is inherently stressful, sometimes for both the therapist and youth. To help ease the anxiety and reticence associated with the introduction of exposure tasks, therapists can encourage the youth's full participation in the process, welcoming questions and collaboration along the way. Providing a clear and developmentally sensitive rationale for the use of exposure tasks will further help to facilitate rapport.

Once rapport has been established (Step 1), the second step in conducting exposure tasks is to generate a list of anxiety-provoking situations with the child to facilitate the creation of the fear hierarchy (see Box 2.1 for a task analysis of exposure tasks). The fear hierarchy consists of a list of anxiety-provoking situations generated by the child that are then ordered by the amount of anxiety that they produce. Situations that produce mild levels of anxiety are listed first, while events that evoke high levels of anxiety are listed last. Once children learn skills to cope with their anxiety, they will practice the skills learned in therapy in each of the situations listed on the hierarchy (see Figure 2.1 for a sample hierarchy).

Children with anxiety disorders often present with multiple diagnoses. To keep things manageable, it might be helpful to separate the

## BOX 2.1. Task Analysis of Exposure Tasks

1. Facilitate the youth's engagement in exposure tasks by providing a clear and developmentally sensitive rationale and by being open to the youth's questions throughout the initial discussion and the entire process.

2. Generate a list of anxiety-provoking situations.
   a. Encourage the youth to list all situations that make him or her anxious, regardless of the level of anxiety.
   b. Consider creating separate hierarchies if the youth has fears/anxieties that span numerous themes (e.g., social situations, fear of germs). Another option is to create a second hierarchy, if needed, after successful completion of the first.
   c. Separate the situations into easy, medium, and hard.
   d. Assign a numerical rating to each situation within each category from 0 to 8 based on how anxiety-provoking the situation is (SUDS [subjective units of distress] ratings).
   e. Complete the hierarchy by listing by increasing level of difficulty all situations that were generated.

3. Decide in a collaborative manner which exposure task the youth will complete first.
   a. Assist the youth with this decision to help maximize the chance of success.
   b. Secure props, if necessary, or otherwise plan on how the exposure will be carried out logistically.

4. Generate a plan for completion of the exposure task.
   a. Facilitate the youth's use of learned coping skills during the exposure task by providing reminders and gentle prompts as needed.
   b. Practice or role-play the exposure tasks with the youth.
   c. Generate a list of potential outcomes for the exposure task and problem-solve possible difficulties.

5. Conduct the exposure task.
   a. Assess the youth's SUDS ratings before beginning the exposure.
   b. Continue to assess SUDS ratings periodically throughout the exposure task if possible, to determine an optimal stopping point.
   c. End the exposure task when it is successfully completed (e.g., it naturally ended) or when SUDS ratings have decreased from preexposure levels.

6. Process the exposure task once it is completed.
   a. Reward the youth for his or her effort in completing the exposure task, even if it was not completed exactly as intended.
   b. Encourage the youth to identify helpful coping strategies as a means of increasing a sense of control over the situation, and self-efficacy.
   c. Assist the youth in identifying parts of the exposure task that were particularly challenging and generate potential solutions for future tasks.
   d. Encourage the youth to challenge maladaptive cognitions regarding the feared situation using evidence from the exposure task.

7. Collaboratively choose the next exposure task.
    a. Consider choosing an easier exposure task if anxiety in the first exposure task was much greater than anticipated, to help secure the youth's engagement in the task.
    b. Choose exposure tasks that will be completed out of session as well as tasks to be completed during the next therapy session.
    c. Be sure to consider logistical issues when planning exposure tasks.

child's fears or anxieties based on themes. For instance, if a child has both separation fears and socially related ones, the therapist and child can decide which to focus on first, perhaps by identifying which is causing the most impairment. Next, the youth can generate a list of situations that are anxiety-provoking. Initially, the therapist can encourage the child to generate the situations without considering the level of anxiety produced; the goal of this first step is to generate as many situations as possible. The therapist can also assist the child by raising related situations as potential sources of anxiety; doing so will help him or her gain a better understanding of the nature of the child's anxiety. For instance, perhaps a child with separation anxiety notes that he gets worried if his mother goes somewhere in the evening without him. The therapist might then ask if the child also gets worried when his mother goes out during the day. In this case, learning about the particular times of day

| Situation | SUDS rating |
|---|---|
| Spend the night at a friend's house | 8 |
| Stay with a babysitter while the caregiver goes out at night | 7 |
| Take the bus to and from school | 6 |
| Play in a different room of the house than the caregiver is in during the evening hours | 5 |
| Refrain from calling the caregiver while she is at work | 4 |
| Go to a friend's house to play during daytime hours for a brief period of time without the caregiver | 3 |
| Play in a different room of the house than the caregiver is in during daytime hours | 2 |

FIGURE 2.1. Example of an exposure hierarchy for a child with separation anxiety disorder.

when the anxiety is greatest will facilitate properly developing the fear hierarchy. The therapist can also use pretreatment assessment data as a source of information about anxiety-provoking situations. Examining assessment data may be particularly helpful in cases where the child has difficulty generating situations or is reluctant to do so.

Once a list has been generated, the therapist can assist the child in classifying the situations into easy, medium, and hard categories (Kendall et al., 2009). Easy situations are likely to be those that the child acknowledges elicit anxiety, but at mild levels. Medium situations create more anxiety for the child, whereas hard situations may be so anxiety-provoking that the child cannot imagine ever facing them. Once the situations have been sorted into broad categories, the child and therapist can collaboratively assign subjective units of distress (SUDS) ratings to each situation (Wolpe, 1969). SUDS ratings can be captured using whatever scale the child is most likely to understand, though popular treatment programs for anxious youth (e.g., Coping Cat; Kendall & Hedtke, 2006) use a 0- to 8-point scale in which increasing numbers reflect greater anxiety. A feelings thermometer that visibly demonstrates increasing anxiety with corresponding number anchors can also assist in assigning SUDS ratings to the situations.

Sometimes children will have difficulty in differentiating the SUDS ratings and assigning numbers to each situation. A variety of strategies that can be used to assist the child with assigning accurate ratings are reviewed in the "Developmental Adaptations" section of this chapter. Sometimes it is difficult for the child to assign ratings or to rank-order particular situations, even after using a variety of strategies to assist with the process. In cases such as this, the ratings may become clear after exposure tasks have been started and the therapist has observed the child's behavior in a particular situation. At other times, the child may give a rating to a situation that the therapist feels fairly confident is inaccurate. For instance, a child might minimize the anxiety he or she would likely feel in a given situation. Or, a child might provide a very low rating (0 or 1) for a situation because, by reporting no anxiety, he or she hopes that it might not be placed on the hierarchy (and thus the youth would not have to practice that situation!). When a child seems to be minimizing his or her anxiety, the therapist might initially include the situation and then encourage the child to *really imagine* what the situation might be like, to obtain a more accurate SUDS rating. Or, the therapist might have the child recall a recent similar situation where the he or she experienced high levels of anxiety. Often, using such questioning and imagining will help the child to generate more realistic expectations. If it does not, however, the therapist could move forward with the ranking provided by the child but modify the exposure slightly by breaking the task down into smaller steps to ensure that the child has a successful experience. For instance, if a child who is separation anxious indicates very low SUDS ratings for a sleepover but has not yet even played at a friend's house, the therapist can encourage a daytime and then an evening playdate before attempting the sleepover. In the few cases in which the child says that a clearly anxiety-provoking situation does not cause anxiety for him or her, the therapist might encourage the child to just try the experience out after they have successfully completed at least a few other exposures. In both instances, however, the goal is to help the child create a relatively accurate fear hierarchy to facilitate success with the exposure tasks. Once each situation has a corresponding SUDS rating, the situations can be arranged in order of difficulty in a pyramid style or in the format of a ladder, with each rung representing an anxiety-provoking situation.

Once the hierarchy has been created, the child and therapist can work together to decide which situation should be used for the very first exposure task (Step 3). This collaborative approach is particularly important when several situations receive the same rating or when the child could not decide on a precise rating for a particular situation (e.g., in the case of social anxiety, a child assigned answering the phone at home a "2–3"). The important issue here is to choose an exposure task that has a high likelihood of success, which is most likely to be one from the bottom of the fear hierarchy. The therapist also needs to consider potential logistical issues (e.g., arranging for an interaction with another child). He or she will also need to be mindful of liability issues. For instance, if a child has a fear of driving over bridges, the therapist might drive with the child over a bridge during an exposure task. But if there is an accident during the exposure task, who is liable? Sometimes, clinic or university policy will dictate the exposure tasks that can actually be carried out. When policy precludes exposure tasks being completed outside of the office, then the therapist will need to be creative when designing the tasks. For example, the child could watch a video of someone driving over a bridge during the session and then actually experience the *in vivo* exposure with his or her family outside of the session.

At times, an exposure task may be effective only if the child cannot anticipate it, such as with a child who fears that her caregiver will be late picking her up from school. In such instances, an effective exposure task might be to have the child's caregiver deliberately pick her up a few minutes late from the therapy appointment or from school, with no particular warning to the child. So as not to violate the child's trust, the therapist can let both the child and parent know in advance that sometimes exposure tasks will be unplanned and occasionally even unpleasant. The therapist can emphasize that the therapist will give the child an exposure task only when he or she is confident that the child can successfully manage the experience.

Evidence on the amount of preparation needed for exposure tasks with children is mixed (Hedtke et al., 2009; Tiwari et al., 2013). Even so, some advance preparation appears to be wise—if for no other reason than to engage the child and maintain rapport. In preparing for an exposure task, the therapist can practice or role play the situations with the child (Step 4). He or she can encourage the child to use coping skills during the practice exposure and have the child identify which skills were most helpful. The therapist can also help the child to suggest potential difficulties that might occur during the exposure and assist with problem solving them. For instance, during an exposure that requires a youth to give a speech, the child might worry what would happen if he or she forgot what to say. The therapist can help the child generate a list of strategies to successfully manage the experience. For instance, the therapist could encourage the child to briefly glance at a note card that includes a cue to remind him or her what to say, or even to use a coping thought such as "Many kids who give speeches forget what to say sometimes—it's not the end of the world!"

Following preparation, the therapist and child conduct the exposure task (Step 5). The therapist should assess the child's SUDS ratings before the exposure task begins and throughout the task, if it is possible to do so. Sometimes it will not be possible to assess SUDS ratings throughout, or doing so may interfere with the actual task. When it is possible to collect the ratings during the task, however, the child should stay in the situation until the SUDS ratings have decreased—for however long it takes for the anxiety to decrease, if feasible. If the child does not stay in the situation long enough for the SUDS ratings to decrease, then he or she will have escaped (i.e., avoided) the source of anxiety. Because the child will most likely experience a decrease in SUDS ratings once he or she leaves the situation, the child will be reinforced for avoiding the situation, which will serve to maintain the anxiety. When it is not possible to gather ratings during the exposure task, the therapist can collect SUDS ratings after the task is finished.

Importantly, the therapist and youth should process the exposure task fully once it has been completed (Step 6; Ollendick et al., 2009;

Tiwari et al., 2013). Processing the experience provides an opportunity for the youth to identify helpful and potentially unhelpful coping strategies, to challenge anxious thoughts, and to build self-efficacy. If the youth has difficulty in processing the exposure, the therapist can guide the processing, but he or she should encourage the child's reactions. Theoretically, exposure tasks work in part by providing corrective information to the fear structure (Foa & Kozak, 1986); thus, it is important that the child make appropriate conclusions regarding the exposure task. Facing fears is a stressful task! Processing the experience in a positive way will also help the child to remain a willing participant in treatment. The youth should also be provided with rewards that are commensurate with the difficulty of the exposure task. For completing comparatively mild anxiety-provoking tasks, the child should choose from a list of small rewards, whereas for those that evoke higher anxiety the child can receive a very special reward (see Chapter 9 for greater elaboration on rewards).

Following the processing of the latest exposure task, the therapist and youth can decide which exposure to complete by the next therapy session (Step 7). Sometimes, the therapist and child realize that the child's anxiety is more severe than originally anticipated, and an easier exposure task is chosen. At other times, it might be clear to the therapist that the child is ready for a more difficult task. Either way, the therapist should use behavioral observations from the previous exposure tasks, along with the child's input, to collaboratively choose the next task.

Importantly, the assignment of exposure tasks for homework has been associated with positive treatment outcomes (Tiwari et al., 2013), so the therapist and child should also agree on which tasks to do for homework. Note that throughout this discussion there has been an emphasis on collaboration, and as Kendall, Robin, et al. (2005) observe, one should consult with the child—"but not in the 'Negotiation Trap'" (p. 142). In short, encourage the child to be part of the process, but be clear on what must be completed. For instance, it is not an option to not do an exposure task; however, the therapist can let the child choose which exposure task to do, whether in session or for homework. Likewise, if a youth shows much more anxiety than was anticipated during an exposure, stopping midway through is not an option, but modifying the exposure task might be. It can be upsetting for therapists to observe a child's distress during an exposure task. Therapists should seek support from colleagues as needed, because it will be crucial for the therapist to stay calm, firm, and warm throughout the process of completing exposure tasks.

## Developmental Adaptations

Unlike some CBT strategies that are used more frequently with older or more developmentally mature youth, exposure tasks can be used with youth of all ages. There is some preliminary data, however, suggesting that exposure therapy may be less effective with adolescents (Drysdale et al., 2014). In particular, Drysdale and colleagues suggest that adolescents experience emotion regulation difficulties, in part because of an imbalance in the development of brain structures involved in emotional reactivity and regulation. The amygdala, which mediates fear learning, is functional early in life—in contrast to the prefrontal cortex, which is not fully developed until young adulthood. The result of this imbalance is heightened emotional reactivity that is difficult to regulate. In both rat and human samples, Drysdale and colleagues found that the rate of extinction was significantly lower in adolescent, than in child or adult, samples. A *post hoc* analysis of treatment outcome data also revealed a pattern (albeit not a significant one) in which adolescents benefited the least from CBT, compared to child and adult groups (Drysdale et al., 2014). As the authors emphasize, the *post hoc* analysis of the treatment data could not isolate the effects of exposure tasks only; however, in combination with the experimental work described previously, the data do provide indirect support for their hypothesis that adolescents may be less responsive to exposure therapy.

Further research will help to clarify the ways in which development can influence the impact of exposure tasks. For now, exposure tasks are a core element of anxiety, trauma-based, and obsessive–compulsive disorders for youth of all ages. Because the use of exposure tasks taps a variety of skills and abilities, attention to a youth's developmental level will help the exposure task to proceed smoothly and will maximize its effectiveness. Attention to developmental level begins when explaining the rationale and logistical aspects of exposure tasks. Younger children will likely benefit from a simple explanation, whereas adolescents may appreciate a more nuanced discussion surrounding the use of exposure tasks. When describing the fear hierarchy, terms such as "fear ladder" may be used with younger youth. Keep in mind that tailoring the discussion of exposure tasks based on developmental level will hopefully serve to engage the youth in the therapy process. Consequently, therapists can assess the youth's understanding along the way, being sure to invite questions and clarifications.

SUDS ratings provide the basis of the fear hierarchy, and, thus, accurate ranking of situations is important. Youth with anxiety disorders have been shown to experience their emotions with greater intensity than typically developing youth (Suveg & Zeman, 2004), which may make differentiation between the ratings difficult. Younger or cognitively delayed youth may also have difficulty in differentiating SUDS ratings (Suveg, Comer, Furr, & Kendall, 2006). For instance, a younger child may not be able to differentiate a SUDS rating of 4 from a 6. To help youth assign ratings most accurately, a "feelings thermometer" can be used (Kendall, Robin, et al., 2005). The feelings thermometer has a simplified SUDS scale from 0 to 8, and each number has a descriptor (e.g., 0 = *this is a cinch*). The therapist can also model situations in which he or she felt "a little" nervous, versus those where he or she felt "very very nervous." For instance, the therapist can describe a time when he felt nervous at about a "3," focusing on the physiological, cognitive, and behavioral components. The therapist can then contrast the experience with a time when he felt anxious at about a "5." In each example, the therapist can vividly describe the situation to help the child see the differences in the ratings. The therapist can also directly ask a child about a situation to help with the accuracy of SUDS ratings. For instance, a therapist can ask a child who has a fear of going for a playdate to a friend's house to imagine the situation and then describe what his or her body feels like and what he or she is afraid will happen. Sometimes children have difficulty generating situations and ratings without prompts, but with direct questioning they can provide accurate responses. Even with these modifications, providing accurate SUDS ratings may still be difficult for some youth. In such cases, youth can categorize situations into easy, medium, and hard without assigning ratings. Then the therapist can use behavioral observations and reports from others to help arrange items on the fear hierarchy.

Preexposure preparation and postexposure processing may also vary by developmental level. Whereas therapists often lead the design of exposure tasks for younger youth, older youth can be encouraged to take a primary role (Kendall, Choudhury, Hudson, & Webb, 2002). Exposure planning and processing often involve a discussion of anxious thoughts. As noted earlier, one theory of exposure tasks is that they help to challenge maladaptive beliefs about anxiety-provoking situations, which would require the youth to be able to identify thoughts. However, younger or cognitively delayed youth may have difficulty with the cognitive component of exposure tasks. In such cases, therapists can greatly simplify this component of exposure tasks by using the cognitive strategies discussed in Chapter 3. Therapists can also place greater emphasis on the physiological rather than the cognitive components of anxiety before and after exposure tasks. For example, therapists can help the youth identify whether they had "butterflies in their stomach" before, during, or after the exposure task. They can also encourage the youth to compare his or her physiological state before versus after the task. Some CBT programs include a workbook that the child uses to facilitate learning the skills and to document out-of-session activities (e.g., Coping Cat; Hedtke & Kendall, 2006). Documenting the exposure tasks, where the child writes each step of the coping plan and then documents the outcome, might be tedious for younger youth or those with specific developmental challenges (e.g., writing problems, learning disabilities). In such cases, the therapist can think about the purpose of the activity and make modifications as necessary. For instance, the child could audio record herself while verbally processing the out-of-session exposure task and bring it to the next session for the therapist. Alternatively, some children may prefer drawing (rather than writing about) the experience. For children who do prefer to write, the focus should be on processing the exposure task, not spelling, grammar, or similar issues. As outlined in Coping Cat (Hedtke & Kendall, 2006), out-of-session tasks should be "Show That I Can" activities designed to encourage the practice of skills out-of-session and to build self-efficacy rather than typical school-like homework activities. These modifications can also be made for adolescents, who may be hesitant to complete tasks that are similar to typical homework tasks.

Social development should also be assessed, particularly given some research that suggests that youth with social phobia show less of a response to CBT programs than youth with other disorders (Crawley, Beidas, Benjamin, Martin, & Kendall, 2008). Youth with delays in social development may need education and practice in basic social skills prior to engaging in exposure tasks. The literature suggests that exposure-based treatments that incorporate social skills may result in improved outcomes for youth with social phobia (Beidel et al., 2007; Masia-Warner et al., 2005). Recently, Sarver, Beidel, and Spitalnick (2014) reported on the use of a virtual reality experience for youth with social anxiety to practice social skills. The virtual reality experience targeted greetings and initiating conversations, giving and receiving compliments, assertiveness, and maintaining conversations. The environment could be adjusted for the level of interactional difficulty, and the skills were practiced in the context of interactions with a range of characters (e.g. principal, school bully, popular classmate). Overall, both children and parents were satisfied with the virtual reality experience and found it easy to use. Programs such as this allow the therapist to modify important treatment components in developmentally sensitive ways that may be best received by the child.

Developmental modifications may also involve the family. The empirical literature is widely mixed as to whether there are treatment outcome benefits to including families in treatment (see Breinholst, Esbjørn, Reinholdt-Dunne, & Stallard, 2012, and Wei & Kendall, 2014, for reviews). However, there may be practical reasons to involve the family in treatment. For instance, in the case of youth with separation fears, exposure tasks will almost always involve the caregivers. Similarly, some youth might need parental assistance to complete out-of-session exposure tasks and to reinforce the skills that are learned in therapy. Adolescents, who often desire increased autonomy (Allen, Hauser, Bell, & O'Connor, 1994), may prefer that caregivers not be involved in treatment. For motivated teens, it may not be necessary to have much parental contact except for occasional check-ins to which the teen is privy. Undermining an adolescent's developing autonomy may be harmful to the therapeutic relationship, which may then negatively influence treatment engagement and outcomes. In cases where a therapist believes it is necessary to involve the caregivers in some way despite the teen's resistance, a warm, yet direct and genuine, conversation with the teen may be best.

## Diversity Considerations

The vast majority of randomized clinical trials that included an evaluation of exposure-based treatments have been conducted with primarily Caucasian samples (Huey & Polo, 2008). However, emerging evidence supports the use of exposure-based strategies with racially and socioeconomically diverse youth (Ginsburg, Becker, Drazdoweski, & Tein, 2012; Gordon-Hollingsworth et al., 2015; Huey & Polo, 2008; Mifsud & Rapee, 2005; Silverman et al., 1999). Exposure-based CBT has been shown, for example, to be effective for treating Hispanic/Latino youth with anxiety disorders generally (Pina, Silverman, Fuentes, Kurtines, & Weems, 2003; Silverman et al., 1999) and trauma in African American and Hispanic youth specifically (Cohen et al., 2004). Ginsburg and Drake (2002) likewise found that exposure-based CBT delivered in the school setting was effective in reducing anxiety in 14- to 17-year-old African American adolescents living in an urban setting, but that a psychoeducation control condition was not. To accommodate delivery of the treatment in the school setting, the length of treatment was reduced from 12 to 10 sessions, the length of individual sessions was also reduced by 15 minutes, and parents were not included in treatment. Additionally, therapists used examples that participants were likely to encounter in their daily lives, such as neighborhood violence and economic stress, as a meaningful percentage of the adolescents lived in poverty and/or a single-parent household.

Issues of transportability of CBT treatments are important to consider, given that ethnic minority youth living in socioeconomically disadvantaged environments may not have access to empirically supported treatments. Ginsburg et al. (2012) further examined the transportability of CBT to the school setting by testing whether it would be similarly effective when administered by school personnel to 7- to 17-year-old youth, the majority of whom were African American. School-based therapists had a variety of educational backgrounds and years of schooling and used exposure-based CBT strategies, to varying degrees. CBT was modified to a modular format that included detailed information on each module and handouts. All modules could be used as needed, based on the therapist's judgment, except for psychoeducation and exposure, which both had to be implemented. CBT resulted in similar outcomes to a usual-care condition, though treatment response rates for CBT were comparable to those in the published treatment outcome literature. An examination of predictors of response found that higher baseline anxiety, a greater number of urban hassles, maladaptive cognitions, high levels of parenting stress, and strained parent-child relationships related to poorer outcomes, whereas therapist use of CBT session structure (e.g., agenda setting) and competence in using the CBT components related to better treatment response.

Most recently, Gordon-Hollingsworth et al. (2015) examined therapy process and outcome variables in a sample of African American and Caucasian children ages 7–17 years who received exposure-based CBT for anxiety disorders. Regarding treatment process variables, African American youth showed lower treatment attendance and less mastery of therapy material than Caucasian youth, after controlling for demographic (socioeconomic status, child living situation) factors. African American youth were also rated as less engaged and compliant in treatment, which was particularly meaningful in the context of other analyses, which showed that treatment engagement predicted a better treatment response. Though there were no racial differences in overall response rates as assessed by measures of improvement, African American youth were less likely to be free of all targeted anxiety disorders than Caucasian youth at posttreatment.

Emerging support exists for the use of exposure-based treatments for diverse youth with anxiety disorders, but support for cultural modifications of the programs is mixed (Huey & Polo, 2008). As reviewed in Huey and Polo (2008), though cultural sensitivity is warranted when applying EBTs to diverse youth, the extent to which the programs are modified should be carefully considered to preserve fidelity. The studies reviewed previously suggest that modifications of exposure-based therapy for use with diverse youth can be effective. For instance, shortening the length of treatment overall, as well as the length of individual sessions, did not negatively impact treatment outcomes. This is consistent with the notion that the evidence base for the use of exposure tasks is strong, even when they are implemented early in treatment (Gryczkowski et al., 2013). Thus, perhaps when working with diverse youth with anxiety disorders, therapists can consider implementing exposure tasks early, given the risk of attrition. Because diverse youth are also at risk for poor treatment engagement, therapists should also be sensitive to alliance issues, particularly when introducing exposure tasks early in the treatment process. Exposure tasks are always created with regard to the individual youth's specific anxiety symptoms and types of avoidance, and this is true when working with youth of all backgrounds. Exposure tasks lend themselves well to modification based on individual differences, and therapists need only show creativity and sensitivity to meet those needs.

## CONCLUSIONS

The use of exposure tasks has a long and rich history in the treatment of anxiety, trauma- based, and obsessive–compulsive disorders in youth. Although exposure tasks are a very powerful core treatment element, debates are still ongoing regarding how this strategy exerts its effects. Exposure tasks may work chiefly by building self-efficacy, modifying maladaptive cognitions or fear structures, and/or, counterconditioning, among various factors. Understanding the principles that underlie exposure tasks will help therapists to use this strategy flexibly and more astutely. Exposure tasks can be readily used with youth of all developmental levels, and emerging empirical support suggests that they can also be used effectively with ethnically diverse youth. Therapists who remain sensitive to the individual needs of the youth will likely have the most success in using exposure tasks.

## BOX 2.2. Illustrative Case Example

Lucas was a 9-year-old Hispanic boy with separation anxiety disorder when he presented to the clinic for treatment. The therapist explained to Lucas and his mother that individual CBT would be implemented over the course of about 12 sessions. Lucas and his mother were attentive during the therapist's explanations, though they both appeared to have reservations about the exposure tasks part of treatment. In particular, Lucas's mother, "Mrs. M.," noted situations in which Lucas became nervous (e.g., sleeping alone, being in any room in the house by himself, attending sleepovers), and the therapist explained that after learning coping skills Lucas would actually practice using the skills in the real-life situations that Mrs. M. described. Mrs. M. appeared hesitant about the value of exposure tasks overall and seemed particularly concerned when the therapist noted that Lucas could even learn to sleep on his own. Lucas's mother quickly noted that, though Lucas was afraid to sleep away from her, they both really enjoyed sleeping in the same bed. It was difficult for the therapist to ascertain whether sleeping together was simply a family value or whether Lucas chose to sleep with his mother because of anxiety. The therapist replied that it was not necessary to decide about the sleeping issue right away—that there were plenty of other situations involving separation fears that the child and the therapist could work on together first. Once both Lucas and his mother seemed on board with CBT and the use of exposure tasks, in particular, treatment commenced.

Beginning in the second session of treatment, the youth and therapist worked together to build the fear hierarchy. Given Lucas's relatively young age, the therapist referred to the hierarchy as a "fear ladder." Each week during the first portion of treatment, the child and therapist added new situations to the fear hierarchy, until the ladder included approximately 15 situations. On the lower rungs of the ladder Lucas included such items as being in the family room while his mother was in the kitchen (the rooms were connected) and playing with a friend in his bedroom upstairs while his mother was downstairs. Items on the middle rungs of the ladder included going to his cousin's house to play without his mother and staying in aftercare at school, whereas the most difficult items included riding the bus to school and going on sleepovers.

Note that the therapist initially decided not to add sleeping alone to the fear hierarchy. Each time the issue came up, both Lucas and his mother became defensive, noting that Lucas's cousins also slept with their parents. Because they were very willing to address other items, and because it was still not clear whether sleeping together was a cultural value or a sign of avoidance related to Lucas's separation anxiety, the therapist chose to press ahead with the many other issues that could be addressed. Despite Lucas's defensiveness about sleeping with his mother, he was actively engaged when creating the fear hierarchy. He generated situations very easily and was amenable to adding potential situations that the therapist suggested. For instance, Lucas did not indicate that he would like to spend the night at his cousin's house but readily agreed upon the therapist's suggestion. The therapist also invited suggestions from Mrs. M., who was eager to be involved in the process.

For the first exposure task, the therapist and child agreed that, instead of having Lucas's mother wait for him in the waiting room, she would wait for him in the car. Though Lucas was easily able to separate from his mother in the therapy clinic, he was often worried about whether she was still in the waiting room during the therapy session. The therapist and Lucas practiced an imaginal exposure task in which his mother waited for him in the car rather than the waiting room. Lucas readily engaged in the practice session and implemented coping skills (e.g., taking deep breaths, repeating coping thoughts to himself) with little prompting from the therapist. During the following week, the therapist and Lucas did the exposure task *in vivo*. When the therapist took Lucas to the therapy room, he was visibly anxious. The therapist encouraged Lucas to use the coping skills that he had learned to manage his anxiety. Lucas was readily able to generate several coping thoughts, such as "My mom has never been late to pick me up, she will probably be here when I am done" and "She has a parking pass, so it is very unlikely that she will be asked to leave the parking lot." The therapist assessed Lucas's SUDS ratings throughout the session, which started at an 8 and gradually decreased to a low of 1. When Lucas went out to the parking lot, his mother was there, as expected. At that point, Lucas and the therapist went back into the therapy room, where they processed the exposure task. Lucas recognized that his anxiety went up as he thought of all the potential negative outcomes but went down as he used coping thoughts. Lucas's affect was visibly brighter, and he noted that the exposure task was easier than he thought.

Over the next several weeks, Lucas and the therapist continued to complete the exposure tasks that were listed on his fear hierarchy. Most exposure tasks went as planned, though as they became more difficult Lucas began to exhibit some resistance. For instance, after Lucas successfully went over to a friend's house several times by himself, the therapist suggested a sleepover. Lucas was resistant to this suggestion, noting that he was no longer interested in doing a sleepover. The therapist had Lucas generate a list of all of the positive outcomes of sleeping at his friend's house. Lucas was still resistant but agreed to consider the exposure while he was working on other tasks. In the meantime, Lucas completed nearly every exposure task on his hierarchy, including sleeping independently from his mother.

Over the course of treatment, as Lucas and his mother internalized the principles of anxiety treatment, they decided that they both wanted for Lucas to be able to sleep in his own room. Lucas and his mother first moved to his bedroom to sleep. Initially she slept in the bedroom with him, but gradually she moved farther away from him until she was outside of his door and then eventually in her own room. Mrs. M. was sure to reward Lucas appropriately with each step. Given Lucas's progress, it was clear that therapy was coming to a close. With just a few sessions left, Lucas agreed to the sleepover; he chose a close friend with whom he had played many times before. A coping plan was generated, and the therapist and Lucas worked together to write it down on a small card that he could keep under his pillow in case he needed reminders during the night. Lucas's mother was actively engaged in the coping plan, and when Lucas asked her if she would pick him up if he became anxious, she declined and assured him that he had all of the skills

(continued)

## BOX 2.2 (*continued*)

he needed to cope with his anxiety. The therapist also normalized the experience of anxiety that Lucas was likely to experience. Lucas successfully completed the exposure task for homework, as planned.

When processing therapy with Lucas during his final session, it became clear that he had developed a repertoire of coping skills he felt confident in using as a result of much practice. Lucas understood that, once therapy ended, it would be important for him to continue to engage in exposure tasks. In fact, he seemed to appreciate the power of exposure tasks by noting that whenever he felt nervous in the future about a situation the best thing to do would be to just face the fear!

# 3

## Cognitive Strategies

with Matthew P. Mychailyszyn and Monica R. Whitehead

### BACKGROUND OF THE ELEMENT

Cognitive strategies are a key component of manualized CBT programs for internalizing disorders among children and adolescents. Clinicians use these strategies to help youth become more aware of negatively distorted and/or unrealistic thoughts that are maintaining their anxiety or depression. Once maladaptive thoughts are identified, cognitive restructuring is then used to help youth challenge the validity of these thoughts and generate more positive or realistic alternatives (Kendall & Suveg, 2006). To do this, clinicians employ specific cognitive strategies, such as Socratic questioning, testing the evidence, cognitive modeling, reattribution of responsibility, decatastrophizing, and the downward arrow technique. For example, a child with separation anxiety disorder may have maladaptive thoughts such as "What if something terrible happens to my mom and dad and they never come back?" and "I'll be all alone forever with no one to take care of me." These thoughts may affect the child's willingness to stay with a babysitter when his or her parents go out, participate in playdates without a parent present, or even attend school regularly. A clinician could help this child to increase her (or his) awareness of the negative thoughts about harm befalling her parents, identify distortions that characterize her thinking (e.g., always expecting the worst possible outcome when separated), gather evidence to show that the facts do not support this prediction (via Socratic questioning and other cognitive strategies), and develop more adaptive thoughts to cope with these situations (e.g., "They're just out for dinner and will be back soon"). This chapter begins with coverage of the historical and theoretical background and the empirical support for the use of cognitive strategies, followed by guidelines for the practical implementation of this element with anxious and depressed youth.

## Brief History

The early roots of cognitive strategies can be traced back to the 1940s and 1950s, when researchers in psychology and related fields began challenging behaviorist views that human personality and behavior were solely conditioned responses to environmental stimuli and that psychologists should study only that which is observable. John Dollard and Neal Miller (1950) observed that rats would imitate one another under certain conditions, indicating that they were learning by cognitively mediated processes rather than solely through stimulus–response conditioning. Based on their observations, they developed a theory of social learning postulating that a great deal of human learning involves social interaction and is facilitated not only through basic drives and needs but also cognitive processes (Dollard & Miller, 1950).

Rotter (1954) modified this social learning perspective, placing further emphasis on "the importance of conscious thought processes in mediating human behavior" (Masters, Burish, Hollon, & Rimm, 1987, p. 387). Rotter hypothesized that individuals develop general cognitive expectations based upon which specific behaviors are rewarded and which are not. For example, a student who studies hard and is rewarded with a good grade develops a general expectation that hard work will lead to positive results, whereas a student who studies hard but earns a poor grade develops an expectation that hard work does not necessarily produce the desired result.

Further developments related to social learning theory occurred during the 1960s and 1970s. Based upon his research on observational learning, Bandura developed his own version of social learning theory (Bandura & Walters 1963), often viewed as the bridge between behavioral and cognitive learning theories. According to his theory, individuals develop mental representations of their environments and themselves through various social experiences, including exposure to models and verbal discussions (Bandura, 1977a). Bandura (1977a) made a distinction between expectancies of *self-efficacy* (i.e., anticipating mastery of a behavioral challenge) and expectancies related to *response outcome* (i.e., expecting that a behavior, if enacted, will have a rewarding outcome). Bandura asserted that perceived *self-efficacy* is a crucial ingredient for behavior change and that an individual's belief in probable success mediates the chances that new behaviors will be performed outside of the therapy context. This hypothesis was supported in several studies using modeling to treat phobias in adults (e.g., Bandura, Adams, & Beyer, 1977; Bandura, Reese, & Adams, 1982). In these studies, self-efficacy beliefs (e.g., "I know that I'll be able to pick up this spider") affected the participants' level of anxiety toward feared objects and also their actual performance. In 1986, Bandura renamed his theoretical approach (i.e., from social learning theory to social cognitive theory) to more accurately describe the emphasis on the cognitive mechanisms underlying behavioral change; this theory remains highly influential today.

Motivation and emotion research in the 1960s and 1970s also emphasized cognitive influences. For example, Schachter and Singer (1962) developed the cognitive theory of emotional arousal, which posited that individuals cannot label emotions based solely upon the physical sensations that they experience. Rather, the mind must *interpret* external cues to identify the physical symptoms as a particular feeling (e.g., anger, fear). In their early research, the two researchers injected participants with adrenaline, thereby generating physical symptoms similar to those associated with strong emotions (e.g., racing heart, flushed face, trembling hands). Some participants were told about the side effects of the injection, and others were not. Following the injection, participants completed a questionnaire in the same room as a confederate who acted either happy or angry. Participants who had not been informed of the injection's effects exhibited behaviors and endorsed feelings similar to those of the confederate. Those who had been told about the adrenaline did not exhibit those responses, as they already had a cognitive rationale for the physical symptoms. Schachter and Singer concluded that when individuals experience physiological arousal that cannot otherwise be explained, they report feelings consistent with their cognitive interpretation of the situation. Not only did the cognitive theory of emotional arousal highlight the influence of cognition on human emotion and behavior, but it also prompted a great deal of further research on this topic for several decades.

Finally, a discussion of the historical roots of cognitive approaches would not be complete without highlighting the work of Albert Ellis and Aaron Beck. Influenced by the work of Julian Rotter and others, Ellis began to practice and write about his own version of cognitive therapy called rational therapy in 1955. Known today as rational-emotive behavior therapy (REBT), Ellis's confrontational approach reflected his belief that therapists needed to directly challenge irrational thoughts when helping clients replace those thoughts with more rational ones (Ellis, 1971). At approximately the same time, Beck, then a psychiatrist at the University of Pennsylvania, noticed patterns of cognitive distortions reflecting pervasive negative views of the self, world, and future in his work with depressed patients. He believed that depression could be alleviated if the cognitive distortions could be corrected through logical reasoning and helping clients develop more accurate perceptions of reality, which formed the basis for his cognitive theory of depression (Beck, 1967). Beck is considered by many to be the founder of cognitive therapy.

## Theory Base

The theoretical foundation of cognitive strategies posits that the ways in which people interpret situations can lead to feelings of distress and dysfunctional behavior (Spiegler, 2016). Early pioneers of cognitive therapy, such as Beck (1976) and Ellis (1971), postulated an A-B-C paradigm not only as an explanation of emotions and behavior but also as a way of conceptualizing psychopathology more broadly. In this paradigm, A refers to the activating event; B, the related beliefs and thoughts about the event; and C, the consequences of such beliefs. For example, an adolescent who is rejected by a potential girlfriend (activating event) may conclude he is unlovable (belief), thus resulting in feelings of disappointment or sadness and subsequent avoidance of social interactions (consequences). This example demonstrates that it is not the event itself that may cause distress; rather, it is the interpretation of the event. If an individual interprets an event in a maladaptive (e.g., irrational, negatively distorted) way, it is likely that he or she will experience a corresponding negative emotion and then perhaps engage in maladaptive behaviors.

Beck's cognitive model (1967, 1987) focused specifically on depression, emphasizing that depressed individuals tend to think in self-deprecating ways and view themselves in terms of inadequacy, failure, and worthlessness. Beck (1976) placed particular emphasis on the role of *automatic thoughts*, which are thoughts that come to mind reflexively or very rapidly without prior planning, which may then develop into a pattern of thinking over time. During times of negative emotion, these maladaptive thoughts appear valid to the individual who is experiencing them. However, once the thoughts are evaluated, it becomes clear that they are distorted; yet, they function to maintain or intensify negative emotions and unhelpful behaviors. According to Beck and Shaw (1977), the content of depressed individuals' automatic thoughts centers around three themes: negative views of the self (e.g., viewing the self as undesirable and worthless), negative views of the world (e.g., seeing the world as placing unreasonable demands on oneself or obstacles that interfere with achievement of life goals), and negative views of the future (e.g., believing that current difficulties will continue indefinitely). In addition to these themes, depressed individuals tend to misinterpret their experiences, exhibiting a *systematic bias* against themselves—for example, blaming the causes of events on personal failure, exaggerating negative information about themselves, and consistently making negative predictions about the future (Beck & Shaw, 1977). Beck viewed this overemphasis on negative information to the exclusion of positive as logical errors in thinking, which he called *cognitive distortions*. He identified six cognitive distortions that often characterize the thoughts of individuals experiencing psychological distress, including drawing conclusions without sufficient evidence, focusing only on the negative and ignoring positive details, thinking in an all-or-nothing fashion, and generalizing the outcome of one incident to similar future situations (Beck, 1976). Other distortions include beliefs of personal worthlessness, "musturbation" (e.g., "I ought to be able to do this task," or "I should have known that was going to happen"; Ellis & Dryden, 1987), and "awfulizing," or perceiving events as being unbearable or extremely distressing (Ellis, 1977).

Whereas automatic thoughts are tied to specific situations, the more generalized cognitions that underlie these thoughts are core beliefs, or the central ideas that individuals have about themselves, others, and the world (J. S. Beck, 2011). These beliefs, which begin to develop during childhood, shape the way that individuals perceive and react to their environment. According to Judith Beck (2011), Aaron Beck's daughter, core beliefs are "enduring understandings so fundamental and deep that [individuals] often do not articulate them, even to themselves," frequently viewing them as "absolute truths" (p. 32). Moreover, individuals tend to interpret situations in ways that are consistent with their core beliefs, selectively attending to information that is consistent with these beliefs and ignoring conflicting evidence. The concept of schemas is often used interchangeably with that of core beliefs. However, the elder Beck (1964) had differentiated these two concepts, positing that schemas are cognitive *structures* in the mind and core beliefs are the *content* within those structures. Several categories of core beliefs have been identified, including those related to helplessness, unlovability, and worthlessness (J. S. Beck, 2011). For example, a depressed college student who holds a core belief related to helplessness (e.g., "I can't do anything right") may respond to one low exam grade with negative automatic thoughts (e.g., "I'm terrible at math and won't ever pass this class"), which may reflect one or more cognitive distortions (e.g., focusing only on the negative while discounting positive performance on recent assignments, generalizing the outcome of this one exam to all future exams in the course). According to Judith Beck (2011), focusing on modifying core beliefs early in treatment can lead to more rapid improvements in mood and functioning and thus help clients to interpret new problems that may arise during treatment in a more adaptive way.

Beck (1976) also emphasized that the negative beliefs held by individuals prone to depression can become reinforced through stressful or negative life events. According to Rose and Abramson (1992), individuals who experience traumatic events, such as maltreatment during childhood, are placed at risk for developing a negative cognitive style, which can lead to feelings of hopelessness (i.e., expectation of negative outcomes combined with feelings of helplessness) and symptoms of depression. This negative cognitive style is characterized by the tendency to consider negative life events as internal (i.e., their fault), stable (i.e., the situation will not get better), and global (i.e., negative outcomes will occur in all situations; Sweeney, Anderson, & Bailey, 1986). Alternatively, youth with anxiety disorders tend to have danger-focused cognitions, such as "I cannot escape," "I am going to get hurt," or "I am going to be attacked" (Bell-Dolan & Wessler, 1994). Accompanying these danger-focused thoughts is the belief in an inability to cope with danger or the unknown (i.e., low confidence in generating a positive outcome of a situation; Wilson & Hughes, 2011) and a feeling of being out of control (Bell-Dolan & Wessler, 1994). Because of these underlying beliefs, youth with anxiety disorders tend to have distorted thoughts not only about the environment but also about their personal safety and abilities (Kendall, Howard, & Epps, 1988). Understanding internalizing disorders through the lens of cognitive theory and being aware of the types of cognitions that characterize anxiety and depression among youth can help guide the therapist when implementing cognitive strategies during treatment.

## Evidence Base

There is considerable empirical support for the use of cognitive strategies with anxious and depressed youth. However, relatively few studies have evaluated this element by itself, as it is most frequently examined as part of multicomponent CBT protocols. Based on definitions for empirically supported treatments published by Division 12 of the American Psychological Association, CBT is regarded as being "probably efficacious" as a treatment for childhood depression, "well-established" for adolescent depression, and "probably efficacious" for child and adolescent anxiety disorders (e.g., David-Ferdon & Kaslow, 2008; Silverman, Pina, et al., 2008). In addition, interpersonal psychotherapy (IPT) is a "well-established" treatment for adolescent depression (Verdeli, Mufson, Lee, & Keith, 2006). Table 3.1 includes a description of cognitive strategies utilized in several empirically supported CBT protocols for depression and anxiety among children and adolescents.

In one of the first randomized trials examining cognitive strategies for youth with depression, Reynolds and Coats (1986) compared CBT, relaxation training, and a waitlist control among a small sample ($N = 30$) of moderately depressed adolescents. The CBT intervention included three phases, self-monitoring, self-evaluation, and self-reinforcement. Cognitive components included challenging the depressive tendency to maintain a negative view of the future and examining unrealistic assumptions about personal responsibility for events. At posttreatment, CBT was equivalent to relaxation training in terms of reductions in depression as compared to the waitlist control, and the gains were maintained at 5-week follow-up.

Another multicomponent CBT protocol that incorporates cognitive strategies is the Adolescent Coping with Depression (CWD-A) course (Lewinsohn, Hoberman, Teri, & Hautzinger, 1985). This group-based approach is founded on a multifactorial model of depression that posits that automatic, maladaptive, and irrational beliefs are a contributing factor to youth depression. Several cognitive strategies are used in this program, including heightening awareness of thought patterns, identifying frequent and intrusive negative thoughts, learning about triggers for negative thoughts, and developing adaptive counterthoughts. In the first randomized trial evaluating the CWD-A program (Lewinsohn, Clarke, Hops, & Andrews, 1990), 59 youth with major depression or dysthymia were randomly assigned either to the CWD-A course without parent therapy, the CWD-A course with caregivers participating in a parallel parent group, or a waitlist comparison control condition.

**TABLE 3.1. The Cognitive Strategies Element in Representative EBT Manuals**

| | |
|---|---|
| *Coping Cat* (Kendall & Hedtke, 2006) | • The clinician explicitly teaches cognitive strategies as part of the E (expecting bad things to happen) step of the FEAR plan (Feeling frightened, Expecting bad things, Attitudes/actions to help, Results and rewards). During the first half of treatment, the youth learn how anxious thoughts affect anxiety. They identify their own anxious self-talk and common thinking traps and learn how to change anxious self-talk to coping self-talk. The youth practice this skill during the second half of treatment during exposure tasks. |
| *C.A.T. Project* (Kendall, Choudhury, Hudson, & Webb, 2002) | • The clinician explicitly teaches cognitive strategies as part of the E (expecting bad things to happen) step of the FEAR plan. The youth are taught to identify and challenge anxious self-talk and to change anxious thoughts to coping thoughts. They continue to practice this skill when completing exposure tasks. |
| *Family-Based Treatment for Young Children with OCD* (Freeman & Garcia, 2009) | • Cognitive strategies are explicitly taught and viewed as tools for the youth to use during exposure tasks. Specific cognitive strategies include teaching the youth to "boss back" OCD (e.g., telling OCD that "I don't believe what you're telling me") and to use positive self-talk (e.g., "I can do this"). Cognitive strategies are reviewed throughout the program and implemented during exposure tasks. |
| *OCD in Children and Adolescents* (March & Mulle, 1998) | • The youth learn and practice several cognitive strategies to counteract negative self-talk surrounding OCD symptoms. Cognitive techniques include changing unhelpful self-talk to constructive self-talk, restructuring beliefs about the probability of danger and perceived responsibility for negative events, and cultivating detachment from OCD (e.g., "It's *just* OCD again"). These skills are practiced throughout treatment as the child works to "boss back" OCD. The parents are taught to encourage their child to use these skills during exposure tasks. |
| *CBT of Childhood OCD: It's Only a False Alarm* (Piacentini, Langley, & Roblek, 2007) | • Cognitive strategies are directly taught and practiced throughout the treatment. The role of thoughts in OCD is discussed during the psychoeducation portion of treatment. During the cognitive restructuring phase, the youth are taught to recognize and reframe their obsessive thoughts and to generate more helpful coping thoughts. These cognitive skills are practiced when implementing exposures. |
| *CBT for Social Phobia: Stand Up, Speak Out* (Albano & DiBartolo, 2007) | • The youth are taught the cognitive-behavioral model of social anxiety disorder, how the components of the model influence one another, and the role of coping thoughts. In a group format, the adolescents also learn to identify cognitive distortions and core beliefs, and they "become detectives" in order to challenge their thoughts and generate rational responses. These skills are practiced throughout the exposure phase of treatment. |

**TABLE 3.1.** (continued)

| | |
|---|---|
| *When Children Refuse School: A CBT Approach* (Kearney & Albano, 2007): Chapters 4 and 5 on internalizing symptoms | • Emphasis on cognitive strategies varies by the particular problem area (i.e., the specific reason for school refusal). For avoidance of school-related stimuli that provoke negative affectivity, the youth are taught the CBT model of anxiety, and Socratic questioning is used to identify and change their irrational thinking. For avoidance of social/evaluative situations, in addition to the CBT model, thought bubbles and the STOP acronym (i.e., Feeling Scared? What are you Thinking? Other helpful thoughts? Praise/plan for next time) are utilized to help challenge and change negative thoughts. |
| *Treating Trauma and Traumatic Grief in Children and Adolescents* (Cohen, Mannarino, & Deblinger, 2006) | • Cognitive strategies are explicitly incorporated as part of the C (Cognitive problems) portion of the CRAFTS (i.e., Cognitive problems, Relationship problems, Affective problems, Family problems, Traumatic behavior problems, Somatic problems) acronym for problem domains related to trauma. During the cognitive coping component, the youth and their parents learn about the cognitive triangle, how to identify inaccurate and unhelpful thoughts, and how to generate more accurate and helpful alternative thoughts. Then, the therapist helps the youth to identify and change cognitive errors and other maladaptive thoughts related to the trauma experience. |
| *Adolescent Coping with Depression* (Clarke, Lewinsohn, & Hops, 1990) | • Cognitive strategies are explicitly taught and practiced throughout treatment. The youth are taught to identify negative personal thoughts and develop positive counterthoughts. They also learn to identify and dispute irrational beliefs. Specific cognitive strategies include the C-A-B (consequence–activating event–belief) method of diagramming/analyzing hypothetical (i.e., cartoons) and personal situations and completing a negative thoughts contract. |
| *Interpersonal Psychotherapy for Depressed Adolescents,* 2nd edition (Mufson, Pollack, Dorta, Moreau, & Weissman, 2011) | • Cognitive strategies are occasionally explicitly mentioned but are not considered to be a central component of interpersonal psychotherapy for adolescents (IPT-A). The focus of IPT-A is to target affect (rather than thoughts) to change mood and behavior, though therapists do explicitly work on perspective-taking skills to challenge adolescents' black-and-white thinking related to problem solving and communication. When discussing role transitions, therapists help the youth to "develop a more realistic view of the old role" (p. 153) and correct misconceptions related to family events or dynamics. With respect to role disputes, the youth are encouraged to "look for patterns of nonreciprocal expectations" (p. 132). |
| *Treating Depressed Children: Therapist Manual for "Taking Action"* (Stark & Kendall, 1996) | • Cognitive strategies are explicitly taught and practiced, particularly during the second half of treatment. Girls learn how to "catch and reword" negative thoughts. Therapists use cartoons to teach cognitive restructuring, a sunglasses activity to explain how depression can distort thinking patterns, and various other activities to help the youth to challenge or "talk back" to their negative thoughts. |

*(continued)*

**TABLE 3.1.** (*continued*)

| | |
|---|---|
| *Treating Depressed Youth: Therapist Manual for "Action"* (Stark et al., 2007) | • Cognitive strategies are explicitly taught throughout the treatment. The therapist helps the youth to identify links between thoughts and emotions and to recognize cognitive distortions. The youth also learn about the role of negative thinking and how to develop "coping counters" for pessimistic thoughts and negative self-evaluations. The therapist connects cognitive restructuring with the C (Catch the positive), O (Open yourself to the positive), and N (Never get stuck in the negative muck) steps of the ACTION (Always find something to do to feel better, Catch the positive, Think about it as a problem to be solved, Inspect the situation, Open yourself to the positive, Never get stuck in the negative muck) acronym. The youth are encouraged to be detectives, gathering evidence for their negative thoughts while "sleuthing for the truth," both during sessions and via written homework assignments. |
| *Psychotherapy for Children with Bipolar and Depressive Disorders* (Fristad, Arnold, & Leffler, 2011) | • Cognitive strategies are taught directly during the Thinking, Feeling, Doing portion of treatment. The children are taught to identify hurtful thoughts, make connections between hurtful feelings, actions, and thoughts, and identify helpful thoughts to cope with their hurtful feelings. In a separate session, the parents are taught to identify and change their own negative thoughts related to their child's mood disorder and its impact on the family. |

*Note.* Some book titles are shortened to conserve space. See the References at the back of the book for full titles.

Nearly one-half (46%) of the treatment group demonstrated depression recovery by posttreatment as compared to only 5% in the waitlist control group. Subsequent randomized trials yielded further support for the efficacy of this program (e.g., Clarke et al., 2002; Clarke, Rohde, Lewinsohn, Hops, & Seeley, 1999; Lewinsohn et al., 1990; Rohde, Clarke, Mace, Jorgensen, & Seeley, 2004). Another group-based intervention for depressed youth is the ACTION treatment program (Stark, Streusand, Krumholz, & Patel, 2010). Evidence in support of the efficacy of this program for alleviating depression in adolescent females is promising, though still preliminary (Stark et al., 2008, 2010).

Given that cognitive strategies are typically evaluated in combination with other techniques, it is also important to consider whether they make a unique contribution to the efficacy of CBT for depression. Kaufman and colleagues (Kaufman, Rohde, Seeley, Clarke, & Stice, 2005) explored this question by examining possible mediators of change among depressed adolescents receiving the CWD-A intervention. Results indicated that the *rate of automatic negative thoughts* was a mediator of the relationship between CBT treatment and outcome, with the researchers concluding, "Reducing negative thinking may be the primary mechanism through which the CWD-A intervention reduces depression" (p. 38).

There is also considerable empirical support for cognitive strategies as part of CBT protocols for anxiety disorders, with many protocols targeting youth diagnosed with social phobia, generalized anxiety disorder, and/or separation anxiety disorder. Coping Cat (Kendall, 1990; Kendall, Kane, Howard, & Siqueland, 1990) is one manualized CBT program that focuses on helping youth learn to identify the presence of maladaptive thoughts underlying anxiety, evaluate the nature of those thoughts (e.g., the probability of their coming to fruition, subsequent realities if such feared outcomes did occur), and develop thoughts that are more helpful. Coping Cat has been found to be superior to a waitlist comparison (Kendall, 1994; Kendall et al., 1997) as well as an active control condition (Kendall et al., 2008) and comparable to pharmacotherapy (Walkup et al., 2008). It is also amenable to delivery in group (Flannery-Schroeder & Kendall, 2000) and family-based formats (Kendall et al., 2008). Follow-up studies have demonstrated the maintenance of treatment gains approximately 16 years posttreatment (Benjamin et al., 2013).

There is also evidence for the effectiveness of manualized CBT when implemented for the treatment of other anxiety disorders in children and adolescents. The first randomized controlled trial (de Haan, Hoogduin, Buitelaar, & Keijsers, 1998) to compare CBT to pharmacotherapy for youth OCD assigned participants ($N = 22$, ages 8–17 years) to conditions involving 12 weekly sessions of either exposure and response prevention (ERP) or clomipramine. In addition to behavioral strategies for reducing rituals, the ERP condition included cognitive components, such as explaining the cognitive mechanisms that maintain rituals and avoidance behavior and challenging obsessional beliefs, particularly for older children. Although both treatment conditions yielded significant decreases in OCD-related symptomatology, reductions were more substantial for youth receiving the CBT intervention than for those receiving medication (de Haan et al., 1998). The first randomized trial (Pediatric OCD Treatment Study Team, 2004) to directly compare OCD-specific CBT, sertraline, their combination, and a pill placebo among a sample of 112 youth ages 7–17 years found that CBT and medication alone had comparable outcomes, with the combined treatment showing the most optimal effects. In another example, trauma-focused cognitive-behavioral therapy (TF-CBT) makes use of standard cognitive restructuring techniques as well as a trauma narrative, the latter of which is utilized to identify and process dysfunctional cognitions about a traumatic experience that might not otherwise be disclosed via direct questioning (Cohen, Mannarino, & Deblinger, 2010). Based on a review of randomized clinical trials of TF-CBT conducted with children and adolescents (the majority ranging in age from 8 to 14 years), Cohen and colleagues (2010) concluded that significant evidence exists to support the use of TF-CBT with youth who have experienced sexual abuse and other traumatic events. Notably, although TF-CBT does not target anxiety exclusively, many of these youth struggle with anxiety and related internalizing symptoms.

There is also empirical support for treatments that utilize advanced technology, which offers new possibilities in terms of the medium by which treatment content is delivered and access to treatment. Indeed, "virtual" treatment is likely to be uniquely suited to today's youth, who tend to be technology literate from a very young age. In one example, Wuthrich et al. (2012) reported beneficial effects for the Cool Teens CD-ROM for adolescents (ages 14–17 years) with a primary diagnosis of anxiety. In this study, 43 adolescents were randomly assigned to either the 12-week Cool Teens program or a waitlist control condition. This program, which teaches CBT techniques for anxiety management in eight 30-minute therapy modules, emphasizes cognitive restructuring and gradual exposure. In addition to viewing the program (e.g., text, audio, cartoons, videos) on their home computer, parents were given handouts on key treatment strategies, and the therapist conducted brief telephone calls with parents and the adolescent at various intervals during the 12-week program. Compared to the control group, participants in Cool Teens experienced significant decreases at posttreatment and a 3-month follow-up in the following areas: total number of anxiety diagnoses, primary anxiety diagnosis severity, and mean level of severity across all disorders. Significant improvements were also noted for both mother- and adolescent self-reported symptoms of anxiety, other internalizing symptoms, automatic thoughts, and interference in functioning (Wuthrich et al., 2012). The Cool Teens program was adapted from the Cool Kids group-based CBT approach that had previously demonstrated efficacy in multiple delivery formats (e.g., Lyneham & Rapee, 2006; Mifsud & Rapee, 2005; Rapee, Abbott, & Lyneham, 2006). Similarly, Kendall and Khanna (2008a; 2008b) created the Camp Cope-A-Lot (CCAL) program, a computer-assisted CBT based on Coping Cat. A recent randomized clinical trial of CCAL (Khanna & Kendall, 2010) demonstrated the program's superiority over an education-based control condition as well as its acceptability to participants.

## THE ELEMENT IN PRACTICE

This section includes practical instructions for implementing cognitive strategies with anxious and depressed youth. Step-by-step procedures are outlined in the task analysis in Box 3.1, and expanded information regarding the implementation of each step is included in the following paragraphs. Tips for modifying this element to suit particular diagnoses, varying developmental levels, and youth of diverse racial and ethnic backgrounds are also provided, along with a case example illustrating the implementation of this element with a 15-year-old Caucasian girl with social anxiety disorder (see Box 3.2 at the end of the chapter).

### "Core of the Core" Element

After covering such topics as psychoeducation, pleasant events scheduling, and/or relaxation training, most CBT protocols for internalizing disorders among youth then focus on cognitive strategies (i.e., identifying thoughts related to anxiety or depression, changing these thoughts to coping thoughts) for several sessions. Following this portion of treatment, cognitive strategies are continually practiced and revisited via homework assignments, exposure tasks, and other in-session exercises for the remainder of treatment. As noted in Box 3.1, the clinician begins the cognitive portion of treatment by providing a rationale for cognitive restructuring (Box 3.1, Step 1). Youth are told that the goals of the cognitive phase of treatment are to increase their awareness of thoughts that are maintaining anxiety or depression and learn how to change those thoughts (Cormier, Nurius, & Osborn, 2013). At this point, clinicians typically review the CBT model, which would have been introduced briefly at the beginning of treatment. This discussion focuses on common thoughts, physical symptoms/feelings, and behavior related to anxiety or depression and how these components interact, with particular emphasis on the impact that thoughts can have on behavior and physical symptoms.

Prior to and throughout the cognitive phase of treatment, a detailed assessment of the youth's thoughts in situations related to anxiety or depression is conducted (Step 2). Based upon information obtained during both the initial assessment and subsequent treatment sessions, the clinician may already be aware of some of the youth's thought patterns in challenging situations. However, developing a complete understanding of the child's thoughts related to anxiety or depression is an ongoing process that continues throughout treatment. During

## BOX 3.1. Task Analysis of Cognitive Strategies

1. Provide a rationale for cognitive restructuring, and review the CBT model, emphasizing how thoughts influence feelings/physiological responses and behavior.

2. Conduct a detailed assessment of the youth's cognitions related to anxiety or depression via the initial pretreatment assessment, information obtained during weekly sessions, ongoing homework assignments, and/or self-report measures.

3. Teach youth to become more aware of their thoughts in various situations, and explain the role of negative self-talk (i.e., automatic thoughts) in anxiety or depression:
   a. First, use obvious and/or nonthreatening situations and ask youth what they would be thinking, to increase overall awareness of self-talk.
   b. Next, discuss ambiguous situations (e.g., those that could provoke positive or negative thoughts) to help youth understand the difference between negative self-talk and coping self-talk as well as how these thoughts can, in turn, lead to different behaviors and feelings.

4. Help youth to identify thoughts in anxiety- or depression-provoking situations and to identify patterns of cognitive distortions.
   a. Model identifying negative self-talk in problematic situations by using cartoon strips and/or personal examples.
   b. Through role play or imagery exercises, help youth to identify and verbalize their thoughts in problematic situations by answering such questions as "What is my self-talk?" and "What do I think is going to happen?"
   c. Teach youth to look for common cognitive distortions or "thinking traps," and help them identify underlying schemas, or core beliefs, about the self, others, and the world that can be challenged in subsequent sessions.
   d. Provide ongoing practice with identifying thoughts via homework assignments that require youth to record thoughts in specific situations related to their anxiety or depression between sessions.

5. Assist youth in challenging their negative thoughts and generating coping thoughts:
   a. Use various cognitive strategies, including logical, empirical, or functional disputes delivered via direct teaching, Socratic questioning, and/or metaphorical or humorous styles.
   b. Teach youth to "test the evidence" by gathering facts that support and refute their beliefs (e.g., "Do you know for sure that this is going to happen? What else might happen in this situation?"). By reviewing the facts, youth can reach a new conclusion, which leads to coping thoughts.
   c. Practice in changing negative thoughts to coping thoughts occurs through clinician modeling, role-play exercises, and discussion of situations recorded in thought diary homework assignments.
   d. For homework, youth should continue to monitor their thoughts in particular

situations and now also work on developing coping thoughts for situations related to anxiety or depression.

6. Teach youth to praise/reward themselves for progress in successfully employing coping thoughts.

the cognitive portion of treatment in particular, a great deal is learned about these thoughts through in-session discussions and activities as well as self-monitoring homework assignments that require the youth to record thoughts in specific situations between sessions (see Chapter 11). Cognitions can also be assessed by using self-report inventories and think-aloud procedures. Several self-report measures have been developed to monitor the cognitions of anxious and depressed youth, such as the Children's Negative Affectivity Self-Statement Questionnaire for anxiety (Ronan, Kendall, & Rowe, 1994) and the Children's Negative Cognitive Error Questionnaire for depression (Kingery et al., 2009). During think-aloud procedures, youth participate in role-play exercises or listen to audio recordings of simulated scenarios (Spiegler, 2016). While imagining themselves in these situations, children are prompted to verbalize their thoughts.

Following the assessment process, youth are taught to become more aware of their thoughts (i.e., self-talk) in various situations and to develop a more in-depth understanding of the role of negative self-talk in anxiety or depression (Step 3). This process often begins by presenting obvious and/or nonthreatening situations (e.g., a child opening a birthday gift, dropping a pencil; Kendall & Hedtke, 2006) and asking youth to generate possible thoughts associated with each situation. Once youth can readily identify thoughts for more straightforward scenarios, they are presented with ambiguous situations that could provoke either positive or negative thoughts and are guided through the process of generating possible thoughts. For example, in the Coping Cat program (Kendall & Hedtke, 2006), youth are presented with a drawing of a child who is ice skating and are asked to report what children with varying levels of prior skating experience (i.e., beginner vs. more experienced) might be thinking by filling in two different thought bubbles above the picture. While working through similar examples, youth begin to understand the difference between negative self-talk and more realistic, or positive, coping self-talk and how the type of thoughts that an individual has in a given situation can lead to different behaviors and feelings.

After gaining a greater awareness of self-talk and its role in anxiety or depression, youth learn to identify their own thoughts in problematic (i.e., anxiety- or depression-provoking) situations and to recognize common cognitive distortions that characterize their thinking (Step 4). This process typically begins with modeling the identification of negative self-talk through the use of cartoon strips or personal examples. For instance, a clinician working with a socially anxious adolescent could describe a time when he or she had to give a speech and felt very nervous, placing particular emphasis on the thoughts that were going through his or her mind in this situation. The use of personal examples not only models the process of identifying negative thoughts for the adolescent but also builds rapport, helps to normalize the experience of anxiety, and enables the teen to feel more comfortable sharing his or her own thoughts in anxiety-provoking situations. Through discussion, role play, imagery, and/or think-aloud procedures, youth describe their thoughts in challenging situations by answering such questions as "What is my self-talk?" or "What do I think is going to happen?" Ongoing practice with identifying thoughts is provided via homework assignments that require youth to record thoughts in specific situations related to their anxiety or depression. Completed self-monitoring sheets (also called thought diaries or daily thought records) are reviewed each week, providing realistic examples for clinicians and youth to discuss in subsequent sessions.

Once youth have become more adept at identifying their own negative self-talk in problematic situations, they learn how their thoughts match up with common cognitive distortions. For example, the group treatment program for social phobia in adolescents by Albano and DiBartolo (2007) focuses on identifying different types of negative automatic thoughts (i.e., negative cognitions that often come along with anxiety), including all-or-none thinking, catastrophizing, and disqualifying the positive. Treatment programs for depression use similar strategies for helping youth to identify distortions in their thinking. The CWD-A course (Clarke, Lewinsohn, & Hops, 1990) emphasizes that many negative thoughts are irrational, or overreactions to a particular situation. Youth learn about categories of irrational beliefs, such as exaggerations and unreasonable expectations, and are encouraged to look for these patterns in their own thinking. Over time, youth become better at catching themselves when they begin falling into a "thinking trap," which serves as a signal to implement cognitive restructuring strategies.

In the next step, youth are guided through cognitive restructuring (Step 5), a process that involves challenging the validity of their negative thoughts and predictions and generating more positive or realistic counterthoughts (i.e., coping thoughts). Clinicians begin by asking youth questions directly, gradually helping them develop the ability to challenge their own thoughts. Beal, Kopec, and DiGiuseppe (1996) outline various methods that clinicians can use to challenge distorted thinking and help them to develop more rational thoughts. *Logical disputes* focus on challenging children's illogical reasoning patterns, and *empirical disputes* aim to gather factual data or evidence for the child's predictions. *Functional disputes* target the costs and benefits of particular ways of thinking (e.g., "What are the advantages of thinking _____?"). Questions can also be delivered in a variety of different styles, such as didactic (i.e., direct teaching), Socratic (i.e., guided questioning), metaphorical (e.g., using an analogy based upon change that occurs in nature, such as asking children to change a negative "caterpillar thought" to a coping "butterfly thought"), or humorous (Beal et al., 1996; Friedberg & McClure, 2015).

As part of the Socratic questioning process, a variety of more specific cognitive strategies are implemented, such as *decatastrophizing* and *reattribution of responsibility*. *Decatastrophizing* is helpful for children who expect the worst possible outcome for a given scenario or tend to overestimate the probability of danger or harm. Youth are asked questions such as "What is the worst thing that could happen?"; "What is the best thing that could happen?"; and "What is most likely to happen?" Decatastrophizing is often paired with problem solving, particularly for youth who believe strongly that catastrophic outcomes have a high likelihood of occurring (Friedberg & McClure, 2015). In such cases, therapists help youth problem-solve to develop a plan for coping with the feared outcome (see Chapter 4). Then, this plan becomes part of the decatastrophizing, as youth can generate a coping thought such as "Even if the worst does occur, I have a plan for dealing with it." Another cognitive strategy to help restructure children's thoughts is *reattribution of responsibility*, which can be facilitated through discussing a responsibility pie exercise (Greenberger & Padesky, 2015). This task involves the therapist and child working together to generate a list of possible causes for a distressing event and drawing a pie chart to allocate a certain percentage of responsibility to each factor. All other factors must be accounted for before the child can assign a portion of the pie to him- or herself. This exercise helps youth to rethink the amount of responsibility they are taking on for events outside of their control and to view the situation in a different way.

Many treatment manuals for anxiety and depression use the

*metaphor of a detective* who is working to gather evidence for negative thoughts, a cognitive strategy referred to as *testing the evidence*. Through this process, therapists ask key questions to help youth to gather facts that support their beliefs (e.g., "What facts absolutely support your conclusion?"; "What makes you 100% sure that your prediction is true?") and to compile facts that do not support their beliefs (e.g., "Do you know for sure that this is going to happen?"; "What facts make you doubt your prediction?"; "What else might happen in this situation?"; Friedberg & McClure, 2015; Kendall & Hedtke, 2006; Stark & Kendall, 1996). After gathering the facts, youth are asked how else they might view the situation, in contrast to what they originally thought. By reviewing the facts and coming to a new conclusion, youth develop coping thoughts. They begin to realize, for example, that a negative outcome is less likely to occur than they first predicted, that a positive (rather than negative) result might actually occur, or that even if the situation does not go well, they can cope and try again next time. Similar to other skills learned during the cognitive phase of treatment, youth practice generating coping thoughts through clinician modeling, role-play exercises, and discussion of situations recorded in the thought diary homework assignments (see Box 3.2 at the end of the chapter for a case example). Coping thoughts generated in session can be written down on cards that youth can either post in key places at home (e.g., bulletin board, mirror, refrigerator) or carry in a pocket, notebook, or backpack for a tangible reminder of coping thoughts to use during challenging situations. For homework, youth continue to monitor their thoughts in specific situations throughout the week, recording both negative and coping thoughts. Youth learn to praise and reward themselves when they have made progress in changing negative self-talk to coping self-talk (Step 6).

There are several additional key issues to keep in mind when implementing cognitive strategies. Cognitive restructuring can be extremely difficult if a feared outcome has a high likelihood of occurring for a particular child or adolescent (Albano & DiBartolo, 2007). For example, youth who have poor social skills may have realistic worries about being teased by other children. In such cases, it is necessary to provide social skills training before moving forward with the cognitive portion of treatment. To promote treatment gains, it is also important to uncover the core beliefs or assumptions underlying an adolescent's negative automatic thoughts (Albano & DiBartolo, 2007). For example, a teen who worries about making mistakes when giving a speech at school may have a core belief that if his or her performance is not perfect that means that he or she is stupid, which is the belief that the clinician needs to focus on during cognitive restructuring. To identify these core beliefs, clinicians can use the downward arrow technique described by Judith Beck (2011), which involves identifying a negative automatic thought and then asking several follow-up questions, such as "What would that mean to you?" and "And then what would happen?" Once the core assumption is uncovered, the teen can challenge it by gathering evidence and generating coping thoughts, as described earlier in this section.

Although the cognitive strategies used across various internalizing disorders are similar, there are minor modifications for particular diagnoses. For example, in treatment programs for OCD, the cognitive restructuring portion of treatment focuses on OCD symptoms that are fueled by negative emotion, such as fear, guilt, or disgust, and the cognitive training is conducted to help children develop tools to successfully "boss back" OCD during ERP tasks (March & Benton, 2007; March & Mulle, 1998). The cognitive training portion of treatment includes constructive self-talk (i.e., changing unhelpful thoughts to more realistic self-talk, generating coping thoughts by "talking back to OCD"), restructuring beliefs related to overestimation of catastrophic events and perceived responsibility for these events by learning to identify and disregard "what OCD says," and developing detachment from OCD through simple self-statements (e.g., "It's just OCD again"; "My brain is hiccuping again"). Parents learn about these cognitive techniques so that they can encourage youth to use them during exposure and response prevention tasks outside of therapy sessions (March & Mulle, 1998).

Cognitive strategies play a very prominent role in treatments for depressed youth. In fact, some programs, such as Taking Action (Stark & Kendall, 1996), incorporate cognitive elements into nearly every session throughout treatment. Although not universally the case, many manualized treatments for depressed youth, such as the CWD-A course (Clarke & DeBar, 2010) and the ACTION program for depressed youth (Stark et al., 2007), are designed for a group rather than individual format. According to Stark et al. (2006), youth can more readily recognize and restructure negative thoughts in other group members first and then develop the ability to identify and change their own negative self-talk. The ACTION program also uses the unique metaphor of the "Muck Monster," who fills youth with negative thoughts. One particular cognitive restructuring activity involves "talking back to the Muck Monster"—that is, challenging negative thinking in a more concrete and depersonalized way that helps youth to stop being "stuck in the negative muck" (Stark et al., 2006, p. 198). This program includes many other hands-on activities to facilitate cognitive restructuring, such as putting dark lens covers over a pair of sunglasses to show how negative thinking is similar to wearing dark glasses.

## Developmental Adaptations

Early cognitive therapy practices were developed for use with adult populations (A. T. Beck, Rush, Shaw, & Emery, 1979) and rested on the foundational construct of *metacognition* (see Vasey, 1993; Wells, 2004), which is commonly defined as "thinking about thinking." When working with adults, it is generally assumed that individuals have the ability to consciously examine the content and nature of their thoughts. Developmental psychology research has demonstrated that the acquisition of cognitive skills tends to occur in specific stages, with the capacity for metacognition typically emerging during middle to late childhood (Siegler, 1998). Indeed, Grave and Blissett (2004) point out that 5- to 8-year-old children (i.e., in the preoperational stage) have normative developmental limitations in such cognitive capacities as causal reasoning, metacognition, memory capacity, and attention span. Furthermore, these youth experience smaller gains than older children and adolescents, according to both individual CBT efficacy studies and meta-analytic reviews (see Grave & Blissett, 2004, for a review). However, a very small number of studies have focused specifically on this age group, and additional research is needed to determine the extent to which children's level of cognitive development impacts the effectiveness of CBT. Paula Barrett (2000) offers an insightful reflection on the issues related to this topic, emphasizing that a fundamental error is made when youth are simply considered "little adults" (p. 481) for whom adult-derived interventions can be applied with little to no developmental modification.

So what, then, can be done to ensure that clinicians attend to each child's developmental level and deliver cognitive skills appropriately across age groups? First, Kingery and colleagues (2006) underscore that each client must be considered individually to provide the most developmentally appropriate intervention possible. One of the most important ways to accomplish this goal is by evaluating each youth's cognitive abilities. Clinicians can engage in this type of assessment through formal and informal means. Therapists should inquire whether the child has had any prior psychological or educational evaluations. In the absence of such data, clinicians may conduct their own evaluation as part of their routine pretreatment assessment. A review of school records that document the child's academic performance may provide a means for estimating cognitive abilities (Neisser et al., 1996). When these options are not available or practical, clinicians can use initial treatment sessions to engage in informal assessment of the youth's cognitive developmental level. Through early rapport-building activities (e.g., asking about the youth's family, friends, attitudes toward school, favorite activities) and psychoeducation exercises (e.g., learning awareness of somatic signs of emotional distress, affect identification, recognition of thoughts), the clinician can take note of the youth's cognitive maturity and level of insight into his or her own internal experience.

Using information obtained from this assessment, the therapist can implement cognitive strategies in a way that is tailored to the youth's ability. One of the most common obstacles is the difficulty that younger youth often have with identifying their own thoughts and experiences. Kane and Kendall (1989) found that youth in middle to late childhood (e.g., ages 9–13 years) struggled to identify problematic thoughts in imaginal and *in vivo* contexts, though they were able to consider what might happen to another child in a similar situation. These authors conclude that there may be a developmental threshold below which disorder-relevant cognitions cannot be targeted directly through a straightforward question-and-answer format. However, such a hypothetical cutoff point does not necessarily mean that cognitive content cannot be accessed by younger youth. Cognitive strategies may simply need to be adapted to fit their developmental level. For instance, Eisen and Silverman (1993) describe adjusting a cognitive therapy protocol for a 6-year-old child who had difficulty identifying anxious thoughts: cartoon strips of favorite superheroes were utilized, through which troubling cognitions could be more concretely conveyed. This technique also served as a vehicle for therapist-guided generation of coping thoughts and ultimately, through practice, helped the child to be able to independently practice the cognitive skills.

It is also important to recognize that an apparent lack of awareness of maladaptive cognitions can sometimes reflect avoidance of discussing difficult thoughts and feelings (Kane & Kendall, 1989). For younger children, one way to approach this challenge is to externalize the source of upsetting thoughts to a fictional entity of their choice (e.g., "Worry Monster," "Nervous Bug," "Sadness Cloud"). In this way, the child is absolved of the responsibility for having the thoughts and is provided with an opponent figure whose negative influence will be battled against by the child and his or her support "team" (e.g., parents, therapist, teachers, etc.). The developmentally attuned therapist will acknowledge that, even for older youth, it is less threatening for an individual to imagine someone else dealing with a target situation, and this tactic can be a productive avenue for generating alternative adaptive cognitions. This approach carries the added benefit of helping youth to realize that they are not the only one dealing with this difficulty. Kingery and colleagues (2006) describe an example in which an adolescent with an affinity for dance was asked to brainstorm coping thoughts that her favorite dancer might use when experiencing distress. Another possibility would be to have the youth imagine attempting to assist a friend in generating coping-focused thoughts.

Numerous other techniques can facilitate the implementation of cognitive strategies with youth across various ages. One suggestion for helping young children grasp the influence of thoughts on emotions and behaviors is to juxtapose the child's attitude toward a stimulus that could either be anxiety-producing or exhilarating with the experience of a contrasting peer. For example, the child can be asked whether he or she enjoys riding roller coasters or is afraid of them; whatever the response, the therapist then inquires about a peer who holds the opposite attitude. The child is then asked to imagine being at an amusement park and approaching a very large roller coaster. Because the stimulus itself (e.g., the roller coaster) is the same, the therapist can explore how it is the difference in thoughts and expectations about the roller coaster that differentiates the child from his or her peer in terms of associated feelings (e.g., excitement vs. anxiety) and subsequent behaviors (e.g., running to get in line vs. running the other way).

Metaphors can also be a powerful way for children and adolescents to develop a greater understanding of their own cognitive processes. For older youth, an important lesson is that troubling thoughts are only a sampling of a multitude of thoughts that occur over the course of the day. Middle childhood to adolescent clients who are particularly interested in sports can be encouraged to consider the coming and going of thoughts like the ticker that runs along the bottom of the screen on ESPN providing sports news and player performance statistics. In the same way that youth might latch onto a particular piece of unfortunate news (e.g., favorite team has lost a game or favorite player has been injured) and forget all of the other information continuously passing by, so too do negatively biased thoughts attain greater saliency and thus become the focus of worry and rumination.

It is also important for clinicians to be aware of methods for effectively guiding youth of various ages through the process of iden-tifying thoughts. When presenting questions, Friedberg and McClure (2015) recommend using a "gentle and curious stance" so that the child or adolescent does not feel bombarded with questions (p. 91). These authors also suggest using open-ended questions that promote imag-ery (e.g., "What popped/flew into your mind?"; "What did you say to yourself"; "What raced through your head?") rather than "What thoughts are you having about _____?" or "What are you thinking?" (p. 91). Finally, it is important to recognize that many youth will need direct instruction surrounding the completion of the daily thought records (see Chapter 11).

Given developmental differences in cognitive awareness and maturity, caregivers are expected to be more involved in the treat-ment process with young children than with adolescents. Piacentini and Langley (2004) offer recommendations for how caregivers can be instrumental in this role for youth with OCD. Rather than accommo-date the self-perpetuating cycle of OCD, either through verbal reassur-ances or facilitation of anxiety-avoidant rituals, caregivers can offer brief supportive statements, for example, "It sounds like your OCD is giving you a hard time" (p. 1192). Such an approach signals to the youth that the use of cognitive coping strategies may be helpful for combating the cycle of obsessive thinking. For youth struggling with depressive symptoms, caregivers can help youth recognize when they are engaging in cognitively biased thinking patterns and subsequently help them to challenge those thoughts.

## Diversity Considerations

When implementing manualized treatments with anxious or depressed youth, it is also important to be mindful of cultural and ethnic differ-ences. In relation to cognitive strategies, sensitivity to culture must be observed when evaluating the validity of an individual's thoughts. For example, when working with a Hispanic child with separation anxiety disorder who is worried about family members' safety outside of the home, the therapist must explore cultural factors such as family beliefs and experiences with safety that could help the therapist determine whether the child's fears are realistic or whether the thoughts are mal-adaptive and should be challenged. Although the evidence base is rela-tively small, this section reviews extant empirical support for cognitive strategies as an acceptable and helpful intervention for internalizing disorders across various ethnic groups.

Research evaluating the cognitive strategies element individually with youth from diverse ethnic backgrounds is lacking; however, several studies evaluating CBT programs that include a cognitive component have reported similar levels of improvement across racial or ethnic groups. In one study involving 56 children (6–16 years old; 46% Caucasian, 46% Hispanic, 8% other), a group CBT condition was compared against a waitlist control to evaluate the effectiveness of this treatment for anxiety disorders (Silverman et al., 1999). The CBT condition included a cognitive training component in which children were taught to be aware of and modify their maladaptive thoughts. At posttreatment, 64% of the children in the CBT condition no longer met diagnostic criteria, compared to 13% in the waitlist control group. Reductions in symptoms were also noted on parent and child measures. Race/ethnicity was not a moderator of treatment effects, demonstrating that similar gains were found across groups. Notably, in their review of EBTs for ethnic minority youth, Huey and Polo (2008) identified group CBT as a treatment that is *possibly efficacious* for Hispanic/Latino and African American youth with anxiety disorders, based upon criteria outlined by Chambless and Hollon (1998).

With respect to depression, the Treatment for Adolescents with Depression Study (TADS) was a multisite study involving 439 youth, ages 12–17 years (73.8% Caucasian, 12.5% African American, 8.9% Hispanic), that compared the relative efficacy of individual CBT, fluoxetine, a combination of CBT and fluoxetine, and placebo (Treatment for Adolescents with Depression Study [TADS] Team, 2003, 2005). The CBT in TADS incorporated cognitive strategies throughout treatment, including increased awareness of thoughts, understanding cognitive distortions, and challenging automatic thoughts, attributions, and beliefs (Curry et al., 2000). At posttreatment, the combination treatment was significantly more effective than either of the single treatments and the placebo (Curry et al., 2006). Moreover, race was neither a predictor nor a moderator of outcome, indicating that findings were applicable across groups. Based upon the low number of minority children relative to Caucasian children involved in this study, however, additional research on the effectiveness of these treatments with more diverse samples of youth is needed before firm conclusions can be drawn.

IPT for depression is a manualized treatment that has been evaluated with Puerto Rican adolescents (Rosselló & Bernal, 1999; Rosselló, Bernal, & Rivera-Medina, 2012). In one study, it was found to be equally as effective as CBT, and both treatments were superior to a waitlist control condition. At posttreatment, 82% of adolescents receiving IPT were no longer considered clinically depressed, compared to 59% of adolescents in the CBT condition. In both conditions, efforts were made to incorporate cultural elements and adaptations whenever possible. In an extension of this study that added comparison conditions of group IPT and group CBT, Rosselló et al. (2012) found that both group and individual CBT produced significantly greater levels of improvement in depression than the IPT conditions. In explaining their findings, the authors hypothesized that perhaps overall CBT was more effective than IPT because the CBT treatment is more structured, concrete, and directive, which speaks to the cultural value of *respeto* (respect; Rosselló et al., 2012). Given that very few studies have evaluated the relative efficacy of different types of manualized treatments for depression with particular ethnic groups, additional research is needed. That said, based upon studies published thus far, Huey and Polo (2008) conclude that CBT can be considered *probably efficacious* for the treatment of depression among Latino youth, and IPT meets the status of *possibly efficacious.*

The results of several studies support the use of CBT with Asian and Pacific Islander (Chorpita, Taylor, Francis, Mofitt, & Austin, 2004), Chinese (Lau, Chan, Li, & Au, 2010), and Brazilian youth (de Souza et al., 2013), demonstrating superiority to a waitlist control with significantly fewer youth in CBT meeting criteria for an anxiety disorder at posttreatment. Lau and colleagues (2010) also found that a reduction in anxious cognitions and improvement in coping skills served as mediators of treatment outcome for Chinese youth.

Until the research foundation on this topic is strengthened, there are several important guidelines for clinicians to consider when implementing cognitive strategies with diverse populations. Wood, Chiu, Hwang, Jacobs, and Ifekwunigwe (2008) offer several principles for administering CBT with Mexican-American youth that likely apply to other diverse groups, including taking time to learn about the family's cultural practices (e.g., language proficiencies) and respecting the family's conceptualization of mental health difficulties. When implementing cognitive strategies, explaining the rationale for such strategies may be indicated so that families understand the extent to which such strategies fit in with their values and conceptualization of the problem. Wood et al. (2008) also recommend engaging the extended family in treatment, as extended families may be considered to be as equally important as the nuclear family in some cultures. Sherry Cormier and colleagues (2013) point out that other professionals who are central figures in the client's cultural background can be incorporated into treatment (e.g., traditional healers in Native American communities). When working with diverse clients and addressing maladaptive cognitions, it is also important to be mindful of the language used. For example, some individuals may prefer not to label thoughts as "irrational" or "distorted." Treatment providers should be sensitive about what terminology is used when assisting clients with evaluating and labeling thoughts. Finally, it is important to consider the cultural context of each individual client when evaluating his or her thoughts and beliefs rather than evaluating thoughts solely based on the majority culture's values, goals, and schemas (Cormier et al., 2013).

## CONCLUSIONS

The cognitive strategies treatment element is based upon foundational principles of cognitive theory, with historical ties to social learning theory and cognitive theories of emotion. The evidence base supporting the effectiveness of this element includes studies evaluating cognitive strategies as part of multicomponent CBT programs that include cognitive restructuring and related techniques, with a small number of studies also demonstrating that changes in anxious or depressed cognitions serve as mediators of treatment gains. To implement this core treatment element effectively, it is essential to understand theoretical principles related to the role of negative/biased cognitions in internalizing distress. The step-by-step procedures outlined in this chapter can serve as a practical resource to guide implementation of this treatment element. Clinicians should be mindful of various ways to adjust cognitive strategies to meet the needs of particular diagnoses, developmental levels, and children and adolescents from diverse backgrounds.

## BOX 3.2. Illustrative Case Example

Sally, a 15-year-old Caucasian female who met the criteria for social anxiety disorder, was seen for 12 sessions of individual CBT. She was in the 10th grade and lived with her mother, father, and 17-year-old sister. Regarding social anxiety symptoms, Sally avoided activities such as going to the mall, attending school events (e.g., dances, pep rallies), and going to friends' houses for get-togethers or sleepovers. When around peers and adults other than her family members, Sally constantly worried that she would do something stupid or embarrassing. She avoided answering the telephone or calling friends, even if she needed important information such as details of a homework assignment. Her parents and sister reported a tendency to "rescue" Sally from her distress by completing anxiety-provoking tasks for her, including ordering food at restaurants and making phone calls. Sally occasionally invited a few close friends over to her house, but she reported not enjoying this very much due to constant worries about what her friends must be thinking about her. Although a straight A student with no attendance problems, Sally constantly worried about what others thought of her throughout the school day, experiencing frequent headaches and stomachaches, and avoiding activities such as eating lunch while at school because of her social worries. At the beginning of treatment, Sally expressed a strong desire to feel less anxious, have more friends, and participate in more social activities. She regularly attended weekly sessions and practiced CBT skills outside of the therapy sessions each week, with support and encouragement from her family.

To address Sally's extreme shyness with the therapist at the beginning of treatment, several extra "get to know you" activities were incorporated into the initial treatment session (e.g., cards with questions about favorite music, television shows, etc., that the therapist and adolescent took turns answering). Gradually, Sally became more comfortable discussing situations that were anxiety-provoking for her, and an anxiety hierarchy was created. Items on the hierarchy included situations such as calling to order a pizza, calling a friend to ask about a homework assignment, initiating a conversation with an acquaintance at school, inviting a friend to go to the mall or watch a movie, ordering food at a restaurant, asking an unfamiliar adult for directions, and giving a presentation in front of an audience.

At the beginning of the cognitive portion of treatment, the therapist reviewed the CBT model and explained the role of thoughts in maintaining anxious feelings and behavior. For the next several weeks, the therapist asked Sally to complete self-monitoring sheets for homework to record thoughts connected to various anxiety-provoking situations that she faced throughout the week. Given that Sally was a bright and highly motivated adolescent, she quickly caught on to the idea of identifying thoughts. She also readily understood the difference between anxious and coping thoughts as well as the connection between anxious thoughts and feelings. However, Sally was initially reluctant to share her thoughts verbally during sessions with the therapist, indicating that she felt "stupid and embarrassed." The therapist addressed this challenge by sharing some of her own thoughts surrounding personally anxiety-provoking situations (e.g., giving a speech), providing gentle

*(continued)*

## BOX 3.2 (*continued*)

encouragement, and using activities such as cartoon strips and role-play exercises to help Sally feel more comfortable elaborating upon her anxious thoughts. The therapist also shared information gathered during the initial assessment (e.g., questionnaires, the clinical interview) with Sally to remind her of the types of thoughts that she had endorsed and to help her make connections between these thoughts and the situations on her self-monitoring logs.

After monitoring and discussing thoughts for several weeks, the therapist helped Sally to identify patterns in her thoughts related to anxiety-provoking situations and to match those patterns with common "thinking traps" (i.e., cognitive distortions). Sally's prominent thinking traps included expecting that the worst was going to happen, mind reading (i.e., making assumptions about what others are thinking), and jumping to conclusions before having all of the facts. Given Sally's advanced cognitive skills, the therapist also used Socratic questioning to help uncover some of her core beliefs surrounding social situations. For example, when discussing her thoughts surrounding the task of calling a friend to ask a question about a homework assignment, Sally revealed believing that the friend would think that her question was silly or she would not know what to say when her friend answered the phone. The therapist asked such questions as "If your friend thinks that your question is silly or you don't know what to say, how or why does that matter?" Sally indicated that then her friend might no longer like her or would think that she is stupid. Similarly, when faced with giving a presentation in front of the class at school, Sally worried about doing something embarrassing or making a mistake and being laughed at by her peers. The therapist asked, "And if you make a mistake or people laugh at you, why does that matter?" Through a series of similar questions, it became clear that Sally held several core beliefs related to extremely high standards for her social performance, including believing that everyone must like her and she must appear intelligent all the time.

Once the cognitive distortions and core beliefs had been identified, the therapist taught Sally how to challenge her anxious thoughts and change them to more realistic coping thoughts. The therapist encouraged Sally to work like a detective, "gathering the evidence" to determine the validity of her anxious thoughts. For example, when Sally jumped to the conclusion that her friend would refuse her invitation to come over and watch a movie, Sally was encouraged to ask such questions as "Do I know for sure that this will happen?" and "What else might happen—other than what I originally thought?" Over time, Sally was able to recognize that she was jumping to conclusions without having all of the facts and that usually social situations had a better outcome than she originally anticipated. This process of challenging thoughts occurred hand in hand with the completion of exposure tasks, allowing her to "test" her predictions in real-life situations. For example, one week Sally set a goal of calling three friends and raising her hand to ask a question in class at least once a day. Prior to completing these tasks, she used a self-monitoring sheet to record her anxious thoughts, generate coping thoughts to use in the situations, and then relate what actually happened. In many cases she received a positive response, which helped her to recognize that her once firmly held core beliefs were not always true.

Through the process of challenging her thoughts, Sally generated various coping thoughts, such as "Most of the time, interactions with my friends and other kids at school go pretty smoothly," "I don't have to be perfect," and "Everyone makes mistakes, I just have to try my best." As Sally worked her way through the lower portion of her anxiety hierarchy and had success with simpler social interactions (e.g., calling a friend), this gave her the confidence to face more challenging tasks (e.g., asking an unfamiliar adult for directions, introducing herself to a new peer). When planning exposure tasks, it was often helpful for Sally to role-play anticipated social scenarios with the therapist, which allowed the therapist to provide feedback (e.g., specific social skills) and cue Sally to implement the problem-solving and relaxation skills learned during earlier phases of treatment. By the end of treatment, Sally had made excellent progress in challenging her anxious thoughts and accomplishing the majority of the items on her hierarchy. Although still a bit shy, Sally added a few new friends to her social circle, joined an environmental awareness club at school, and felt much more at ease in various social situations. Following 12 weeks of weekly therapy sessions, she participated in several monthly booster sessions to maintain treatment gains and prevent relapse.

# 4

## Problem–Solving Training

### BACKGROUND OF THE ELEMENT

Depressed and anxious youth tend to see their problems as unsolvable burdens or threats and are less likely to take action as a result. This avoidance often leads to more problems and heightened negative emotions. In problem-solving training (PST), which is sometimes referred to as social problem-solving therapy, the therapist teaches the youth to take a more positive and systematic approach to problems by generating a variety of potentially effective solutions, selecting and implementing the best one, and evaluating the outcome (Spiegler, 2016). By teaching broadly applicable coping skills, PST can enhance the maintenance of treatment effects and generalization of skills learned during the intervention (D'Zurilla & Goldfried, 1971; Spiegler, 2016). In this chapter, coverage of the history, theory, and evidence base for PST is followed by practical guidelines for its use in interventions for youth with internalizing disorders, such as depression and anxiety. Designed to be a useful resource for clinicians, the chapter includes step-by-step implementation suggestions, important developmental and diversity considerations, and a case example of a 16-year-old Caucasian male treated for depression.

### Brief History

PST emerged when cognitive concepts and strategies were incorporated into behavior therapy during the early 1970s (D'Zurilla & Nezu,

2010). D'Zurilla and Goldfried (1971) were the first to introduce PST as an intervention technique with a set of formal procedures. In a widely cited article, these authors proposed that PST be included among the existing behavior modification techniques. While hard to imagine in today's context, this was somewhat of a bold proposition, given that PST targeted primarily cognitive—and thus largely covert—processes.

D'Zurilla and Goldfried (1971) defined problem solving as a conscious effort to generate a variety of potentially effective response alternatives and increase the likelihood that the most effective response would be selected from among them. Bridging research and theory from a variety of literatures, including experimental psychology, education, and industry, the two researchers distilled the problem-solving process into five—now widely known—stages: (1) general orientation (e.g., attitudes toward the problem), (2) problem definition and formulation, (3) generation of alternatives, (4) decision making, and (5) verification. In their intervention model, they proposed that the therapist use well-established behavior modification procedures, including verbal instruction, modeling, and reinforcement, to teach the client the skills most relevant to each stage. Upon meeting acceptable performance thresholds, the client was to progress from stage to stage and eventually assume more autonomy in the problem-solving process, with the therapist adopting more of a consultant role. Despite their proposed stage theory framework, D'Zurilla and Goldfried (1971) acknowledged that real-life problem solving need not be sequential and that some movement back and forth between stages would be expected.

Directly targeting the cognitive process offered a number of advantages for behavior modification efforts. First, it provided a new way to view effective responding in problem situations. According to the prevailing social learning theories, effective responding could be attributed to trial-and-error learning, instruction, or the observation of others. Adding another option, D'Zurilla and Goldfried (1971) suggested that the person might instead "figure out" what to do through effective problem solving, essentially by mentally combining previously learned behaviors to form a novel response pattern, considering its consequences, and making value judgments about those consequences. A distinction was made between this mental problem-solving process and the actual implementation of a selected response. Specifically, an individual might be able to solve a problem cognitively but yet not be able to carry out the solution because of a skills deficit, anxiety, or lack of motivation (D'Zurilla & Goldfried, 1971). Second, the problem-solving approach held much promise for improving the maintenance and generalization of interventions. Unlike most of the existing behavior modification techniques (e.g., relaxation training) that targeted discrete responses in specific situations, the goal of PST was not to help clients solve particular problems but rather to teach them how to solve problems more generally. Once acquired, this new "learning set" could be independently applied to a wide variety of problem situations and thereby enhance maintenance and generalization. Indeed, D'Zurilla and Goldfried (1971) saw problem solving as having the potential to train a client to function "as his own therapist" (p. 111).

Spivack and Shure were also highly influential in the development of problem-solving interventions. In a very productive research program that ran parallel to, yet surprisingly independent of, D'Zurilla and Goldfried's efforts, Spivack and Shure drew connections between problem-solving skills and behavioral adjustment in young children and evaluated a related training program (e.g., Shure, Spivack, & Gordon, 1972; Shure, Spivack, & Jaeger, 1971; Spivack, Platt, & Shure, 1976). In a study with Head Start preschoolers, Shure et al. (1971) found that, irrespective of verbal productivity and intellectual functioning, children rated as less well adjusted (e.g., higher emotionality, aggression) by their teachers generated fewer possible solutions and a narrower range of solutions to hypothetical problems than their more well adjusted peers. Subsequently, Shure et al. (1972) demonstrated the effectiveness of a comprehensive PST intervention targeting preschoolers. Improvements on the problem-solving measures were not accompanied by changes in teacher-rated behavior in this study, but Shure and Spivack (1980) later provided support for a mediational role of problem-solving skills.

This early work in problem solving has inspired a tremendous amount of intervention research. Whether delivered as a sole intervention or as part of a packaged treatment, PST has been applied to a wide range of clinical disorders, including depression, schizophrenia, anxiety, and substance abuse, as well as health problems, including cancer and obesity (see D'Zurilla & Nezu, 2007, for a review). For youth with internalizing disorders in particular, PST ranked in the top 10 most frequently used practice elements in a recent quantitative review of evidence-based treatments for children and adolescents with anxiety and depression (Chorpita & Daleiden, 2009).

## Theory Base

Understanding how to apply PST with youth experiencing internalizing distress starts with a grounding in its fundamental assumptions.

PST arose as part of a movement rejecting the medical model of psychopathology. From a social learning perspective, abnormal behavior was not a symptom of underlying disease but rather a learned response that was ineffective and led to negative consequences (D'Zurilla & Goldfried, 1971). An inability to cope with problem situations was viewed as a necessary and sufficient condition for an emotional or behavioral disorder. Thus, from this perspective, the best way to "treat" the disorder was to teach problem-solving skills, with the goal of facilitating more effective responding. By helping individuals develop broadly applicable coping skills, PST can also be helpful in preventing disorders and/or relapse (Spiegler, 2016).

Nezu (1987) applied these social learning concepts in his problem-solving formulation of depression. In this formulation, he posited that depression is activated by the interaction of stressful events, problems, and problem-solving deficits. Ineffective responding in problem situations results in negative consequences that serve to make the existing problem worse and increase the probability of future problems. By decreasing reinforcement and motivation for future problem-solving attempts, ineffective responding also increases vulnerability for a depressive episode. For example, already feeling overwhelmed, an adolescent is worried about an upcoming exam and also having to work afternoons for her part-time job. Faced with this problem, she decides to skip work and is fired as a result, which leaves her with a new set of problems, including the distress of being fired, conflict with her parents, and a lack of spending money. Her mood worsens, problems increase, and her ability to solve them is further diminished in the process. An important aspect of this formulation is the reciprocal nature of events, problems, and problem solving. Problem-solving ability moderates the nature and number of problems arising from negative life events, and, in turn, ineffective problem solving can lead to negative life events and future problems.

In Nezu's (1987) formulation, ineffective responding arises from deficiencies in any or all of D'Zurilla and Goldfried's (1971) five problem-solving stages (i.e., general orientation, problem definition and formulation, generation of alternatives, decision making, and verification). Critical to the *general orientation* stage is the adoption of a positive problem-solving attitude or response set. To the contrary, negative thinking characterizes depression, and affected youth may be more likely to see problems as unique to them, magnify their extent, engage in self-blame, and feel unable to respond (Nezu, 1987). The *problem definition and formulation* stage emphasizes the importance of taking a systematic, orderly, and comprehensive approach to problems (D'Zurilla

& Goldfried, 1971; D'Zurilla & Nezu, 2010). Negative thinking patterns may make it more difficult for depressed youth to be objective and specific when addressing their problems (Nezu, 1987). For example, an adolescent who tends to blame him- or herself for everything will be less able to accurately define a problem, identify its true source, and generate possible solutions.

The *generation of alternatives* stage involves coming up with possible solutions to a particular problem in a way that maximizes the likelihood that the most effective response is included among them (D'Zurilla & Goldfried, 1971). Depression is associated with the generation of a restricted range of response alternatives that results in ineffective responding (Nezu, 1987). The goal of the *decision-making* stage is to select the most effective response alternative. Effective responses alter the situation, maximizing positive consequences while minimizing negative ones. Depression hampers decision making. Cognitive biases, such as selectively attending to the negative, can lead to the inaccurate assessment of response alternatives and their potential consequences (Nezu, 1987). Of course, having fewer quality response options to choose from makes ineffective responding more likely for depressed youth regardless of their decision-making abilities.

The final stage of problem solving occurs after the chosen response alternative has been enacted. *Verification*, later referred to as *solution implementation and verification* (D'Zurilla & Nezu, 1982), involves an assessment of the actual outcome and whether any self-correction is needed (D'Zurilla & Goldfried, 1971). The key question is whether the actual consequences of a solution match those anticipated during the decision-making stage (Nezu, 1987). For youth experiencing depression, biased thinking may preclude objectivity in assessing outcomes. They may focus on the negative, set very high expectations for themselves, and be more swayed by the short-term, rather than long-term, consequences of their actions (Nezu, 1987; Rehm, 1977).

Overall, despite ample evidence relating depression and more general problem-solving deficits in child and adolescent samples (e.g., Mullins, Siegel, & Hodges, 1985; Sacco & Graves, 1984), there is surprisingly little empirical support for the particular stage-related deficits proposed by Nezu (1987) other than that found for orientation variables in studies of adolescents. Positive problem orientation has been found to moderate the relation between negative life stress and depression, and, conversely, negative problem orientation and impulsive and avoidant response styles predict depression (e.g., Frye & Goodman, 2000; Reinecke, DuBois, & Schultz, 2001). Beyond that, there is some evidence linking depressive symptoms and the generation of fewer solutions (Frye & Goodman, 2000; Levendosky, Okun, & Parker, 1995). Though the types of deficits proposed by Nezu (1987) may well exist, researchers have tended not to assess them, instead relying on self-reports of more global attitudes and abilities.

Research examining problem solving and anxiety is much less advanced, but the Nezu (1987) formulation seems readily adaptable. Studies with adults have documented links between anxiety and less effective problem solving (e.g., Dugas, Letarte, Rheaume, Freeston, & Ladouceur, 1995) and evidence of a moderating role for problem-solving ability in the relationship between negative life stress and anxiety (Nezu, 1986). Anxious youth present with a range of cognitive biases that would appear to adversely impact their problem-solving ability. For example, Chorpita, Albano, and Barlow (1996) found that anxious children had a distinct tendency to interpret ambiguous situations as threatening, endorse more avoidant plans in response, and assign higher probability to the occurrence of threatening events. Problem situations are inherently ambiguous, and perceiving them as threats may impede the ability to objectively define them, discourage the generation of solutions, and prevent decision making and implementation (Dugas et al., 1995).

## Evidence Base

Most evidence supporting the efficacy of PST for youth is indirect, deriving from studies evaluating multimodal treatments that include it as one component (see Table 4.1 for a summary of PST applications in evidence-based treatment manuals for internalizing disorders in youth). More specifically, in efforts to identify evidence-based treatments, PST is a component of those labeled as "well established" for depression (David-Ferdon & Kaslow, 2008), "probably efficacious" for bipolar disorder (Fristad & McPherson, 2014), and "probably efficacious" for anxiety disorders (Freeman et al., 2014; Silverman, Pina, et al., 2008).

In the closest approximation of a stand-alone evaluation, Stark and his colleagues compared behavioral problem-solving therapy (BPS), self-control therapy (SC), and waitlist conditions in a sample of 29 children (mean age = 11.17 years) scoring in the moderately to severely depressed range on a self-report measure of depression (Stark et al., 1987). The initial four sessions of both active 12-session group treatments were quite similar (e.g., rationale, self-monitoring, group

TABLE 4.1 The Problem–Solving Training Element in Representative EBT Manuals

| | |
|---|---|
| *Coping Cat* (Kendall & Hedtke, 2006) | • Problem solving is explicitly mentioned and integrated throughout this treatment, with a specific session dedicated to developing problem-solving skills. The therapist is also encouraged to model problem solving in anxiety-provoking situations of increasing intensity. |
| *C.A.T. Project* (Kendall, Choudhury, Hudson, & Webb, 2002) | • As with *Coping Cat*, problem solving is integrated throughout the treatment and is also the focus of a particular session about coping and problem solving. The therapist is encouraged to help adolescents acquire skills for problem solving in anxiety-provoking situations. |
| *Family-Based Treatment for Young Children with OCD* (Freeman & Garcia, 2009) | • Problem solving is explicitly incorporated into parental scaffolding for teaching ERP in one section of the treatment.<br>• The parents also problem-solve potential barriers to homework completion (child and parent assignments) with the therapist. |
| *CBT of Childhood OCD: It's Only a False Alarm* (Piacentini, Langley, & Roblek, 2007) | • Although problem solving is not a specific skill taught in this treatment, the parents and/or the therapists are encouraged to help the youth use it in several places throughout this treatment (e.g., in problem solving obstacles to homework compliance or engaging in exposure exercises). |
| *CBT for Social Phobia: Stand Up, Speak Out* (Albano & DiBartolo, 2007) | • Problem solving is explicitly mentioned in a section on "problem solving and skills training," a series of three sessions, one of which is dedicated jointly to social problem solving and cognitive restructuring (the other two sessions focusing on social skills training and assertiveness training). |
| *When Children Refuse School: A CBT Approach* (Kearney & Albano, 2007): Chapters 4 and 5 on internalizing symptoms | • Though covered in detail as part of parent–child negotiation and contracting in a chapter devoted to reward-based school refusal (Chapter 7), there is no clear teaching of problem-solving skills in the two chapters on internalizing symptoms. |
| *Treating Trauma and Traumatic Grief in Children and Adolescents* (Cohen, Mannarino, & Deblinger, 2006) | • Problem solving is explicitly mentioned, with one section devoted to enhancing problem solving and social skills, including related worksheets for youth to complete.<br>• Problem solving is also referenced at other points in the treatment through the use of an acronym (i.e., CRAFTS) for the types of problems addressed in treatment (Cognitive, Relationship, Affective, Family, Traumatic behavior, Somatic). |
| *Adolescent Coping with Depression* (Clarke, Lewinsohn, & Hops, 1990) | • Problem solving is an explicit focus of this treatment, with an entire section devoted to learning negotiation and problem solving. |

**TABLE 4.1.** (*continued*)

| | |
|---|---|
| *Interpersonal Psychotherapy for Depressed Adolescents,* 2nd edition (Mufson, Pollack Dorta, Moreau, & Weissman, 2011) | • Teaching problem solving is an explicit component of this treatment, with the therapist assisting the client in each of the formal steps involved in problem solving. |
| *Treating Depressed Children: Therapist Manual for "Taking Action"* (Stark & Kendall, 1996) | • Problem solving is explicitly discussed in this treatment, with a specific section dedicated to it. The therapist is also encouraged to model the use of problem solving to overcome impediments the client encounters. |
| *Treating Depressed Youth: Therapist Manual for "Action"* (Stark et al., 2007) | • Problem solving is an explicit component of this treatment, with a section focused on this skill and the steps one takes to learn it, as well as a separate appendix describing the steps. |
| *Psychotherapy for Children with Bipolar and Depressive Disorders* (Fristad, Arnold, & Leffler, 2011) | • Problem solving is explicitly discussed and integrated throughout this treatment, including several related activities and handouts.<br>• Additionally, there are separate problem-solving skills chapters intended to address parents' and children's problem-solving deficits. |

*Note.* Some book titles are shortened to conserve space. See the References at the back of the book for full titles.

problem solving to increase frequency of pleasurable activities). The remaining sessions in the BPS condition were devoted to teaching problem-solving skills and developing strategies for increasing the occurrence of pleasant activities. In the SC condition, the remaining sessions targeted self-monitoring of pleasant activities and positive self-statements, setting more realistic performance standards, adaptive attributions, and self-consequating. Both of the active treatments were effective relative to the waitlist condition, producing statistically and clinically significant improvements in depression. The BPS condition fared a bit better than the SC condition on the parent ratings, with mothers reporting significant improvements in internalizing behavior at posttreatment and in social withdrawal, depression, and internalizing behavior at an 8-week follow-up.

Multimodal treatments that include PST as a component are effective in treating child and adolescent depression (e.g., Clarke et al., 1999; Kahn, Kehle, Jenson, & Clark, 1990; Lewinsohn et al., 1990; Mufson et al., 2004; Mufson, Weissman, Moreau, & Garfinkel, 1999). Most of these are cognitive-behavioral treatments that also include psychoeducation, cognitive restructuring, pleasant events scheduling, and skills training (e.g., coping, emotion regulation, and social skills). For example, in a study with 59 depressed adolescents (mean age = 16.23 years), Lewinsohn and colleagues compared adolescent-only and adolescent and parent versions of their CWD-A (Lewinsohn et al., 1990). The CWD-A consisted of 14 group skills training sessions targeting teaching of relaxation skills, increasing pleasant events, controlling negative thoughts, and improving social skills, as well as a conflict resolution component addressing communication and problem solving with parents. In the PST component, adolescents were taught to concisely define problems, brainstorm alternative solutions, decide on one or more mutually satisfactory solutions, and specify the details for implementing the agreed-upon solution. In the adolescent-and-parent version, seven parent sessions overviewing what was taught to the teens were added to promote acceptance and support for the intervention. Both versions resulted in significant reductions in depression that were maintained at a 2-year follow-up assessment, whereas adolescents in the waitlist control condition showed very little improvement. No significant differences between the two versions of the CWD-A course were found.

PST is also included in the only "first line" psychosocial treatment for pediatric bipolar disorders (Fristad & McPherson, 2014). Family psychoeducation plus skill building interventions provide families with information on the symptoms, course, and treatment of bipolar disorders while also teaching coping skills helpful in symptom management (e.g., Fristad, Verducci, K. Walters, & Young, 2009). Fristad et al. (2009) conducted a randomized controlled trial (RCT) with youth ($N = 165$; ages 8–12 years) meeting the criteria for depression or bipolar disorder that compared multifamily psychoeducational psychotherapy plus treatment as usual (MF-PEP + TAU) and waitlist control plus treatment as usual (WLC + TAU) conditions. MF-PEP was evaluated as an adjunctive intervention, and all youth were allowed to continue with TAU, including medication. The MF-PEP condition consisted of eight 90-minute sessions with concurrent parent and child groups. After two sessions devoted to psychoeducation, the remaining six sessions targeted a variety of coping skills, including emotion regulation, problem solving, and nonverbal and verbal communication. In the problem-solving skills sessions, children and parents were taught five basic steps: "Stop" (Take a moment to calm down), "Think" (Define the problem and brainstorm strategies), "Plan" (Decide which strategy to use), "Do" (Carry out the strategy), and "Check" (Evaluate the outcome; Fristad, Arnold, & Leffler, 2011). The MF-PEP + TAU condition resulted in a significantly greater decrease in mood symptom severity at the 1-year follow-up that was maintained at an 18-month follow-up. The WLC + TAU condition showed similar improvements after receiving the MF-PEP intervention.

Multimodal interventions including problem-solving training are also effective in treating youth with anxiety disorders (e.g., Barrett, Dadds, & Rapee, 1996; Barrett, Healy-Farrell, & March, 2004; Beidel, Turner, & Morris, 2000; Freeman, Sapyta, et al., 2014; Kendall, 1994; Kendall et al., 1997, 2008; Walkup et al., 2008). These are all variants of CBT that also include some combination of psychoeducation, cognitive restructuring, exposure, relaxation, and contingency management. With three RCTs demonstrating its effectiveness, Coping Cat has garnered much empirical support as a packaged treatment (Kendall, 1994; Kendall et al., 1997, 2008). In Coping Cat, problem solving is taught as a strategy used to generate specific action plans (i.e., FEAR plans) for coping with anxiety-provoking situations (e.g., take deep breaths, think positive, do something distracting).

The C.A.T. Project is an adaptation of Coping Cat for adolescents (Kendall et al., 2002). It is quite similar to Coping Cat, but there are a number of adjustments to better accommodate the developmental needs of older youth (e.g., more sophisticated psychoeducational information, age-appropriate pictures and examples, less emphasis on affect recognition, point system rather than stickers, encouragement of independence). As in Coping Cat, problem solving is used as a strategy for generating alternative plans for coping with anxiety. Both versions of this treatment were tested in the Child/Adolescent Anxiety Multimodal Study (CAMS), a large federally funded multisite randomized placebo-controlled trial (Walkup et al., 2008). Youth ($N$ = 488, ages 7–17 years) diagnosed with an anxiety disorder were randomly assigned to one of four conditions: CBT (Coping Cat for children or the C.A.T. Project for adolescents), sertraline (an antidepressant medication), combined (CBT + sertraline), and placebo pill. All three active treatments outperformed the placebo on clinician ratings of improvement and, although the combination proved superior to both of the individual treatments, CBT was equally as effective as sertraline but with fewer physical side effects. Though there were no direct comparisons between the TWO Coping Cat versions, the fact that age did not moderate treatment response (Compton et al., 2014) does lend some support for the efficacy of the C.A.T. Project.

In an RCT evaluating an Australian adaptation of Coping Cat (Coping Koala), Barrett et al. (1996) tested a family-based supplement that included parent instruction in problem-solving skills. Youth

($N$ = 79; ages 7–14 years) diagnosed with an anxiety disorder were assigned to one of three conditions: CBT (Coping Koala); CBT+FAM (i.e., CBT plus parent–child sessions targeting parent instruction in contingency management and anxiety management, communication, and problem-solving skills), or WL (waitlist). Each of two active treatment conditions consisted of 12 sessions with matched therapist-contact time. The problem-solving component of the CBT+FAM condition included skills training for parents and encouragement for the family to schedule weekly discussions aimed at addressing child and family problems. Both active conditions were superior to the waitlist condition at posttreatment, but the CBT+FAM outperformed CBT on diagnostic recovery rates, and this difference was maintained at a 1-year follow-up. It is worth noting, however, that the two treatments were found to be equally effective at a 6-year follow-up assessment (Barrett, Duffy, Dadds, & Rapee, 2001), and more recent studies have yielded mixed support for family-based treatments (e.g., Kendall et al., 2008).

## THE ELEMENT IN PRACTICE

The focus of this chapter now shifts to the practical implementation of problem-solving training with anxious and depressed youth. The key PST steps are outlined in the task analysis in Box 4.1, and added detail(s), examples, and issues to think about along the way are described in this section along with suggested developmental adaptations and diversity considerations. An illustrative case example involving a 16-year-old Caucasian male treated for depression is also provided in Box 4.2 at the end of the chapter.

### "Core of the Core" Element

Before implementing PST, the therapist should consider several factors that can impact its effectiveness (Box 4.1, Step 1). First is whether the youth has the minimal language and cognitive abilities to participate. Can he or she identify and talk about problems? Think of alternative solutions? Understand cause and effect? These are not "yes or no" questions. PST has been used with very young children, and there are many ways to help support learning for youth who may be having difficulty in one or more of these areas (see the next section of this chapter). Second, problem solving offers no quick fixes, instead requiring commitment and a willingness to delay gratification long enough to

## BOX 4.1. Task Analysis of Problem–Solving Training

1. Consider the characteristics of the youth that may impact his or her problem-solving abilities, such as developmental, motivational, and family factors, as well as skills deficits affecting the solution's implementation.

2. Provide a rationale for problem solving.
   a. Introduce it as a coping skill.
   b. Distinguish between adaptive and maladaptive styles, using the provided example.
   c. Emphasize the importance of a positive problem-solving orientation.

3. Define the problem.
   a. Problems are typically either an obstacle to a goal or the presence of competing goals or demands.
   b. Generate a list of current problems, and select one to define.
   c. Help the youth define the problem clearly and objectively.

4. Set a goal.
   a. Determine what the youth would like to have happen.
   b. Goals should be realistic, attainable, and defined using observable outcomes.

5. Generate alternative solutions.
   a. Use the "brainstorming" method to help the youth come up with as many solutions to the problem as possible.

6. Select the best solution.
   a. Help the youth engage in systematic decision making (e.g., discard unrealistic solutions, identify potential consequences, weigh pros and cons).

7. Implement the solution.
   a. Consider whether the youth has the skills needed for implementation.
   b. Help the youth make a plan for implementation.
   c. Identify and discuss any potential pitfalls.
   d. Have the youth implement the plan in the natural environment.

8. Evaluate the effectiveness of the solution.
   a. Help the youth determine whether the goal was achieved.
   b. If so, praise and reward him or her (or have the youth self-reward).
   c. If not, either modify the existing plan or return to Step 6 and select a new solution or consider moving back to an even earlier step if needed (e.g., generate more solutions to choose from or a new problem definition or goal).

9. Help the youth recognize the benefits of problem solving, and apply these to additional problems, encouraging increasing levels of autonomy for the youth in the process.

go through all the steps. Third, through early identification, remedial efforts can target any major skills deficits (e.g., social skills deficits) that might impede solution implementation later on in the process. Lastly, the family plays a crucial role in PST with youth. Parents should be willing to give up some control and allow the youth to make choices (Manassis, 2012).

Taking time to provide a rationale for PST helps with motivation and sets a foundation for the importance of adopting a positive problem orientation (Step 2). Problem solving is introduced as a set of coping skills that will help the youth address difficulties and reduce stress. Recognizing problems and taking action is emphasized. As a starting point, the therapist can ask the youth to describe his or her typical approach to solving problems. Using the youth's response, the therapist can contrast adaptive and maladaptive styles. Depressed and anxious youth are more likely to endorse maladaptive styles marked by avoidance and see their problems as unsolvable, threatening, and overwhelming (Chorpita et al., 1996; Nezu, 1987). The therapist counters negative thinking and reinforces the importance of adopting an adaptive approach to problems. For example, in the Taking ACTION Program (Stark & Kendall, 1996), youth are told, "Life is full of bumps in the road and you can either look at them as bumps or nothing more than problems to be solved, or you can look at them as insurmountable mountains. We are going to work on looking at them as problems to be solved" (p. 20). If the cognitive distortions are severe enough to impede progress, the therapist may need to target them with additional cognitive restructuring before continuing with PST (see Chapter 3). The therapist then provides a very brief overview of the major problem-solving steps.

Defining the problem is the third step. The youth must first learn to recognize problems, which might be quite a challenge for those with histories of avoidance. The therapist should help normalize having problems for the youth and offer a basic problem definition, such as being blocked from achieving a goal or having competing goals, and some examples (e.g., cannot find something, conflict with a peer). For youth with internalizing difficulties, experiencing negative feelings may actually *be* the problem. Anger, sadness, or fear can also serve as cues that a problem exists. Now better able to recognize problems, the youth is ready to make a list of current problems and choose one to define. It is best to select an easier problem to start. Problems should be defined as clearly and objectively as possible. The youth is instructed to ask questions and gather information (e.g., What is the problem?

Where does it occur? When does it occur? Who is affected?). Using this information, the therapist helps the youth put the problem into words, rephrasing and reframing as needed.

With a clearly stated problem in place, the therapist then helps the youth set a goal for problem solving in Step 4. Goals should focus on changing the situation and alleviating the problem. They should be realistic, attainable, and concretely defined in observable outcomes. If the problem situation is one that cannot be changed, the youth can instead focus on his or her reaction to the situation. As part of the ACTION intervention (Stark et al., 2007), youth are taught four things to consider when answering the question "What is my goal?": "Ask yourself what you want to have happen. Ask yourself what is the best thing that could happen. Avoid negative thinking. Open yourself to the positive and try to focus on the desired outcome" (p. 39).

Next comes the generation of alternative solutions (Step 5). Solutions are things the youth can do to change, or better cope with, the problem situation. Using the "brainstorming" method, the youth is asked to come up with as many different solutions as possible. Creativity is encouraged, and evaluation is discouraged. In the CWD-A course (Clarke et al., 1990), the following rules are discussed with the group: "List as many solutions as you can. Don't be critical, all ideas are allowed. Be creative. Begin by offering to change one of your own behaviors" (p. 246). Negative thinking can make this step particularly difficult for youth with internalizing problems. If the youth has trouble coming up with ideas or perseverates on reasons why ideas would fail rather than succeed, the therapist can use prompts or suggest alternatives for the youth.

In Step 6, the youth then decides on a best solution. In reaching this decision, the therapist helps the youth engage in a systematic process that involves carefully considering the potential consequences of each generated solution. First, it is helpful to remove any solutions that clearly do not make sense or that are not feasible. The youth is asked to think about the possible short- and long-term consequences of each remaining solution. Using a poster board or form that lists each solution and provides a space for comments (both pro and con) along with a rating can help structure the process for the youth. Pessimism can derail the decision-making process for depressed youth, and the therapist can help by pointing to the positive features of solutions and the limitations or self-defeating consequences of others (Stark et al., 2006). Reminders that even small changes can make a big difference are also helpful. The therapist can address rumination or avoidance by encouraging the youth to write down only the most important advantages or disadvantages, setting a time limit, or reframing the process as a learning opportunity with no wrong choices (Manassis, 2012).

It is now time to implement the chosen solution (Step 7). Before developing an action plan, the therapist should consider whether the youth has the requisite skills (e.g., social, academic). For example, a lack of conversation skills might get in the way of a youth's decision to try to make new friends. In such cases, more thorough assessment and targeted skills training (e.g., see Chapter 8) may be needed before proceeding with PST. The therapist then helps the youth develop a step-by-step plan for carrying out the solution. The plan should be detailed, breaking things down into small achievable steps, and should include a time and place for enactment as well as specifics about needed input or assistance from others. Role playing with the therapist is an excellent way for the youth to practice the plan in a safe environment and also to provide added opportunities for instruction, corrective feedback, and assessment. Asking the youth to anticipate potential pitfalls in the plan and come up with a contingency plan is also helpful.

The therapist assists the youth in evaluating the outcome in Step 8. The goal is to find out whether the plan has been carried out and whether it is having the desired impact. Reviewing the goal set in Step 4 can provide a context for the youth's self-evaluation. If the goal has been met, the therapist offers praise and perhaps other rewards (e.g., stickers, free time) to the youth (see Chapter 9). Teaching the youth to self-evaluate and self-reward is important for promoting the maintenance and generalization of the problem-solving skills. In Coping Cat (Kendall & Hedtke, 2006), children are taught that a reward is something that is given when "you're pleased with the work that was done" (p. 41), and a self-rating is a way to decide whether the child is satisfied with his or her own work. The therapist points out that success leads to rewards, but also that succeeding all of the time is not possible and should not result in punishment. Children are reminded, "All that is asked is that one tries his best" (p. 42). This is an important point. Even if the problem is not solved, the therapist can help the youth look for any signs—even small ones—of improvement in the situation and offer praise for effort and perseverance (Manassis, 2012). Biased thinking is likely to affect the self-evaluations of depressed and anxious youth. As in previous steps, cognitive restructuring techniques, such as normalizing and reframing (see Chapter 3), can be used to counter them. Deciding what to do when an implementation attempt fails is not easy. One option is to modify the existing plan and try again. Another is to return to Step 6 to select a different solution. Sometimes it may be necessary to return to an even earlier step. For example, more solutions to choose from or a new problem definition or goal may be needed. Once the goal has been met, the therapist has the youth apply the problem-solving steps to new problems (Step 9). The benefits of problem solving are emphasized, and the youth is encouraged to assume more autonomy in the process.

There are a variety of ways to teach the problem-solving skills. These include established behavior therapy procedures, such as verbal instruction, modeling, and reinforcement (see Chapters 5 and 9). Prominent among these is *cognitive modeling*, in which the therapist walks through the steps of solving a problem while verbalizing thoughts along the way (Spiegler, 2016). A coping model—one that allows for making mistakes or struggling at times—is suggested. Acronyms can help youth remember the problem-solving steps. In the ACTION program (Stark et al., 2007), girls are instructed to remember the "five P's" (i.e., Problem, Purpose, Plans, Predict and pick, and Pat yourself on the back). Another useful instructional approach is to first have the youth apply the steps in hypothetical situations before moving ahead with actual problems. Role plays allow for practice, modeling, and additional instruction. Because maintenance and generalization are so challenging and relatively few sessions are devoted to PST in the manualized treatments, homework assignments are very important.

Another way to boost maintenance and generalization of PST is to include parents in the intervention. Parents can encourage the use of the trained skills outside of sessions with prompts, provide active instruction, and serve as models. In the C.A.T. Project (Kendall et al., 2002), for example, there are two "meet the parents" sessions. Among the suggestions for parent involvement are fostering independence and confidence, not permitting avoidance, and modeling problem solving in difficult situations. Other programs have more structured and intensive parent components. The PEP (psychoeducational psychotherapy) intervention (Fristad et al., 2011) includes one parent and one child session devoted to PST. The parents learn the steps before the children. They also learn "dos" (e.g., approach child at calm time, empathize with child, ask for child suggestions before offering your own) and "don'ts" (e.g., assign blame, insist on coming up with a solution at an emotional time, choose a parent solution before hearing the child's suggestions) and are given a take-home assignment to identify a problem in the family related to the child's symptoms and use the steps to solve it.

There is a slight difference between treatments for anxiety and depression in the focus of PST. In the anxiety treatments, PST is used to help youth manage their anxiety. In Coping Cat (Kendall & Hedtke, 2006), for example, children learn to develop plans (i.e., FEAR [Feeling frightened, Expecting bad things to happen, Attitudes and actions that can help, Results and rewards] plans) for handling anxiety-provoking situations. In these plans, physical sensations and negative thoughts serve as cues to employ coping strategies, such as positive self-talk and problem solving, to help reduce anxiety and facilitate exposure to feared situations (see Chapter 2). In depression treatments, PST is used to help youth develop plans for changing situations that lead to negative emotions (Stark, Sander, et al., 2006). If the situation cannot be changed, youth are taught to use coping skills designed to enhance mood, such as distraction, talking to someone, or doing something relaxing. Family conflicts are a common problem source for depressed youth, and PST often targets their interactions with parents (e.g., Clarke et al., 1990; Fristad et al., 2011).

## Developmental Adaptations

Problem solving is a fairly complex cognitive process involving the retrieval and processing of information, perspective taking, anticipation of consequences, and planning, among other things. Three core cognitive abilities underlie this process: working memory (i.e., the ability to hold information in mind while solving a problem), selective attention (i.e., the ability to filter out distractions and focus on the most relevant information), and inhibition (i.e., the ability to delay respond-ing; Ropovik, 2014). These abilities fall under the umbrella of executive functioning, which is seated in the frontal lobe and is the last part of the brain to fully mature (Zelazo & Müller, 2002). Paralleling its physi-cal maturation, executive functioning develops gradually throughout childhood and into early adulthood. It does not, however, progress in a stage-like fashion. Rather, the associated abilities exist at some level even in young children but continue to mature at different rates throughout adolescence. For example, the ability to inhibit responding makes its biggest leap in the preschool years and continues to improve between ages 5 and 8 before leveling off to some degree, whereas work-ing memory continues to improve in a linear way between the ages of 4 and 14 (Best & Miller, 2010).

This uneven pattern of development makes it difficult to deter-mine a definitive age at which a child can benefit from PST. The for-mative work of Spivack and Shure shows that children as young as 4 years old can learn the skills (e.g., Shure et al., 1972) and suggests that the skills are capable of mediating behavioral adjustment (Shure & Spivack, 1980). Two cautionary notes are worth considering. One is that a number of other researchers have failed to replicate the mediating effects reported by Shure and Spivack (1980) with preschool samples (e.g., Winer, Hilpert, Gesten, Cowen, & Schubin, 1982). Another is that the Spivack and Shure intervention was much more intensive than PST as delivered in typical therapy settings. In the Shure et al. (1972) pilot investigation, the preschoolers had 50 training sessions devoted to PST that included instruction in a number of foundational skills, such as listening, logic, emotional awareness, and gathering information. Though pinpointing a certain "age of readiness" for PST may not be possible, it is safe to assume that it is more effective with older youth. Consistent with brain maturation and developmental research, Durlak and colleagues found an effect size for older youth (ages 11 years and more) that was almost two times larger than that for younger youth in a meta-analytic investigation of cognitive-behavioral interventions such as PST (Durlak, Fuhrman, & Lampman, 1991).

Especially when working with younger youth or those needing some extra help in learning the problem-solving skills, therapists are encouraged to take a *scaffolding* approach. According to Wood and colleagues, who first used the term, scaffolding is a teaching process in which a child is provided with some assistance in order to reach a learning goal that would normally be out of reach (Wood, Bruner, & Ross, 1976). It is an interactive process in which adult involvement is gradually reduced to the point where it is no longer needed. For example, the therapist might begin with cognitive modeling, talking through each step on the way to solving a hypothetical problem. The child then takes a turn but runs into some difficulty remembering the steps. The therapist uses verbal prompting to help get the child through the steps, gradually fading the prompts as the child demonstrates the ability to move through the steps more independently.

Other useful scaffolding aids include added instruction in basic skills, simplifying the task, and using cues, pictures, games, make-believe, and self-talk. In their seminal work with preschoolers, Shure et al. (1972) taught children basic skills building up to problem solving. For example, children learned about "if–then" thinking in sentence completion exercises (e.g., "If Susan is running, then she is not walking. If Sammy is crying, then he is not _____"). Simplifying tasks by breaking them down into smaller doable steps and remembering to adjust language to the child's level are also helpful. The use of cues, such as acronyms and posters, can be useful supports, especially as the therapist begins to fade prompts. Games and make-believe activities are good scaffolding options because they increase child attention and engagement (Wood et al., 1976). In the ACTION program (Stark et al., 2007), for example, a game is used to illustrate how problem solving can address unpleasant situations. Girls put beads into their shoes and are asked to walk around while eating a piece of candy. They are then asked to take ACTION by using the problem-solving steps (prominently displayed on a poster) to make the situation better. Finally, the use of self-talk is an excellent way to get children to internalize cues. For instance, Shure et al. (1972) emphasized the use of three self-stated questions to help guide children through the problem-solving process (i.e., "What can I do?"; "What might happen if I do that?"; "What else can I do?").

At the other end of the developmental spectrum, adolescents present with their own set of challenges for the therapist. Again, it is hard to judge by age alone, but youth in their teenage years should be increasingly capable of engaging in the type of abstract thinking required in problem solving. Along with their increasing abilities, adolescents may desire more autonomy and control in working through their problems. The therapist must adjust, balancing competing needs for increased independence and structure (Manassis, 2012; Mufson, Dorta, Moreau, & Weissman, 2011). Even with their cognitive advances, adolescents may have a limited perspective on the future and underestimate the longer-term consequences of their current actions, thus requiring that the therapist help point these out to them (Mufson, Dorta, Moreau, & Weissman, 2004). The types of problems experienced by teens will also be different. For example, IPT (Mufson et al., 2011) focuses on major problem areas typically faced by depressed adolescents: grief (loss of a person or relationship), interpersonal role disputes (nonreciprocal expectations about a relationship), interpersonal transitions (developmental life changes, such as puberty), and interpersonal deficits (lack of needed social and communication skills). Parent–adolescent conflict is another common problem area (Clarke et al., 1990). It is important for the therapist to resist getting drawn into these conflicts or attempting to intervene on the teen's behalf (Manassis, 2012).

## Diversity Considerations

There is no direct evidence that PST used alone is effective for ethnically diverse youth with internalizing disorders. One reason is that PST has so rarely been evaluated as a stand-alone treatment. The Stark et al. (1987) study is the closest approximation to an evaluation of pure PST with depressed youth, but the authors did not report on the ethnic composition of their sample. Even indirect evidence is hard to come by because reporting of treatment outcomes by youth ethnicity is the exception rather than the rule (Huey & Polo, 2008). Thus, although there are a number of evidence-based multicomponent treatments for internalizing disorders that include PST, it is often not possible to determine whether they are effective for different ethnic groups. Indeed, in a recent meta-analysis, Huey and Polo (2008) identified only four anxiety and depression outcome studies that met their combined effectiveness and ethnicity inclusion standards (i.e., 75% of sample ethnic minorities or analyses either supporting effectiveness with a subset of ethnic minorities or showing a lack of ethnicity moderation).

Two of the studies identified by Huey and Polo (2008) were evaluations of culturally sensitive adaptations of CBT and IPT interventions for Puerto Rican adolescents (Rosselló & Bernal, 1999; Rosselló, Bernal, & Rivera-Medina, 2008). In adapting the interventions, Rosselló and colleagues used examples based on their experiences with Puerto Rican teens, modified session content to better comport with Puerto Rican culture, and increased the focus on parental involvement. In the Rosselló et al. (2008) study, the parents attended sessions at pre-, mid-, and posttreatment so that the therapist could discuss their teen's progress in therapy, answer questions, and offer recommendations about particular issues. Therapists could also schedule up to two additional sessions with the parents (with or without the adolescent) when more input was needed. Work with the parents was guided by the important cultural values of *familismo* (i.e., strong identification and attachment to the family) and *respeto* (i.e., respect for authority figures). No details regarding adaptations to the PST components, in particular, were provided. Regarding effectiveness, both treatments were similarly effective in reducing depressive symptoms in the initial investigation (Rosselló & Bernal, 1999). Although both treatments proved effective in the later study, CBT was superior (Rosselló et al., 2008). Clinical significance analyses indicated that 62% of the participants in the CBT group and 57% of the participants in the IPT group were no longer in the clinical range at posttreatment.

Cormier, Nurius, and Osborn (2013) offer some general recommendations for implementing PST with diverse clients. Emphasizing that diverse groups will not respond to PST in the same way, they suggest that therapists be sensitive to gender, race, and ethnicity and argue that the traditional problem-solving model is inherently Eurocentric and androcentric. That is, the traditional model is individualistic and may be preferred by Caucasian and male clients, whereas collectivistic approaches emphasizing collaboration may be preferred by clients of color and females (Cormier et al., 2013). For example, inherent in the familism of the Puerto Rican culture is the valuing of family interests over the interests of the individual (Rosselló & Bernal, 1999). Families are at the center and play a predominant role in meeting psychological needs and identity formation. As such, therapists adapting PST for Puerto Rican youth should make efforts to include parents in the process and allow for more dependence on them in the generation of solutions and alternatives (Rosselló & Bernal, 1999). These types of adaptations are consistent with the suggestion of Cormier and colleagues (2013) that PST is more effective when delivered in a culturally sensitive way. Of course, diversity is more than race and ethnicity, and the therapist should consider culture in its broadest sense to include such factors as sexual identity, religion, and socioeconomic status. Religious beliefs, for example, can put restrictions on the range of choices and autonomy granted to youth (Manassis, 2012). The challenge for the therapist is to find a way to teach the problem-solving skills without making the youth feel pressured to assimilate to the norms of the mainstream culture (Cormier et al., 2013).

## CONCLUSIONS

Since its introduction as one of the first formal CBT techniques, PST has been applied to a wide range of clinical disorders and health problems (D'Zurilla & Nezu, 2007) and is one of the most frequently used practice elements in EBTs for youth with internalizing disorders (Chorpita & Daleiden, 2009). In treatments for depression and anxiety, PST is used to teach youth to use problems as cues for action focused on changing the situation or better coping with the resulting negative emotions. By targeting coping skills that can be applied to newly emerging problems, PST offers advantages for maintenance and generalization. The cognitive abilities underlying problem solving develop unevenly, and a scaffolding approach to teaching the skills is suggested. Sensitivity to culture and adapting PST for diverse youth are also important.

## BOX 4.2. Illustrative Case Example

Troy was a 16-year-old Caucasian male presenting with depressive symptoms that had worsened in recent months. After the divorce of his parents about a year earlier, Troy's grades began to decline to the point that he failed two courses. He also withdrew from extracurricular activities, deciding not to rejoin the soccer team despite the fact that he had lettered as a freshman. Troy lived with his father and two younger brothers. His mother lived out of state, but the two remained close by talking on the phone and sharing a 1-month visit at her home during the summer. His father described Troy as "going through a major shift in the wrong direction" over the past several months. Troy had become irritable and sometimes lashed out verbally at his siblings with no obvious provocation. Though they used to get along well, Troy rarely engaged in conversation with his father, resorting instead to nods and simple "yes and no's." Contacted by phone, Troy's mother described him as "just going through the motions" and agreed that he had become very irritable in recent months.

Following a thorough assessment that included a structured interview, Troy was diagnosed with major depressive disorder. His therapist suggested PST in combination with pleasant events scheduling. The goal was to help Troy learn how to better cope with his negative emotions and motivate him to begin engaging in activities that he used to find enjoyable. Troy was clearly able to engage in PST, but he did not appear to be very motivated to participate in the program. His father was very receptive to the proposed treatment plan and demonstrated concern about Troy's recent decline and struggles with anger. Though he was generally open to allowing Troy a role in family decision making, he tended to get more dictatorial at times of stress.

In discussing the rationale for PST with the therapist, Troy acknowledged that it could be helpful "for someone else." He said he "just had too many problems" and that every time he tried to "fix them they just get worse." The therapist contrasted Troy's avoidant style with a more adaptive approach to problems. She told him that it sounded like his problems just seemed so overwhelming that he stopped trying to solve them and that when we stop trying it often causes more problems. Instead, she emphasized how stepping up to take some action could make things better and that the "practice" would make him get better at solving future problems. After some discussion, Troy agreed to give it a try, and the therapist noted that learning any new skill requires effort and persistence, much like what he had shown in refining his soccer skills. To end the initial session, the therapist overviewed the major problem-solving steps and "talked through" each step in solving a hypothetical problem.

Over the next few sessions, Troy was able to identify a few problems to work on and developed an implementation plan to try to solve one of them. The therapist taught Troy to interpret his negative feelings as a cue that a problem existed and some action was needed. As a homework assignment, Troy was asked to make a list of 10 problems he faced during the week. After reviewing the list, the therapist suggested that they start with a problem that was fairly straightforward and not too

(continued)

## BOX 4.2 (*continued*)

emotionally charged. Troy selected a problem that involved calling his mother. Taking time to think it over and gather some information, he observed that he usually thought of calling his mother right after school when he still had energy and "things to talk about." The problem was that his mother was at work during that time and would often return his messages later in the evening when he was too tired to talk. During the brainstorming step, Troy quickly discounted each alternative he came up with. The therapist reminded him that evaluation was not allowed at this point and encouraged him to "just let ideas flow." Eventually, Troy chose to talk with his mother about scheduling their phone calls for early in the evening. As part of his plan, he would record things he wanted to tell her in the notes section of his cell phone. After a couple of practice runs using role play, Troy called his mother, and the two agreed to the plan.

Experiencing some success motivated Troy to apply his new skills to other problems. After Troy noted that he now really enjoyed talking with his mother on the phone, the therapist encouraged him to use the skills to plan more pleasant activities. Troy also devised plans for better coping with his anger and irritability. For example, he established a "cool-off zone" in his room that allowed him space and time to get control of his feelings. As his confidence grew, he assumed more independence in the problem-solving process. He seemed to enjoy reciting the steps for the therapist at the beginning of each session and even attached a copy of the brainstorming rules to the refrigerator at home. Troy's father helped by prompting him to use the skills at home and being more mindful of ways that he might unwittingly support Troy's avoidance. Over time, Troy's family began using the skills to address common problems at home.

Over the course of the 12 sessions, Troy made demonstrable progress. His mood improved, and he reported feeling more confident in his ability to manage his anger and irritability. His father noted that Troy seemed less stressed in general, was talking more at home, and had begun playing in pick-up soccer games with his friends. The two were getting along better but "still had their moments." To address this, the therapist added two joint sessions in which Troy and his father learned some communication and negotiation skills and practiced collaborative problem solving, targeting relationship issues.

# 5

## Modeling

with Jennifer Sauvé and Amber A. Martinson

### BACKGROUND OF THE ELEMENT

Intuitively, we all know that one way in which we learn is by observing others. This is the essence of modeling. More formally defined, modeling procedures involve the use of live or symbolic demonstrations to facilitate client acquisition or performance of a desired behavior. The basic ingredients include a *model*, who engages in a behavior, an *observer*, who attends to the model, *imitation* by the observer, and *consequences* for the imitative response (Spiegler, 2016). For example, a clinician may have an anxious child observe a peer making increasingly bold advances toward a feared object or ask a depressed adolescent with poor social skills to observe another teen engaging others in conversation. The first example involves the use of modeling to get a child to engage in an already learned but inhibited response, whereas the second example is modeling used to teach a new response. Modeling is an efficient and very powerful learning tool and therefore one of the more frequently included practice elements in treatments for youth with internalizing disorders. Modeling has a very rich history, and its use is supported by a large body of conceptual and empirical work. After providing a digestible summary of this background, this chapter turns to practical coverage of how modeling is used in interventions for youth with internalizing disorders, such as anxiety and depression. Included are step-by-step implementation suggestions, a discussion of pertinent developmental and diversity issues, and an illustrative case example of a 9-year-old female treated for extreme dental fears.

## Brief History

Modeling's history can be traced back to the 1940s in attempts to describe imitation from a learning perspective and the 1960s with Bandura's formative work on observational learning. Neal Miller and John Dollard (1941) were the first to offer a comprehensive learning theory account of imitation. Part of a broader movement to recast Freudian concepts in a learning theory framework, they proposed that imitative behavior was an instance of instrumental conditioning. Whether or not imitative responses were reinforced was based on the extent to which responses matched those exhibited by a model. As learning theorists, Miller and Dollard followed this proposal with a series of experimental tests conducted with animals and children showing that the tendency to imitate would increase if reinforced and would then generalize to similar situations. Similarly, Skinner (1953a) explained imitative behavior within a shaping paradigm. That is, as in the acquisition of other behaviors, imitation developed through the contingent reinforcement of successive approximations to a goal response. Key to both of these learning explanations was the notion that imitation was a product of a direct learning process requiring an imitative response and contingent reinforcement.

In contrast, Bandura and Walters (1963) suggested that imitation did not require direct learning, arguing that the prevailing learning theories failed to explain new responses exhibited in the absence of reliable eliciting stimuli. In setting the stage for the observational learning approach, they put forth the idea that imitation could occur in the absence of an overt response by the observer and direct reinforcement during the acquisition period. The notion of vicarious reinforcement was introduced, whereby behavior could be modified as the result of observed consequences to a model.

In summarizing the now famous "Bobo doll" experiments, Bandura and Walters (1963) offered examples of the influences of observational learning on response acquisition and facilitation. When considering these examples, bear in mind that the children's imitation of the model is neither immediate nor directly reinforced, as described in the earlier learning theories (N. Miller & Dollard, 1941; Skinner, 1953a). In one of these studies, Bandura, Ross, and Ross (1961) exposed young children to adult models exhibiting either aggressive (physical and verbal) or nonaggressive (ignoring) responses toward a Bobo doll. When placed in a new situation in the absence of the model, children in the aggressive model condition displayed higher rates of imitative aggression than their counterparts in the nonaggressive model condition. Perhaps most interesting, children exposed to the nonaggressive model also exhibited less aggression than children in a control group who were not exposed to the initial situation. Thus, modeling led to both the elicitation and inhibition of aggressive responding.

In a study illustrating vicarious reinforcement, Bandura (1962) had children view a film-mediated model exhibiting four aggressive responses with varying consequences: model punished, rewarded with approval and food, and no consequences. During the exposure period, the children did not perform overt behaviors or receive direct reinforcement. Postexposure, children in the punished condition exhibited fewer imitative responses than children in the other two conditions. Notably, the imitation was influenced by the perceived consequences for the model's behavior. Seeing the model punished resulted in a decrease in imitative responding.

Over the years, cognitive variables were increasingly emphasized in observational learning theory (e.g., Bandura, 1977c, 1986). For instance, Bandura and his colleagues began to focus more on the fact that modeling experiences could alter the observer's expectancies for performance. In a study evaluating modeling as a treatment for snake phobia, Bandura, Blanchard, and Ritter (1969) noted moderate to high correlations between behavioral (e.g., actually interact with a snake) and attitudinal (e.g., expectations of the capability to interact with a snake) improvements. Of particular interest to Bandura was self-efficacy, or the expectancy that one could master a problem. He came to view such expectancies as driving behavior change. Accordingly, following the cited example, enhancing the participants' expectations for success in touching the snake would have resulted in increases in approach behaviors. Correlational studies, however, do not establish a direction of effect, and the extent to which such expectancies drive behavior change is still an unanswered question.

Turning to its history as a treatment element, the earliest modeling intervention on record is that of Chittenden (1942). After a classwide screening, a group of 10 preschool children identified as most aggressive and domineering viewed a series of short plays in which an adult used dolls to portray both aggressive (resulting in negative consequences for the model) and nonaggressive (resulting in positive consequences) responses in typical conflict situations. When compared to a control group of 9 similarly identified children, the intervention group showed substantial improvements in cooperative behavior and decreases in aggression. One month after treatment, the decreases in aggression were maintained, but the improvements in cooperative behavior were not.

Since that early demonstration, modeling as a sole intervention has been applied to many clinical problems and disorders (see Masters et al., 1987, for a review), including anxiety (e.g., Kornhaber & Schroeder, 1975; Mann & Rosenthal, 1969; Melamed & Siegel, 1975) and depression (e.g., Frame, Matson, Sonis, Falkov, & Kazdin, 1982) in youth. At its peak during the late 1960s and early 1970s, the modeling literature was dominated by comparisons of procedural variations. For example, Kornhaber and Schroeder (1975) evaluated whether model similarity (fear response, age) to observers made a difference in intervention effectiveness. Forty girls (second and third graders) with demonstrated fear of snakes were assigned to one of four modeling conditions: fearless child (appeared unafraid, no reluctance), fearful child (appeared apprehensive, reluctant), fearless adult, and fearful adult. A no-model control group was also included. Fearless and fearful models were equally effective in improving approach behavior, but child models proved to be more effective than adult models and fearful child models produced the greatest improvements on a measure assessing attitudes toward snakes. In a study targeting test anxiety, Mann and Rosenthal (1969) randomly assigned 71 seventh graders to one of six desensitization (i.e., repeated exposure to a feared stimulus in a graded manner) conditions (individual vs. group desensitization, direct vs. vicarious desensitization, vicarious group desensitization observing direct desensitization of a model, control). All treatments produced equally significant decreases on a self-report test anxiety scale as compared to controls. Observing a model being desensitized was just as effective as undergoing direct desensitization.

In sum, highlights of this historical overview include the increasing complexity of the theoretical explanations of modeling, evolving from those requiring direct contact with the contingencies to those incorporating concepts such as vicarious reinforcement and expectancies, and a burgeoning applied literature focused mainly on fear reduction and comparisons of different modeling procedures.

## Theory Base

Few, if any, treatment procedures have as deep a conceptual and empirical base as modeling. Bandura was a prolific scholar whose observational learning theory developed over the course of decades (e.g., Bandura, 1977c, 1986; Bandura & Walters, 1959, 1963). A full account of this vast literature is beyond the scope of this chapter, the hope here being to provide a brief yet informative summary.

Before delving deeper into the treatment of internalizing problems in particular, it is helpful to review some of the more general concepts behind modeling procedures. A good launching point is a summary of modeling effects, component processes, and intervention implications (see Rosenthal & Bandura, 1978, for a comprehensive review). With regard to effects, modeling can result in the learning of a new response or a novel way to sequence already learned behaviors. More commonly, however, the effects are facilitative in that the model's behavior serves as a cue for the observer to perform an already learned response (Masters et al., 1987). Modeling also has inhibitory and disinhibitory effects. Observers are sensitive to the perceived consequences for a model's actions. If those perceived consequences are negative, observers will decrease responses similar to that of the model. Conversely, positive consequences will increase such responses. In fears or anxiety, avoidance results from the inhibition of approach behaviors in light of their perceived negative consequences. Observing a model engaging in approach behaviors in the absence of adverse consequences can result in the "disinhibition" of such responses. Although modeling procedures involving direct exposure to a feared stimulus are considered most effective (Masters et al., 1987), there is evidence that one can become desensitized just by watching a peer engage with a feared stimulus (e.g., Kornhaber & Schroeder, 1975; Mann & Rosenthal, 1969). Modeling can also bring about cognitive changes, such as more positive performance expectancies (e.g., "I know I can do this"). It may also aid in the self-regulation of behavior by providing an internalized "standard" for responding in new situations (Rosenthal & Bandura, 1978). For instance, a child can use the image of a model's approach behavior as a guide for evaluating performance when external feedback is not available (e.g., "It's all right if I looked scared—I kept petting the dog just like the boy in the video"). Finally, as part of its informative function, modeling helps direct attention to important aspects of a situation (Foster, Kendall, & Guevremont, 1988). For example, a modeling demonstration of a social interaction initiation attempt for a depressed adolescent might be paired with therapist prompts to notice encouraging nonverbal cues, such as eye contact and forward lean, exhibited by the intended recipient.

Four component processes govern modeling effects (Bandura, 1977c). Most fundamentally, observers need to *attend* to the modeled behavior. The modeling demonstration should be clear, not overly complex, and have personal relevance (Bandura, 1977c; Rosenthal & Bandura, 1978). Adding to the last point, there is a lot of empirical evidence showing that a model's impact is determined by its similarity and credibility to the observer (Rosenthal & Bandura, 1978). The emotional valence of the stimulus is also important. If the modeling display is too upsetting, the observer may divert his or her attention, a real concern when modeling is used in combination with exposure in anxiety treatments. The second component process is *retention*. The modeled information must be encoded symbolically (e.g., describing a behavioral response in words or use of mental images) in memory to be accessed by the observer at another time. Such encoding is facilitated when the modeled behavior pattern makes sense to the observer (Masters et al., 1987). One way to accomplish this is to accompany the demonstration with verbal comments that help to integrate the sequence for the observer. Rehearsal and practice, imaginal and overt, also aid in retention, and when combined with feedback they can result in progressive improvements in performance. For instance, a therapist can have a child follow a social skill demonstration with practice attempts, providing corrective feedback after each one (e.g., "I liked the way you first made eye contact. Next time, let's see if you can speak a little louder"). *Motor reproduction* involves the translation of the symbolic representations into behavioral enactment (Rosenthal & Bandura, 1978). Imitation requires the physical capabilities for reproduction as well as having all of the needed response elements. Deficits in the needed subskills require remediation. For example, an adolescent may have most of the component skills needed to be assertive but still need to learn how to form "I" statements (e.g., "I feel angry when you . . . ") or some anger control strategies (e.g., deep breathing, counting to 10) to respond appropriately. The final component processes are *motivational*. In line with social learning theory, observers are more likely to adopt a modeled response that has rewarding consequences. Rewards can come in the form of praise after a role-play rehearsal in the therapy context, following successful enactment in the "real world," or vicariously through the observation of consequences for the model (Masters et al., 1987). Rewards function primarily at the cognitive level.

More important than the actual reward is the information transmitted about response–reward contingencies that is encoded and considered before being used to guide action (Rosenthal & Bandura, 1978). Self-evaluation, such as pride and satisfaction, are also important sources of motivation and feedback (Masters et al., 1987).

In the treatment of internalizing disorders, modeling procedures are most frequently used to assist in skill learning (e.g., social skills training) or fear reduction (e.g., exposure). When used to teach skills, it is important to distinguish between an "inhibited ability" and an actual skills deficit (Rosenthal & Bandura, 1978, p. 642). An individual may already have all the needed skills, but anxiety inhibits their use (Masters et al., 1987). Already learned skills may also not appear because of either failure to read cues that should be used (e.g., responding to eye contact with a greeting) or, alternatively, past punishment for their use (e.g., speaking in front of the class previously met with teasing by peers). Although interventions for social anxiety typically include social skills instruction, there is debate over whether certain youth actually have skills deficits (e.g., Cartwright-Hatton, Tschernitz, & Gomersall, 2005). Perhaps their anxiety just inhibits social performance. Regardless, modeling can be effective in the context of an actual skills deficit or inhibition. If the desired response is inhibited, modeling can have facilitative (i.e., cue performance) or disinhibitory (i.e., alter perceived consequences) effects (Rosenthal & Bandura, 1978). Modeling is particularly well suited to addressing actual skills deficits because of its ability to get across needed information more efficiently than trial-and-error learning.

The use of modeling to reduce fear and anxiety is based on the notion of avoidance learning. Bandura (1977c) questioned the then prevailing dual-process theory that described avoidance as resulting from triggered autonomic arousal (e.g., shortness of breath, heart racing) that was reduced by efforts to avoid the feared stimulus. Part of his skepticism arose from the fact that fears could be learned through observation in the absence of any direct experience with the feared stimuli (Rosenthal & Bandura, 1978). Instead, Bandura believed that avoidance depended on the thoughts surrounding fear-related stimuli, such as expectations and the interpretation of social reactions and situational cues (Rosenthal & Bandura, 1978). In a positive feedback cycle, fearful individuals "rehearse" their worries and imagine failure and distress, thus raising autonomic arousal and reinforcing further avoidance and negative self-appraisals. The key to fear reduction, therefore, is to change the underlying thought processes.

Modeling helps to reduce fear through its facilitation of extinction. Observing others engage in approach behaviors in the absence of anticipated negative consequences leads to the vicarious extinction of fear responses. This can be accomplished through overt (e.g., live or filmed) or covert (e.g., imagining a model performing a behavior) demonstrations. A variation referred to as participant modeling gets the client involved in the modeling demonstration. When combined with exposure in the treatment of phobias, the therapist not only models engagement with the feared stimulus but also guides or assists with client participation, thus allowing for more direct extinction of the fear response (Masters et al., 1987; Spiegler, 2016). For example, a therapist might initially hold a child's hand as the child pets a dog. The presence of the therapist is thought to exert a calming effect that functions as an incompatible response (i.e., one cannot be anxious and relaxed at the same time) and is thereby better explained by counterconditioning than extinction per se. Direct contact also allows for the reinforcement of approach behaviors through therapist praise, positive self-feedback, and eventual return to rewarding activities.

As highlighted in the historical overview, Bandura came to see modeling and all other psychological interventions as operating through changes in self-efficacy beliefs (Bandura, 1977b; Bandura et al., 1977, 1982). Self-efficacy, or the expectancy for personal effectiveness, in a given situation was seen as a critical mediator of behavior change. This is different than an expectation that a behavior, if performed, will result in a positive outcome. An individual can believe that a given behavior would likely produce a positive outcome but still have doubts about having the ability to enact the behavior (Masters et al., 1987). For example, an adolescent with a fear of public speaking may be fully aware that giving a class presentation will result in an improved course grade and yet still feel that he is not capable of doing one. Personal mastery experiences, like those targeted in the earlier described participant modeling procedures, are best for improving self-efficacy beliefs (Rosenthal & Bandura, 1978). In other words, continuing with the earlier example, getting the teen to successfully deliver a presentation or two will lead to more positive performance expectancies (e.g., "I can do class presentations, no problems").

## Evidence Base

Modeling is effective as a sole treatment for fears and is also a component of the evidenced-based multimodal treatments for anxiety and depression for children and adolescents (see Table 5.1 for a summary

**TABLE 5.1. The Modeling Element in Representative EBT Manuals**

| | |
|---|---|
| *Coping Cat* (Kendall & Hedtke, 2006) | • Modeling is explicitly mentioned and integrated throughout this treatment. The therapist acts as a coach, using modeling to help teach many of the skills (e.g., modeling recognizing anxious feelings, being a coping model by disclosing a prior fear or situation which caused anxiety, as well as many others). |
| *C.A.T. Project* (Kendall, Choudhury, Hudson, & Webb, 2002) | • Modeling is explicitly discussed and integrated throughout this treatment. As in the closely related *Coping Cat*, the therapist acts as a coach, using modeling to help teach many of the skills (e.g., being a coping model during *in vivo* exposure, modeling the recognition of the physical symptoms of anxiety, as well as many others). |
| *Family-Based Treatment for Young Children with OCD* (Freeman & Garcia, 2009) | • Modeling is explicitly mentioned and integrated throughout this treatment. Parents serve as coping models, and parent modeling is encouraged throughout the treatment, such as during ERP exercises. There is a separate chapter devoted to exposure and response prevention and modeling. |
| *OCD in Children and Adolescents* (March & Mulle, 1998) | • Modeling is explicitly discussed as a supplemental treatment component. It is described as potentially useful in exposure exercises, with the therapist demonstrating more appropriate or adaptive behaviors during the exposure. |
| *CBT of Childhood OCD: It's Only a False Alarm* (Piacentini, Langley, & Roblek, 2007) | • Modeling is explicitly mentioned as part of the ERP exercises. The therapist is told that desired behaviors will need to be modeled or shaped during the ERP exercises. |
| *CBT for Social Phobia: Stand Up, Speak Out* (Albano & DiBartolo, 2007) | • Though rarely explicitly mentioned, modeling is clearly present in this treatment. The therapist and cotherapist serve as models during many of the role plays initially to teach skills, such as cognitive restructuring. As treatment progresses, other group members are encouraged to serve as models for one another. |
| *When Children Refuse School: A CBT Approach* (Kearney & Albano, 2007): Chapters 4 and 5 on internalizing symptoms | • Though rarely mentioned explicitly, modeling is fully integrated throughout this treatment. The therapist and parent are both encouraged to model, such as during exposure exercises, thought challenging, and relaxation training. |
| *Treating Trauma and Traumatic Grief in Children and Adolescents* (Cohen, Mannarino, & Deblinger, 2006) | • Though rarely explicitly discussed, modeling is clearly present in this treatment. The therapist is encouraged to demonstrate a limited number of techniques, such as belly breathing, and encourages the parents to model praising behavior by noticing or remarking on the child's helpful behavior. |

*(continued)*

**TABLE 5.1.** (*continued*)

| | |
|---|---|
| *Adolescent Coping with Depression* (Clarke, Lewinsohn, & Hops, 1990) | • Modeling is explicitly mentioned and fully integrated throughout this treatment. The therapist is instructed to model during communication and skill training, such as in active listening and providing constructive feedback. Group members also serve as models for one another in guided skill practice (e.g., providing introductions, joining a conversation). |
| *Interpersonal Psychotherapy for Depressed Adolescents,* 2nd edition (Mufson, Pollack, Dorta, Moreau, & Weissman, 2011) | • Modeling is encouraged as one of a number of therapeutic techniques to aid in behavior change, though the therapist is cautioned that such techniques must be balanced with less active and more client-driven activities. |
| *Treating Depressed Children: Therapist Manual for "Taking Action"* (Stark & Kendall, 1996) | • Modeling is explicitly discussed and fully integrated throughout this treatment. The therapist is encouraged to model and discuss the process of problem solving to illustrate ways to cope with unpleasant emotions, sharing emotions, problem-solving strategies, and ways to prolong the experience of pleasant emotions. |
| *Treating Depressed Youth: Therapist Manual for "Action"* (Stark et al., 2007) | • Modeling is presented as one strategy that therapists may use to help the youth engage in positive behavior, such as learning to manage their emotions and dealing with teasing. Therapists are also encouraged to watch for opportunities to demonstrate how the group members may help one another to achieve their goals. |
| *Psychotherapy for Children with Bipolar and Depressive Disorders* (Fristad, Arnold, & Leffler, 2011) | • Modeling is present in this treatment but restricted to therapist demonstrations of nonverbal communications, such as facial expressions, or problem-solving strategies. |

*Note.* Some book titles are shortened to conserve space. See the References at the back of the book for full titles.

of modeling applications in selected EBT manuals for internalizing disorders in youth). In fact, efforts to identify empirically supported treatments have found participant modeling to be "well established" for the treatment of phobias and multimodal treatments incorporating modeling to be either "well established" or "probably efficacious" for the treatment of anxiety disorders and depression (Chambless & Ollendick, 2001; David-Ferdon & Kaslow, 2008; Ollendick & King, 2004; Silverman, Pina, et al., 2008).

Modeling is effective in treating fears across gender and age in both individual and group formats (e.g., Davis, Rosenthal, & Kelley,

1981; Faust, Olson, & Rodriguez, 1991; Klingman, Melamed, Cuthbert, & Hermecz, 1984; Kornhaber & Schroeder, 1975; Melamed, Hawes, Heiby, & Glick, 1975; Peterson, Schultheis, Ridley-Johnson, Miller, & Tracy, 1984; Ritter, 1968; see Chorpita & Southam-Gerow, 2006, for a comprehensive review). In an example intervention with children between the ages of 4 and 10 (mean age = 5.5 years), Faust et al. (1991) found evidence for the superiority of participant modeling relative to a standard hospital procedure in the preparation for elective ear tube surgery. In the hour preceding surgery, children in the active treatment condition viewed a tape depicting a 5-year-old girl undergoing surgery while modeling appropriate levels of anxiety and the use of coping skills (i.e., deep breathing, imagining floating on a cloud) and encouraging the children to practice these skills during the demonstration. With a group of preadolescents (ages 5–11 years), Ritter (1968) compared vicarious and contact desensitization procedures in the treatment of snake phobia. The vicarious desensitization condition included the observation of the experimenter and five peer models engaging in increasingly brave interactions with a large snake, whereas the contact desensitization condition added opportunities for the adolescents to have physical contact with the models and the snake. Though both active treatments proved superior to the control condition, the contact desensitization group experienced the greatest overall improvement in behavioral avoidance test performance. In comparing variations of participant modeling procedures used to treat female adolescents with spider fears, Davis and colleagues determined that the combination of a rationale, prolonged immediate exposure, and the use of real spiders was most effective (Davis et al., 1981).

Modeling is also an important element in a number of evidence-based multicomponent interventions for anxiety disorders (e.g., Barrett et al., 1996, 2004; Beidel et al., 2000; Deblinger & Heflin, 1996; Kendall, 1994; Kendall et al., 1997, 2008; see Table 5.1 for examples). These are typically manualized CBTs that use some combination of psychoeducation, cognitive restructuring, exposure, relaxation, problem solving skills training, and contingency management. For instance, Kendall and colleagues have demonstrated the effectiveness of Coping Cat, a packaged treatment for children with anxiety disorders, in three randomized control trials (Kendall, 1994; Kendall et al., 1997, 2008). Modeling is integrated throughout this treatment. Therapists are encouraged to act as coaches who actively engage children, structure learning activities, and provide encouragement. Therapists model the completion of self-ratings of anxiety levels, recognition of anxious feelings, deep breathing and relaxing, as well as problem-solving and other cognitive skills. They also act as coping models, demonstrating the various skills in anxiety-provoking situations by using imagined and role-play scenarios.

Multicomponent treatments incorporating modeling also have demonstrated success in the treatment of depressed children and adolescents (e.g., Clarke, Hops, & Lewinsohn, 1992; Clarke et al., 1999; Kahn et al., 1990; Lewinsohn et al., 1990; Liddle & Spence, 1990; Mufson, Moreau, Weissman, & Garfinkel, 1999; Mufson, Pollack, Dorta, et al., 2004; Stark et al., 1987). Like the anxiety interventions, these treatments tend to be cognitive-behavioral packages that include some combination of psychoeducation, cognitive restructuring, and skills instruction (e.g., coping, emotion regulation, problem solving, social skills), in addition to pleasant events scheduling. An example is the Coping with Depression course shown to be effective in the treatment of depressed adolescents (Clarke et al., 1999; Lewinsohn et al., 1990). Modeling is a key component of skills instruction. Group leaders model the instructed skills and provide feedback on student performance. Peers also serve as models during group exercises and paired practice periods. Interpersonal therapy adapted for depressed adolescents by Mufson and her colleagues is an evidence-based alternative to the CBTs (e.g., Mufson et al., 2011; Mufson, Moreau, et al., 1999). In this treatment, the therapist and teen identify particular problem areas (e.g., grief, interpersonal role disputes, and role transitions) and develop plans to address them through a variety of therapeutic techniques, including role plays and therapist modeling to aid in affective expression, communication, and decision making. The evidence base for IPT as an effective treatment for depressed adolescents includes a randomized control trial (Mufson, Pollack, Dorta, Wickremaraine, et al., 2004).

## THE ELEMENT IN PRACTICE

With the historical, theoretical, and empirical foundations set, the focus of this chapter now turns to the use of modeling in practice. The key steps of modeling are outlined in the task analysis in Box 5.1. More detailed coverage of the steps is included in this section, along with important developmental adaptations and diversity considerations. An illustrative case example of a 9-year-old female treated for extreme dental fears is also provided in Box 5.2 at the end of the chapter.

## BOX 5.1 Task Analysis of Modeling

### PHASE 1: PLANNING

1. Consider youth characteristics that may affect the effectiveness of the modeling:
   a. Assess for prerequisite skills and abilities for learning to take place (e.g., displays generalized imitative response, sensory capabilities, and physical abilities for motor reproduction; has cognitive abilities needed to understand rationale, engage in covert rehearsal).

2. Carefully identify the precise goal behavior or response pattern to be taught through modeling:
   a. If the behavior is complex, consider breaking it down into more manageable steps, subskills, or tasks;
   b. Arrange the steps, subskills, or tasks into a coherent sequence to maximize retention;
   c. Graduated presentations work best (e.g., increasing in complexity or difficulty).

3. Ensure that the consequences to be used are effective:
   a. Carefully identify what is reinforcing for the youth;
   b. Consider whether the goal behavior is one that will be reinforced in the youth's natural environment (e.g., parents, peers).

4. Select a model and consider modeling stimuli:
   a. Consider the relevance, similarity, and credibility of the model for the youth (e.g., age, gender, ethnicity, and scenarios);
   b. Determine whether a coping model or a mastery model will be used;
   c. Consider the demonstration modality (e.g., live, film or video).

### PHASE 2: IMPLEMENTATION

5. Provide a rationale for the modeled behavior:
   a. Ensure that the value and relevance of the modeled behavior are clear to the youth;
   b. Consider adding concepts, rules, or strategies for using the behavior.

6. Before the modeling demonstration, be sure that the youth is attending and alert (and that the learning environment is conducive to learning):
   a. The arousal level of the learner should be considered—either too much or too little arousal can impede learning;
   b. Past reinforcement for behavior may also affect the current learning environment (e.g., more difficult to teach in face of a previously punished response).

7. Instruct the youth as to what behavior to observe as well as any relevant contextual cues (e.g., discriminative stimuli signaling performance):
   a. Emphasize the absence of negative consequences for the model's engagement in the behavior;                                          (*continued*)

## BOX 5.1 *(continued)*

  b. Emphasize the presence of positive consequences for the model's engagement in the behavior.

8. Clearly and consistently model the desired behavior:
   a. Adjust the speed of the modeling demonstration for the youth, and consider slowing down and pausing as needed. Slowing down may improve encoding and retention.

9. Prompt the youth to reproduce and rehearse the behavior:
   a. The goal is a visible behavioral response;
   b. Rehearsal may be aided by the youth's engaging in self-observations of the desired behavior;
   c. Retention of the modeled behavior is crucial for subsequent rehearsals.

10. Aid initial practice attempts through joint practice or verbal coaching, as needed:
    a. Fade these induction aids with continued practice attempts;
    b. Remember that the client must be motivated to reproduce the behavior;
    c. External reinforcement and self-reinforcement may both be used.

11. Capitalize on vicarious reinforcement (e.g., praising the model's behavior, emphasizing the positive consequences to the model).

12. Provide immediate positive or corrective feedback after each practice attempt to reinforce goal-directed behavior. Additional reinforcers may be needed to ensure that the practice attempt is performed.

13. Rehearsal is essential for successful retention. It may be either overt (e.g., viewing others actually engaging in the behavior) or covert (e.g., imagining a model performing the behavior).

### PHASE 3: PLANNING FOR GENERALIZATION

14. Alternate between rehearsal and feedback until the youth is able to master the desired behavior.

15. Consciously plan for generalization:
    a. Identify situations in the youth's natural environment in which the behavior can be implemented, and rehearse whenever possible;
    b. Consider the potential obstacles to successful performance in the natural environment, and plan work-arounds for them;
    c. Identify implementation aids that may be helpful in carrying out assignments in the natural environment (e.g., ask a parent or teacher to attend to the performance and offer praise);
    d. Schedule booster sessions or follow-up as needed.

## "Core of the Core" Element

Although modeling typically involves having the client replicate a modeled behavior just after a demonstration with the therapist providing feedback, there are a number of procedural variations. In following the general guidelines offered in Box 5.1, the clinician will have to make decisions about which formats work best for a particular situation. Graduated modeling refers to the use of modeling sequences in which behaviors are presented in an increasingly difficult manner. For example, a modeling demonstration might progress from a social interaction initiation with one child to an initiation involving a group of children engaged in an ongoing activity. Graduated modeling is most often used in combination with either guided or participant modeling. Whereas guided modeling involves a demonstration accompanied by therapist provision of information and instruction, participant modeling pairs the demonstration with encouragement for the child to engage in the target behavior (Foster et al., 1988). For example, after viewing a filmed depiction of the use of coping skills during a medical procedure, a child may be given instructions to actively practice the skills during or just after the demonstration. With covert modeling, the youth constructs an image of a model engaging in a desired behavior. This procedure is purely imaginal and often aided by therapist instruction and description. For example, an adolescent might be instructed to imagine detailed scenarios in which he or she uses assertion skills in a variety of conflict situations. Modeling demonstrations themselves can be either live (i.e., using an actual person in real time) or symbolic (e.g., film, book, or cartoon). A final variation is self-modeling, or the review of one's own performance, combined with feedback. Following up on the example above, the teen might also be asked to watch videos of him- or herself engaging in an assertive behavior, with or without the therapist present.

The *planning* phase incorporates Steps 1–4. The therapist should consider whether the youth has the required prerequisite skills and abilities. For example, the youth must have certain sensory (e.g., can see or hear the demonstration) and motor (e.g., has the ability to imitate the modeled response) capacities to perceive the demonstration and reproduce the goal behavior. Another consideration is whether the cognitive abilities needed for encoding, covert rehearsal, and understanding the rationale are present. Asking the youth questions or to narrate or "talk through" the modeling scenario can be helpful in informally assessing understanding. Covert rehearsal requires fairly advanced imagery abilities and thus may be better suited for adolescents (e.g., Pentz & Kazdin, 1982). The goal behavior must be identified and carefully defined in exact, observable, and measurable terms. In other words, two or more people should be able to observe the performance and agree as to whether it occurred. The behavior may have to be simplified by breaking it down into more manageable steps, subskills, or tasks. As is done in shaping procedures, the steps should begin at a level that can be readily performed by the youth and then gradually increase in difficulty. Therapists should also assess the youth's motivation. In cases where motivation is lacking, extra efforts to identify meaningful rewards may be especially important (see Chapter 9). Interviews with the youth and parents can be useful in identifying potentially effective reinforcers. Another consideration is the degree to which the goal behavior is one that is likely to be reinforced in the youth's natural environment. For instance, a newly taught assertive response may follow all of the steps prescribed in the literature but yet not be effective when used in the youth's peer group. This may require some rethinking about the appropriateness of the goal behavior. In any event, discussing the possibility that even the right goal behavior enacted in a perfect way may not always result in the desired reaction from others with the youth is important. The therapist should also consider the degree to which the model is relevant, similar, and credible to the observer. In particular, the therapist should think about not only model characteristics, such as age and gender, but the actual scenarios used in the demonstrations as well. This can be accomplished by working with the youth to identify relevant situations and generate descriptive details. Despite these considerations, the therapy context often dictates that the therapist serve as the model, as is done in most of the multicomponent treatment packages (e.g., Cohen, Mannarino, & Deblinger, 2006; Kendall & Hedtke, 2006). In group formats, the use of peer demonstrations may also be an option (e.g., Clarke et al., 1990).

The *implementation* phase includes the actual modeling demonstrations, initial practice attempts, and subsequent rehearsal (Steps 5–13). The modeling process and expectations are described for the youth. Whether the youth has any concerns and is willing to proceed can also be assessed. Efforts should be made to engage youth in modeling by discussing the relevance and value of the procedure. Before the actual demonstration, the therapist should make sure that the youth is attentive and provide instructions for exactly what to observe. Noting that the model will be engaging in the behavior in the absence of any negative consequences is also helpful. The demonstrations should be clear and consistent. The pace should be adjusted to the youth's needs, and only one step or skill should be demonstrated at a time. Having the model verbalize the thoughts and feelings that go along with the overt response may also be helpful. Prompts for the youth to perform the behavior should be followed by immediate praise and corrective feedback as needed. Induction aids, such as joint practice or verbal coaching, may also be helpful in getting the youth to engage in initial attempts, but these should be faded. Rehearsal, praise, and corrective feedback continue until mastery has been attained. Self-directed practice (i.e., youth engaging in rehearsal attempts on their own, outside of the therapy session) is likely to have a greater influence on self-efficacy perceptions and should also be encouraged (Rosenthal & Bandura, 1978).

Of course, the ultimate goal is to get the youth to continue using the learned behaviors after treatment has ended. As such, the final phase (Steps 14–15) involves planning for generalization. The therapist should work with the youth to identify relevant situations for skill use and rehearse them. Problem solving to identify potential obstacles and ways to get around them is helpful. Other suggestions include starting the youth with an easier behavior performance goal and taking action to ensure that initial attempts are met with success. The importance of repeated practice and feedback is worth reemphasizing. Practice in a variety of situations helps with generalization and instills a sense of mastery (Rosenthal & Bandura, 1978).

Beyond these more universal features, there are additional considerations when using modeling to reduce fears and anxiety. Because efforts are most often intertwined with exposure, the therapist should become familiar with such procedures (see Chapter 2). Another important consideration is whether to use a mastery or coping model. A coping model, which at first displays undesirable or fearful behavior and then becomes more competent, is generally considered to be more effective than a mastery model, which displays desired behavior from the start (Masters et al., 1987). At least with children, however, this convention may be based more on the idea that similarity is central to model effectiveness than actual empirical findings. Despite ample support for the effectiveness of coping models with children (e.g., Faust et al., 1991; Klingman et al., 1984), direct comparisons with mastery models have failed to find differences (e.g., Chertock & Bornstein, 1979; Kornhaber & Schroeder, 1975). For example, in the Kornhaber and Schroeder (1975) study, fearless and fearful child models were equally effective in treating snake fears. The arousal level of the youth during a modeling demonstration should also be considered. If the arousal is too high, the youth may engage in distraction or other covert coping methods that detract from the learning process (Rosenthal & Bandura, 1978). Guided participation and induction aids may also be required to motivate initial performance attempts. For example, the therapist could accompany a child as he or she climbs a ladder, or a glove could be worn by an adolescent as he or she touches a snake for the first time.

Lest the therapist new to modeling become overwhelmed by the number of steps and considerations, it is important to bear in mind that modeling is a very robust procedure capable of withstanding some variation in techniques. Indeed, studies comparing different active modeling treatments (e.g., symbolic vs. live, participant vs. nonparticipant) generally show that all are effective relative to controls (e.g., Bandura, Grusec, & Menlove, 1967; Bandura & Menlove, 1968; Faust et al., 1991; Gresham & Nagle, 1980; O'Connor, 1972).

## Developmental Adaptations

Modeling procedures work for youth of all ages and abilities, but little is known about the impact, if any, of developmental differences on effectiveness. Bandura (1977c) wrote extensively about the developmental implications of observational learning theory, but his suppositions have not been empirically examined. Though only an imperfect proxy for estimating developmental levels, age is often ignored in modeling intervention studies. For example, two studies evaluating the use of modeling in the reduction of presurgical anxiety blended children ranging in age from 2 to 11 years without examining age as a factor in outcomes (Peterson et al., 1984; Peterson & Shigetomi, 1981).

Although Bandura (1977c) did not put forth a stage theory per se, he emphasized that observational learning evolved with maturation and experience. For example, modeling was thought to progress from instantaneous to delayed reproduction. Even very young children can engage in instant imitation, but the capacity for delayed imitation increases along with the ability to symbolize experiences and translate them into motor behavior. In fact, Bandura believed that the ability to form mental representations of the modeling demonstration was critical for delayed imitation. With continued development, children begin to form abstractions from modeling observations that aid in the development of more general principles underlying observed performances (e.g., aggressive behavior with peers will usually be punished).

The power of observational learning is evidenced by the fact that even 2- and 3-year-olds with fears and anxiety benefit from modeling demonstrations (Bandura & Menlove, 1968; Peterson et al., 1984;

Peterson & Shigetomi, 1981). Further, young children with severe mental retardation can be trained to engage in imitative responses, and modeling is often used to teach language to children with autism (e.g., Baer, Peterson, & Sherman, 1967; Lovaas, Berberich, Perloff, & Schaeffer, 1966). Frame et al. (1982) used instructions, modeling, role play, and feedback to successfully improve four depressive behaviors (inappropriate body position, lack of eye contact, poor speech, and bland affect) exhibited by a boy diagnosed with both depression and mental retardation. Collectively, the results show that modeling can be used with children from a range of developmental levels.

Though youth at all ages can benefit from modeling, a number of interventions have relied on puppets or dolls as models in an effort to help attract and maintain child attention. For example, Lizette Peterson and colleagues (1984) used puppet models in a modeling demonstration designed to reduce adverse reactions in children preparing for elective surgery. Children in the puppet condition watched a "Teddy Bear" model depict a typical hospital visit, including admission, blood test, preoperative injection, anesthesia, recovery room, and discharge. In a study evaluating a CBT for young children with anxiety disorders, Hirshfeld-Becker et al. (2010) used puppet play to help children learn and practice various coping skills. In other notable adaptations, these authors presented the rationale in age-appropriate story form, incorporated games, used contingency management, and added parent-only sessions. Symbolic modeling procedures are also frequently used with youngsters (e.g., Bandura & Menlove, 1968; Keller & Carlson, 1974; O'Connor, 1972; Peterson et al., 1984). In an example with 3- to 5-year old children exhibiting extreme fear of dogs, Bandura and Menlove (1968) presented a graduated series of films depicting child models engaging in approach behaviors. One group observed one model, whereas the second observed a variety of models interacting with the dog. Though both conditions resulted in fear reduction, only those in the multiple models condition were subsequently able to perform the most threatening approach behaviors.

With increased cognitive and verbal abilities, older children and adolescents might be expected to acquire greater benefit from covert modeling than younger youth, but there have been few studies evaluating this procedural variation. In a rare side-by-side comparison of overt and covert procedures, Pentz and Kazdin (1982) found that overt modeling resulted in notably greater improvements in assertive behavior and self-efficacy in a group of adolescents. Yet in studies with college students, Kazdin demonstrated that imaginal techniques were effective in treating snake fears (Kazdin, 1973, 1974c). At the very least, when considering the use of covert modeling with children or adolescents, one should first assess their ability to engage in imagery.

In an interesting adaptation capitalizing on the developing abstract thinking and self-evaluation abilities of young adolescents, Kahn et al. (1990) used a self-modeling procedure to treat depression. The authors reasoned, based on research with adult samples, that the repeated observation of oneself on edited or rehearsed videotapes engaging only in responses incompatible with depression should result in behavioral, cognitive, and affective improvements. After receiving an explanation and rationale, the participants in this group rehearsed and were eventually filmed engaging in "nondepressed" behaviors (e.g., appropriate eye contact, pleasant voice tone, and verbalizing positive self-attributions). In brief sessions (10–12 minutes) conducted twice a week over 6–8 weeks, the participants were simply instructed to watch the tapes without the therapist present. The self-modeling treatment was equal to two other active treatments (i.e., the CWD-A course and relaxation training) in producing improvements on self-report measures of depression and self-esteem relative to a waitlist control group.

The intervention literature has not made the most of the rich developmental theory base provided by Bandura. Potential developmental differences have most often been overlooked. A question of particular interest is the extent to which efforts to better incorporate increasing verbal and abstract thinking abilities into interventions might enhance the effectiveness of modeling with older children and adolescents. Though clearly expected, based on Bandura's (1977c) theory, there is little evidence that the addition of verbal descriptions or use of mental images is more effective for older and more developmentally sophisticated youth.

## Diversity Considerations

Not surprisingly, given its robust nature, modeling appears to cut across ethnic and racial lines in its effectiveness (e.g., Constantino, Malgady, & Rogler, 1986; Lewis, 1974; Malgady, Rogler, & Constantino, 1990). Nonetheless, cross-cultural applications may require adaptations to ensure the similarity and relevance of the model. Sherry Cormier and colleagues (2009) suggest that models be culturally compatible with the client's background (e.g., using an African American model if developing an intervention targeting African American youth), the content of the modeling demonstrations be culturally relevant and not just reflective of mainstream values (e.g., assertiveness skills may be more valued in some cultures than in others), and that possible cultural differences in observational learning styles be considered (e.g., the degree to which having or seeing a model is valued).

In an excellent example of cross-cultural adaptations, Constantino et al. (1986) incorporated the use of *cuentos*, or folktales, in their modeling therapy for Puerto Rican children. Characters in the folktales served as therapeutic peer models in conveying the theme or moral of the stories. The original themes were altered to better tailor the intervention to the goals of reducing anxiety and disruptive behavior (e.g., social judgment, control of anxiety and aggression, and delay of gratification). After having the *cuentos* read to them bilingually by therapists and mothers, children engaged in a group discussion of each character's feelings and behavior. Mother–child dyads then acted out the story and resolved the conflict, and the youth were praised for imitation. This was followed by a review of a video of the drama and group discussion regarding the positive and negative consequences of the player's actions. The treatment resulted in improvements in social judgment at posttest and reductions in anxiety at 1-year follow-up.

As suggested by the authors of this study and in line with Bandura's (1977c) theory, the cultural adaptations likely resulted in models that demanded more attention and portrayed more relevant beliefs, values, and behaviors. More studies like the Malgady et al. (1990) investigation are needed to better inform clinicians about possible cultural adaptations in modeling procedures for diverse groups.

## CONCLUSIONS

Modeling is a treatment element that has a deep conceptual and empirical base, and one of its variants, participant modeling, is a "well-established" treatment for phobias. Since its emergence as behavior therapy technique during the 1950s, modeling has been evaluated on its own and as a component in multimodal treatments for a wide range of clinical problems and disorders. In the treatment of internalizing disorders, modeling is most often used to assist in skills acquisition (e.g., social skills training) or fear reduction (e.g., exposure). The extent of related background literature and the many procedural variations suggest that there is a lot to consider when using modeling with children and adolescents. The detailed task analysis and illustrative case example included in this chapter are intended to help guide therapists through this process.

## BOX 5.2. Illustrative Case Example

Iris was a 9-year-old Caucasian female referred for psychological services by her mother because of an extreme dental fear. The family dentist suggested the referral because Iris had missed three successive scheduled examinations. During her last dental visit almost 2 years earlier, Iris became disruptive, refusing to open her mouth, squirming in the chair, and crying. Shortly after that visit, she refused to accompany her younger brother to his dentist appointment even though she would only need to sit in the waiting room during his visit. On the morning of her next appointment, Iris said that she felt nauseous and pleaded with her mother to cancel. Her mother agreed but insisted that Iris attend the rescheduled appointment. When the time came, however, Iris reportedly refused to get into the car, crying, trembling, and screaming at her mother. Iris's mother admitted to having a fair amount of apprehension about dental procedures herself, though she reported making significant efforts to hide it from her children.

An intake assessment revealed that Iris's fears were restricted to the dental setting. The therapist asked her a number of questions about what aspects of the dental visits caused her the most distress, and her responses formed the basis of a detailed fear hierarchy that was completed during the next session. To construct the hierarchy, the therapist had to determine the relative distress elicited by each scenario. After instructing Iris in the use of SUDS ratings, the therapist helped her conjure up images of comparative anchors (i.e., 0 being completely relaxed, 100 being the most distress she ever experienced). The hierarchy included such scenarios as seeing a toothpaste advertisement on television (SUDS of 10), seeing a dentist appointment reminder postcard (not hers) in the mail (20), thinking about sitting in the dentist office waiting room (30), listening to her mother talk about the importance of her going to the dentist (40), finding out that her brother had an impending dentist appointment (50, but increasing as the date of the appointment approached), smelling the odors of the dentist office (65), opening her mouth for the dentist (70), and receiving an inside the mouth injection (85). This session ended with the therapist and Iris agreeing on a goal for treatment that included Iris being able to undergo a routine dental examination.

In the third session, the therapist taught Iris how to use a variety of coping skills. These included the use of belly breathing (a version of diaphragmatic breathing) and coping self-statements (e.g., "I know I am scared, but I can do it"). The therapist told Iris that these skills would help her to cope with her dental fears and would also be beneficial in other stressful situations. Iris was also told that other children experiencing dental anxiety had found these skills easy to learn and very helpful in getting over their fears. The therapist modeled each coping skill and then asked Iris to practice, providing praise and some corrective feedback. At the end of the session, Iris and her mother were asked if they would be willing to watch a brief video containing depictions of different dental scenarios during the next meeting. Iris was also given a homework assignment to practice her coping skills during the week, checking off a block on a premade chart after each attempt.

The 15-minute video had seven different scenarios. In a graduated manner, these scenarios progressed from scans of an empty dentist office and a dentist explaining simple dental procedures with displays of equipment (e.g., the dental chair, examining light, x-ray machine) to children undergoing dental procedures, modeling the use of coping skills similar to the ones Iris learned. To enhance the coping model demonstrations, a narrative relaying the thoughts and concerns of the model accompanied each scenario. The therapist prompted Iris to attend to the coping model and skill use, emphasizing the fact that the model persisted with the procedure despite the concerns and experienced no untoward consequences. Iris was also told to practice her coping skills as she watched the video and received praise for doing so. SUDS ratings taken at the beginning, middle, and end of the video indicated a midway rise to about 50 and subsequent decline to 20.

This success experience increased Iris's willingness to engage in a live modeling demonstration. The dentist agreed to help set up the observation of a child patient undergoing a routine examination and cleaning. The dentist understood the importance of selecting a child for observation who was similar to Iris in age and known to cope well with the exam procedure. Once a patient was identified, the appropriate parental and child permissions were obtained. On the day of the appointment, the therapist agreed to meet Iris outside the dentist's office. This agreement was a helpful motivator for Iris. The therapist continued to provide encouragement and assess Iris's distress level, using SUDS ratings. Iris was introduced to the patient and asked to find an unobtrusive spot for the observation. The therapist instructed Iris to focus her attention on the patient and to use her coping skills to relieve anxiety during the observation.

Shortly after the live modeling demonstration, Iris agreed to undergo a routine dental examination. On the day before the appointment, she met with the therapist to review the coping skills and discuss any last-minute concerns. The two also reviewed the steps in the fear hierarchy. Appearing very confident and proud of her successes, Iris told the therapist that she could not believe how "stressed out" she used to be "about all this." Though the therapist expressed a willingness to accompany her to the examination, Iris said that she wanted to "go it alone." The exam went well, and Iris reported that she felt that she had finally conquered her fears.

# 6

# Relaxation Training

with Tiffany West and Alayna Schreier

## BACKGROUND OF THE ELEMENT

Relaxation training is a commonly used therapy procedure designed to help individuals reduce anxiety or tension. Broadly defined, relaxation is the "mental and physical freedom from tension or stress" (Titlebaum, 1988, p. 28). Relaxation training involves teaching effective ways to reduce physiological arousal related to tension and stress, thereby helping clients to achieve this freedom. Though many relaxation procedures exist, deep breathing, progressive muscle relaxation (PMR), and imagery are the most common and effective relaxation procedures for children and adolescents with internalizing disorders (Hudson, Hughes, & Kendall, 2004; Morris, 2004). For example, an anxious child who experiences physiological symptoms such as a racing heart and dizziness when having to speak in front of the class can engage in deep breathing prior to public speaking to reduce the intensity of these symptoms. Additionally, a depressed adolescent who has difficulty participating in activities can engage in PMR as a pleasurable activity. Further, a child who experiences flashbacks of a traumatic event can imagine a safe, calm scene through guided imagery to provide distraction from a flashback. This chapter presents a brief history of the use of relaxation skills training, specifically the use of deep breathing, PMR, and imagery, and examines the ways that these techniques have been applied in treatment programs for internalizing disorders in both children and adolescents, and among diverse populations. A case example of a 10-year-old Latino boy with symptoms of anxiety and guilt, and for whom relaxation was a key component of treatment, is presented.

## Brief History

Use of relaxation techniques can be dated back centuries to the Eastern religions of Buddhism and Hinduism, including their practice of meditation and yoga. The goal of these practices was to achieve altered states of consciousness for the purpose of worship, resting the mind, and achieving enlightenment (Samuel, 2008). During the late 19th and early 20th century, Coué (1922) and Freud (Costigan, 1965) used imagery skills to address both medical and psychological ailments. Relaxation techniques expanded beyond imagery during the 20th century with the development of PMR by the physician Edmund Jacobson (1925, 1938). Through the practice of progressively tensing and relaxing various muscle groups, a person develops what Jacobson terms "muscle-sense," or the ability to gain awareness of the difference between feelings of tension and relaxation. This awareness brings a person one step closer to gaining control over feelings of tension in the body. Jacobson went on to develop a training program for PMR for adults, which consisted of 56 sessions and addressed a number of medical conditions, such as ulcers, insomnia, and hypertension (Jacobson, 1938).

Although relaxation procedures, specifically imagery and meditation, were used as therapeutic techniques in psychodynamic and psychoanalytic approaches, it was not until the rise of behavior therapy in the late 1950s through the 1970s that relaxation techniques gained new interest and became a core component of psychotherapy (Walker, 1979). One of the initial uses of relaxation training in behavior therapy was brought about by Wolpe in the development of systematic desensitization, a form of counterconditioning used to treat anxiety-related disorders and phobias. Wolpe (1958) determined that a conditioned fear response could be reversed by eliciting an incompatible response while gradually introducing the feared stimulus. Further, he noted that physiological correlates of relaxation were incompatible with those of anxiety in that a person could not be anxious and relaxed at the same time. Systematic desensitization utilizes relaxation as a natural incompatible response to any feared stimulus.

Since the development of systematic desensitization, relaxation training has been used in psychotherapy with adults to address a number of internalizing disorders (e.g., Cloitre, Cohen, & Koenen, 2006; Craske & Barlow, 2014; Wright, Basco, & Thase, 2006) and was adapted for use with children and adolescents during the early 1970s. In particular, Koeppen adapted the PMR technique developed by Jacobson (1938) for use with children. For instance, Koeppen (1974) used basic images, or what she termed "fantasies," to facilitate children's use of tension and relaxation techniques (e.g., squeezing lemons with the hands, squishing toes in the mud). Ollendick and Cerny (1981) further contributed to the adaptation of relaxation training with children and adolescents by developing additional scripts and conducting research on the efficacy of relaxation training with children. They noted that a developmentally appropriate script, such as the one developed by Koeppen (1974), is valuable in teaching children how to achieve deep muscle relaxation.

More recently, relaxation training has been incorporated as a key component in a number of different treatments for children and adolescents experiencing anxiety (e.g., Kendall & Hedtke, 2006), depression (e.g., Clarke & DeBar, 2010), and trauma (e.g., Cohen et al., 2006). The primary purpose of relaxation training in psychotherapy for children and adolescents is to address the physiological arousal brought on by stress and anxiety in conjunction with other therapeutic techniques to obtain the best outcomes. Relaxation training teaches youth self-soothing behaviors that may help them overcome barriers to particular components of broader treatment. For instance, relaxation can help allay hesitation in anxious youth who struggle to engage in exposures, or anxiety in depressed individuals who struggle to engage in social activities (Clarke & DeBar, 2010). Although relaxation training is commonly used in treatments for depression, the focus is on reducing symptoms of anxiety that accompany depression rather than the depressive symptoms themselves.

## Theory Base

An understanding of the theory underlying the use of relaxation training is valuable for effective use of this element in treatment. The brain elicits autonomic responses throughout the body when perceived threats and stress are imminent (e.g., an elevated heart rate, increased body temperature, perspiration). Relaxation is used to combat these responses, and thus the conceptual foundation of relaxation is grounded primarily in physiological principles. In particular, the autonomic nervous system is composed of the sympathetic ("stress") and parasympathetic ("peace") branches, both of which are involved in regulating physiological arousal in the body. The former works to prepare the body for fight or flight during times of perceived stress, whereas the latter works to calm the body down and maintain homeostasis. Consider the example of a child who developed a fear of large dogs after being bitten. When encountering a dog, the child's sympathetic nervous system is automatically activated, owing to the perceived sense of danger. Her heart begins to beat faster, and her body starts to perspire, preparing her to either fight or flee. As she sees that the dog is wagging its tail and appears friendly, she recognizes there is no imminent danger. Her parasympathetic nervous system is activated, and her heart rate begins to normalize and perspiration decreases.

Cannon (1939) coined the term "fight or flight" to describe the body's primitive, automatic, and innate response to either flee from, or fight, sources of perceived harm or threat. He suggested that this "hard-wired" response initiates a sequence of nerve cell firings and chemical releases that prepares the body for running or fighting by inducing autonomic responses, such as rapid heartbeat and breathing, and increased blood flow to the muscles. Selye (1956) further investigated the fight-or-flight response and determined that the body has a nonspecific reaction to demands placed upon it, coining the term "stress" to describe this phenomenon. Physiologically, the sympathetic nervous system responds to stressors, either positive or negative, and activates the "stress response" that affects one's heart rate, blood pressure, metabolism, and breathing. Selye developed the general adaptation syndrome (GAS) theory to explain the different stages experienced during the stress response. The GAS consists of three distinct stages the body experiences when encountering a stressor: alarm, resistance, and exhaustion. Selye argued that when under stress the body initially becomes alarmed and enters the fight-or-flight mode described by Cannon (1939). The body eventually begins to resist the stressor through some means of coping, and finally, without effective response to the stressor, exhaustion sets in and results in the breakdown of the body, both mentally and physically. In the prior example, the child initially experiences alarm when encountering a large dog. Resistance would occur if he or she employed coping strategies such as deep breathing and muscle relaxation to combat the stressful response. However, if he or she failed to implement effective resistance strategies, exhaustion may occur. Selye (1993) suggested utilizing some form of relaxation on a daily basis in which the eyes are closed, muscles are relaxed, and breathing is steady to both physically and mentally manage stress and prevent the exhaustion phase.

Benson (1975) further advanced our understanding of the body's reaction to stress by identifying what he termed the "relaxation response." He argued that, just as the body has an innate ability to respond to stress (i.e., fight or flight and the stress response) physiologically with an increase in heart rate, blood pressure, metabolism, and rate of breathing, the body has a similar ability to protect itself from stress by decreasing the physiological effects and bringing the body back to a healthier balance (i.e., the relaxation response). Through the relaxation response, there is a decrease in sympathetic nervous system activity in the brain and an increase in parasympathetic nervous system activity, resulting in steady breathing and a decrease in heart rate and blood pressure. Benson noted that a number of techniques can be used to obtain the relaxation response, including deep breathing, muscle relaxation, and meditation.

As mentioned above, rapid and shallow breathing is part of the stress response and can have a significant impact on the ability to reason and adapt to stressors, potentially influencing psychological functioning (Cormier et al., 2013). Too much or too little oxygen can result in impairment of bodily systems and brain functioning. Since the sympathetic and parasympathetic nervous systems are in control of the body's organs and blood vessels, regulated breathing helps to balance these systems and, in turn, aids in their appropriate functioning (Fried, 1993). Thus, when breathing becomes rapid and shallow as a result of overstimulation of the sympathetic nervous system, the use of diaphragmatic, or deep, breathing helps to regain this balance by providing the brain with sufficient oxygen (Cormier et al., 2013).

Behaviorally, the purpose of relaxation in the treatment of anxiety disorders is to combat physiological symptoms of arousal when presented with a feared stimulus so that fear and/or anxiety is no longer associated with the given stimulus. For instance, an adolescent can be taught deep breathing techniques to calm the physiological sensations he (or she) experiences prior to taking a test in school. After he prepares for tests on a number of occasions while engaging in deep breathing techniques, he will learn to associate tests with calm feelings rather than fear and anxiety. When practiced on a regular basis with the body in a calm state, relaxation can also help decrease overall levels of arousal (Morris, 2004).

Avoidance or escape from a feared stimulus results in negative reinforcement; relief from the anxiety upon avoidance or escape reinforces the behavior and makes it more likely to occur in the future (Bouton, 2007). Thus, relaxation skills, when used to provide relief from anxiety, are negatively reinforced by the removal of the aversive stimulus, thus increasing the likelihood that relaxation skills will be used again. For example, the adolescent may experience somatic symptoms prior to tests and may go home sick. These escape behaviors help to reduce or eliminate the adolescent's anxious feelings. However, when she (or he) engages in deep breathing as soon as she thinks about the upcoming test, her anxious feelings are similarly reduced or eliminated, therefore making it more likely that she will engage in deep breathing when she encounters similar situations in the future.

## Evidence Base

Although relaxation has been used in various forms throughout the history of psychotherapy, few studies specifically examine the use of relaxation training for children and adolescents. Initial studies of relaxation techniques stemmed from the literature on systematic desensitization conducted during the 1970s. Van Hasselt, Hersen, Bellack, Rosenblum, and Lamparski (1979) utilized deep muscle relaxation as a treatment component for an 11-year-old child with multiple phobias reporting physiological symptoms, such as dizziness and nausea, and behavioral avoidance of the feared stimuli. The client participated in four sessions of relaxation training and was given relaxation audiotapes to facilitate practice at home between sessions. Improvements in physiological and behavioral/motoric, but not cognitive, outcome measures were noted postrelaxation. The focus of treatment shifted to systematic desensitization after the child demonstrated the ability to engage in prolonged relaxation. Following treatment, cognitive improvements were accompanied by further gains in the physiological and behavioral domains and were maintained at a 6-month follow-up.

The initial deep muscle relaxation script was developed for use in the treatment of anxiety with systematic desensitization (Wolpe, 1969). The script required a person to tense and relax one muscle group at a time (e.g., hands, shoulders, chest, feet) while keeping all other muscle groups still. However, young children struggled to achieve deep muscle relaxation using this script because they had difficulty understanding the adult terminology and targeting the appropriate muscle groups (Ollendick & Cerny, 1981). In response to the need for modification, Koeppen (1974) designed her adaptation of the initial PMR script to be more engaging and effective for children by including imagery of animals and common objects. For example, a child is instructed to pretend to squeeze a lemon with his or her hand and then to pretend to drop the lemon on the floor so that the muscles in the hand are tensed and then quickly relaxed. Although anecdotal evidence speaks to the effectiveness of Koeppen's script, experimental data have not been provided to empirically support its effectiveness (Ollendick & Cerny, 1981). Through unpublished research, Ollendick and colleagues (as cited in Ollendick & Cerny, 1981) found that children became distracted and overly involved with the use of fantasy characters within Koeppen's (1974) script. In response, they developed a script that contained engaging descriptions that better maintained children's attention. An unpublished study by Weisman, Ollendick, and Horne (as cited in Ollendick & Cerny, 1981) compared the effectiveness of Koeppen's (1974) script with that created by Ollendick and Cerny (1981) among 6- and 7-year-old children without clinical symptomatology. Results indicated that, compared to a control group, both scripts reduced muscle tension as measured by electromyography, though neither script differed significantly from the other. Both of these scripts are commonly used in modern clinical settings. These early findings suggest that relaxation training can be an effective component of treatments that seek to reduce anxiety in young children.

Relaxation has also been examined in adolescent populations. Reynolds and Coats (1986) investigated the efficacy of short-term group treatments with depressed adolescents. Adolescents were randomly assigned to relaxation training, CBT, or a waitlist control. No significant differences were found between the CBT and relaxation training conditions, and both active treatments were more effective than the waitlist control. These findings were maintained at 5-week follow-up. In a study of anxious children, Eisen and Silverman (1993) compared cognitive therapy, relaxation training, and their combination. Results indicated that cognitive therapy was more efficacious than relaxation training. However, these authors suggest that treatment should be matched to the client's presenting symptoms. In particular, relaxation training might be more effective for a child with somatic symptoms, while cognitive and behavior therapy may be more effective for a child with cognitive symptoms.

Despite the limited research on relaxation training as a standalone treatment, most empirically supported multicomponent cognitive-behavioral interventions for childhood internalizing disorders include relaxation training (see examples in Table 6.1). In a review of randomized trials of EBTs (Chorpita & Daleiden, 2009), relaxation was

**TABLE 6.1. The Relaxation Training Element in Representative EBT Manuals**

| | |
|---|---|
| *Coping Cat* (Kendall & Hedtke, 2006) | • The clinician explicitly teaches about somatic feelings associated with anxiety during the fifth session. The clinician leads the youth through relaxation skills training, including deep breathing and PMR. These skills are reviewed in the 10th session. |
| *C.A.T. Project* (Kendall, Choudhury, Hudson, & Webb, 2002) | • The clinician explicitly teaches about somatic reactions to anxiety during the third session. The clinician leads the youth through practice, with a focus on breathing, meditation, and PMR. |
| *OCD in Children and Adolescents* (March & Mulle, 1998) | • Relaxation skills are included in a supplemental chapter for use if anxiety management is necessary. The clinician can elect to provide information and skills demonstration of deep breathing, imagery, and PMR. |
| *CBT for Social Phobia: Stand Up, Speak Out* (Albano & DiBartolo, 2007) | • Relaxation skills are briefly discussed and practiced during the third session.<br>• The clinician uses weekly snack time to lead the youth through guided visualization. |
| *When Children Refuse School: A CBT Approach* (Kearney & Albano, 2007) | • The clinician leads the youth through deep breathing and PMR exercises during the first session. The clinician reads from age-appropriate scripts to facilitate the practice of PMR and breathing retraining. |
| *Treating Trauma and Traumatic Grief in Children and Adolescents* (Cohen, Mannarino, & Deblinger, 2006) | • The clinician explicitly teaches how the youth's bodies react to stress and then leads the child through focused breathing and PMR in the third component of the initial, trauma-focused, phase. The clinician reads from provided scripts to facilitate the practice of focused breathing, meditation, and PMR.<br>• Relaxation training is also provided within the parenting skills component of treatment to help manage stress and reinforce skills practice in their children. |
| *Adolescent Coping with Depression* (Clarke, Lewinsohn, & Hops, 1990) | • The clinician explicitly discusses tension and leads the participant through PMR scripts during the third session (Jacobson Relaxation Technique; Benson Relaxation Technique).<br>• Deep breathing is practiced during the eighth session. |
| *Treating Depressed Youth: Therapist Manual for "Action"* (Stark et al., 2007) | • Relaxation skills are provided as a treatment component within the fourth meeting. The clinician can select which relaxation skills to use, based on the needs of the youth. Available skills are imagery and deep breathing. |
| *Psychotherapy for Children with Bipolar and Depressive Disorders* (Fristad, Arnold, & Leffler, 2011) | • The clinician leads the group through relaxation exercises focused on deep breathing including belly breathing, bubble breathing, and balloon breathing. |

*Note.* Some book titles are shortened to conserve space. See the References at the back of the book for full titles.

the second most frequently used practice element (following exposure) for the treatment of anxiety and the ninth most commonly used element in the treatment of depression (with cognitive strategies and psychoeducation at the top of the list). Although the research described below is not specific to relaxation training, relaxation techniques are included as core components of each treatment program.

Relaxation training is consistently used in the treatment of anxiety for children and adolescents (e.g., Albano & DiBartolo, 2007; Kendall et al., 2002; Kendall & Hedtke, 2006). As a form of emotion regulation, relaxation may help the youth to regulate their physiological responses to anxiety and achieve an optimal level of arousal for learning, further helping them engage in additional components of treatment (Hannesdottir & Ollendick, 2007). The recognition of physical symptoms related to anxiety (e.g., heart racing, shallow breathing) allows children to better engage in relaxation and directly addresses physiological arousal (Hudson et al., 2004). Further, the use of relaxation may improve engagement during more demanding aspects of anxiety treatment, such as exposure, because it is an enjoyable activity for children to engage in and may help them feel more in control when experiencing their feared stimulus during exposures (Kendall, Furr, & Podell, 2010).

Techniques such as PMR and deep breathing are utilized in Coping Cat, a treatment for anxiety in children ages 7–13 (Kendall & Hedtke, 2006). The therapist models relaxation to help youth understand the techniques and reduce their physiological symptoms of arousal. Retention of skills is further encouraged by having the youth teach the relaxation skills to their parent(s). Coping Cat has been empirically supported in multiple RCTs (e.g., Kendall, 1994; Kendall et al., 1997, 2008). For example, in a study by Kendall et al. (2008), 161 youth with diagnosed anxiety disorders were assigned to individual CBT (ICBT), family-based CBT (FCBT), both using the Coping Cat manual, and a family education/support/attention (FESA) control group. Both the ICBT and FCBT conditions included relaxation training as a component, while the FESA control group did not learn relaxation skills. Results indicate that, overall, both treatment groups demonstrated better posttreatment outcomes than did the control group, supporting the use of a CBT program that includes relaxation components for anxiety in youth. Recent findings of the CAMS study suggest that relaxation training has only limited impact beyond the cognitive restructuring and exposure elements of Coping Cat, but this may be because the amount of relaxation training provided in the comprehensive intervention is insufficient to engender more substantial change (Peris et al., 2015).

Relaxation also has been shown to be helpful in the development of control over response to stressors and is especially central in the treatment of PTSD symptoms in youth who have experienced trauma. Cohen and Mannarino (2008) have found that youth who have experienced a traumatic event are often deprived of control during and after the event. In TF-CBT (Cohen, Mannarino, & Steer, 2006), control is gained through relaxation training by providing the youth with a "tool kit" of options to utilize in stressful situations to self-soothe and gain mastery over their physiological responses. Relaxation, particularly guided imagery, also helps to provide a distraction from traumatic thoughts, allowing the child to focus on more pleasurable images and activities. An initial multisite RCT assigned 229 participants ages 8–14 years to TF-CBT or child-centered therapy for treating PTSD (Cohen et al., 2004). TF-CBT included a relaxation training component, while the child-centered therapy did not. The findings showed that youth in the TF-CBT condition demonstrated significantly greater levels of improvement on reported symptomatology than those in the child-centered therapy condition. A follow-up study of 183 youth (Deblinger, Mannarino, Cohen, & Steer, 2006) examined symptoms at both 6- and 12-month posttreatment and found that those in the TF-CBT group continued to show significantly fewer symptoms at both assessments.

Relaxation strategies also have been used successfully in treating depressive symptoms in children and adolescents. Depressive symptoms often emerge owing to disturbances in cognitive (e.g., attributional style, self-schema), emotional (e.g., regulation, coping), interpersonal (e.g., limited social support), and family (e.g., negative messages from parents) functioning (Stark et al., 2005). Treatments are designed to address these disturbances, with relaxation skills included to facilitate adaptive emotion regulation. Relaxation may help to dampen the physiological and affective experience of negative emotions, allowing the youth to cope more effectively (Gross & Thompson, 2007). In addition, relaxation may help address tension and anxiety that may prevent depressed youth from engaging in pleasurable activities or social interaction (Stark et al., 2005). For example, the 16-session CWD-A course is a multicomponent treatment program that includes relaxation training as a core element (Clarke et al., 1990). An RCT examining the use of this treatment with adolescents only, with parental involvement, and with a waitlist control found significantly greater declines in depressive symptoms for both treatment groups at posttreatment and 2-year follow-up (Lewinsohn et al., 1990). Additional RCTs by this research group have further demonstrated the efficacy of this treatment with

depressed youth (e.g., Clarke et al., 1999), including school-based samples (Clarke et al., 1995) and youth with comorbid conduct disorder
(Rohde et al., 2004).

## THE ELEMENT IN PRACTICE

This section of the chapter presents practical guidelines for implementing the relaxation training element in treatment. Box 6.1 provides step-
by-step summaries of both shared and specific components for deep
breathing, progressive muscle relaxation, and guided imagery. Box
6.2 (at the end of the chapter) provides a case study illustrating implementation of relaxation training procedures. Basic instructions for the
preparation and conclusion of relaxation training and specific instructions for each individual relaxation technique are discussed in greater
detail below.

### "Core of the Core" Element

Before beginning relaxation training, the therapist should have an
understanding of the youth's developmental level and ability to engage
in the relaxation exercises (Box 6.1, Step 1). If there is uncertainty about
the youth's ability to engage in the relaxation exercises, the therapist
should consider the relaxation readiness test (Cautela & Groden, 1978),
which assesses the ability to follow instructions, imitate behaviors, and
pay attention. Youth with externalizing behavior problems may require
additional modifications. Prior to the relaxation session, it is helpful to
recommend that the youth wear comfortable, loose-fitting clothing to
maximize his or her ability to practice the relaxation skills (Step 2).
      Across relaxation training techniques, the same basic procedures
are used to prepare the youth for the initial relaxation session. First, it
is critical to provide a rationale for engaging in the relaxation exercises,
utilizing developmentally appropriate descriptions of how the exercise
will be beneficial and what the youth should expect (Step 3). Along
with the rationale, and depending on the youth's developmental level,
it is important for the therapist to establish clear guidelines for the
youth to follow, such as listening carefully, following instructions, and
staying quiet. Specific directions allow for a more consistent execution
of the skills. It is important to allow the youth an opportunity to ask
questions and obtain clarification where needed so that he or she feels
completely comfortable and confident in completing the tasks.
      Next (Step 4), the therapist should dim the lights if possible and

## BOX 6.1. Task Analysis of Relaxation Training

### BEFORE THE SESSION

1. Identify the youth's developmental level and ability to participate in the relaxation method chosen. Consider conducting a relaxation readiness test (e.g., Cautela & Groden, 1978) if there are questions regarding the youth's ability to perform the necessary tasks.

2. Ask the youth to wear comfortable, loose-fitting clothing to the session.

### BASIC COMPONENTS AND PREPARATION FOR ALL TECHNIQUES

3. Provide the youth with a clear rationale of the relaxation process, including how it is beneficial and what to expect.
   a. Discuss guidelines for the process, including keeping eyes closed, listening and following instructions, and staying quiet.
   b. Give the youth an opportunity to ask questions and/or discuss concerns.

4. If possible, dim the lighting and reduce any outside noise.

5. Have the youth lie flat on the floor or sit comfortably in a chair and close his or her eyes.
   a. Make sure there are no items nearby that would be distracting or interfere with movements the youth may make.
   b. Encourage the youth to get comfortable and relax.

### SPECIFIC COMPONENTS FOR EACH TECHNIQUE

#### Deep Breathing

1. Demonstrate shallow breathing and deep breathing.
   a. When demonstrating shallow breathing, show how the shoulders and chest move up and down, but the stomach does not move.
   b. When demonstrating deep breathing, show how the stomach expands, but the shoulders and chest do not move very much.

2. Instruct the youth to focus on steadily breathing air in through the nose and out through the mouth for 2–3 minutes.
   a. The youth should breathe in slowly through the nose, watching the stomach expand, while the therapist counts to four.
   b. Instruct the youth to release the air slowly, and watch the stomach move inward.
   c. The youth can place a pillow or light object on his or her stomach to help illustrate its movement.

3. Repeat the deep breathing exercise 5 to 10 times.

4. Provide additional examples as needed for younger children, such as "belly breathing," "bubble breathing," or "balloon breathing" (e.g., Fristad, Goldberg Arnold, & Leffler, 2011).
   a. The therapist should narrate the deep breathing process for the child.

*(continued)*

## BOX 6.1 (*continued*)

### Progressive Muscle Relaxation

1. Obtain a child-friendly script developed for use when conducting PMR with children and adolescents (e.g., Koeppen, 1974; Ollendick & Cerny, 1981; Pincus, 2000).
   a. Prerecorded scripts are available for both children and adolescents in English and Spanish at *http://relax.practicewise.com*.

2. Provide the youth with instructions for effectively tensing and relaxing the different muscle groups that will be targeted.

3. Have the youth focus on deep breathing for 2–3 minutes.

4. Read the script to the youth. If no script is available, make sure the following steps are completed.
   a. Instruct the youth to tense different muscle groups for 5–10 seconds, and then slowly relax for 15–20 seconds.
   b. Have the youth tense muscles as tightly as they can without hurting themselves. It should feel uncomfortable but not painful.
   c. Tense only one particular muscle group at a time. Younger children should tense two to three major muscle groups, while older children can practice with up to 10 muscle groups.
   d. Have the youth focus on the feelings of tension such as being tight, strained, and uncomfortable and feelings of relaxation such as being tingly, warm, and heavy.
   e. Once the muscle groups have been tensed and relaxed separately, have the youth remain quiet with eyes closed and focus on the feeling of relaxation over the entire body for 1–2 minutes.

5. Once completed, have the youth open his or her eyes and slowly sit up. Make sure the youth has become oriented to the room again before moving forward with the session.

### Guided Imagery

1. Have the youth imagine a place where he or she feels relaxed, peaceful, and safe.
   a. Imagery scripts can be used if the youth has difficulty thinking of a place (e.g., Albano & DiBartolo, 2007; March & Mulle, 1998).

2. Ask the youth to describe the details of the imagined place, using all of the senses (e.g., sight, smell, sound, taste, texture).

3. After the script has been completed, the youth should remain quiet and relaxed, focusing on deep breathing for 2–3 minutes.

### AFTER THE SESSION

1. Discuss with the youth his or her impression of the skill. Identify things the youth enjoyed and any possible difficulties he or she had while completing the skills. Modify the procedure to address these difficulties.

2. Recommend that the youth practice these activities daily to help reduce general levels of stress.
    a. Younger children may be instructed to describe the relaxation skills to their parents and/or a sibling. Parents can also be provided with a script and encouraged to read it to their child and/or to help guide the practicing of relaxation skills at home.
    b. Children and adolescents can be given a CD or digital recording and/or a handout of the different scripts to listen to in order to help motivate them to practice the skills.
    c. Children and adolescents can practice these skills in the morning as they are waking up or at night as part of their bedtime routine.

reduce any outside noise. Reducing the amount of light in the room lessens stimulation and can help the youth become calm and achieve a greater level of relaxation. It is important to take the youth's comfort level into consideration before dimming any lights. Some youth, especially those who have been victimized, may prefer to leave the lights on fully throughout the exercise. Reducing outside noise helps to eliminate possible distractions, though, if this is difficult or not possible, playing calm music or using a white noise machine may be beneficial.

The final step in preparation (Step 5) is to have the youth sit or lie down in a comfortable position and close his or her eyes. Note that for some youth—perhaps those who have experienced trauma—closing their eyes may be uncomfortable. Youth should be given the option of closing their eyes. Youth who are initially uncomfortable doing so may become willing once trust is established with the therapist. The therapist should also be cognizant of his or her own position in relation to the youth. Initially, the youth may feel uncomfortable or embarrassed to complete these techniques in front of the therapist. The therapist might consider sitting alongside the youth if he or she is also sitting on the floor, in order to reduce any discomfort. During certain relaxation techniques, the youth is asked to move his or her legs or arms. There should be no objects around the child that may hinder movement. The youth is then instructed to relax as much as possible by allowing his or her body to be supported by the chair or floor and to look forward to taking some time to relax.

Following the general preparation procedures, Box 6.1 includes specific steps for each of the individual relaxation techniques. *Deep breathing* (DB) is suggested as the first technique to implement with youth because it takes the least amount of time to teach, can be used in conjunction with PMR and guided imagery, and is easiest to generalize into everyday activities. PMR and guided imagery can be taught in any order, depending on the individual needs of the client. When teaching deep breathing, the therapist should first demonstrate the difference between shallow and deep breathing (DB Step 1). This is important so the youth can determine when he or she is performing deep breathing appropriately. The youth is taught that during shallow breathing the chest and shoulders move when breathing in and out but the stomach stays still, while during deep breathing the opposite occurs (i.e., the stomach moves in during exhalation and out during inhalation while the shoulders and chest stay still). This can be demonstrated by having the youth put one hand on the chest and one hand on the stomach to more easily detect the difference in movement. Instructing younger children to imagine their stomach filling up and deflating like a balloon may also help them visualize and perform the procedure more effectively.

During DB Step 2, the youth's deep breathing can be facilitated by counting for the child as he or she breathes in through the nose and out through the mouth. It is helpful to continue to remind the youth to breathe steadily in and out and not to breathe too quickly or too slowly. The therapist can demonstrate the difference between steadily breathing in and out versus breathing quickly and hyperventilating. Children can place their hands on their chest and stomach to help facilitate breathing or, if they are lying down, place a light object on their stomach (e.g., small book, stuffed animal) that they try to move up and down. For DB Steps 3–4, the therapist should have the youth continue practicing deep breathing for 3–5 minutes in order to fully allow the youth to relax. To help younger children engage in deep breathing, objects such as a balloon, bubbles, or a pinwheel can be used to provide a more concrete visual example that facilitates the necessary actions of deep breathing.

PMR is the next technique described in Box 6.1. For this technique, the therapist may want to first obtain a developmentally appropriate script to read to the child (e.g., Koeppen, 1974; Pincus, 2000) or adolescent (e.g., Ollendick & Cerny, 1981). For PMR Step 2, before beginning the PMR process the therapist informs the youth that he or she will engage in tensing and relaxing muscles. For older children and adolescents, this can be done by describing and demonstrating briefly how to tense and relax a muscle group, such as the hands. The analogy of a pendulum can be beneficial to the adolescent in that, like a pendulum, the more he or she tenses a muscle, the more that muscle will relax when the tension is released—just as a pendulum swings farther one way after being pulled farther in the opposite direction. For younger children, the therapist can inform the child that he or she will be read instructions and the child is to act out the instructions as described. PMR Step 3 requires the youth to engage in deep breathing for 2–3 minutes prior to beginning the relaxation process. If the youth has not yet learned deep breathing when conducting PMR, instruct the youth to breathe steadily in through the nose and out through the mouth for a few minutes.

If a script has been obtained, the therapist can simply read it to the youth (PMR Step 4). If a script is not accessible, the therapist should make sure the following steps are carried out to fully facilitate PMR. Each muscle group should be tensed for 5–10 seconds and then relaxed for 15–20 seconds. During the tension phase, the youth should tense enough to the point that it is uncomfortable but not painful. Each muscle group should be tensed one at a time, with the number of muscle groups being tensed determined by the child's age and ability. Younger children should tense only two to three major muscle groups in one sitting, while older children may tense up to 10 muscle groups (Ollendick & Cerny, 1981). Each time a child tenses and relaxes a muscle group, encourage the child to focus on feelings of tension and relaxation. This helps the youth to recognize how his or her body feels when it is tense and how it should feel when it is relaxed. Once all muscle groups have been tensed and relaxed, the youth should remain still and focus on breathing for 1–2 minutes, paying special attention to how the body feels when it is fully relaxed. Finally (PMR Step 5), the youth is asked to open his or her eyes and sit up. The youth should be given a moment to orient to the room and become alert again before proceeding forward with the session.

*Guided imagery* (GI) is the final relaxation technique described in Box 6.1. GI Step 1 requires the youth to identify a place where he or she feels safe and comfortable. The therapist can help provide a few examples if the youth has difficulty thinking of a place (e.g., the beach, under a tree, in the youth's bedroom, in the kitchen making cookies with a family member). If the child is still unable to identify a place, there are scripts that can be used (e.g., Albano & DiBartolo, 2007; March & Mulle, 1998). Once a place has been selected, the youth is asked to imagine this place and take a moment to visualize the place as a whole before moving on to the next step. The youth's eyes should remain closed during the process if he or she is comfortable doing so. The youth is asked to describe in detail this place, using all five senses (GI Step 2). For example, a child might first be instructed to describe the scene with much visual detail (e.g., "I see my mom pull out the cookie sheet and ingredients; I see her spread flour on the counter"). Next, the child may be asked to describe different smells in this place (e.g., "I smell the cookies baking in the oven; I smell the dish soap in the sink"). This continues until the child describes the scene by using all five senses. The length of time needed for a guided imagery exercise will depend on the age and attention span of the youth and can range anywhere from 5 to 30 minutes. Finally (GI Step 3), the youth should be allowed some time to sit quietly, focusing on his or her breathing.

Once the relaxation technique(s) has been practiced during session, the therapist concludes by facilitating a discussion with the youth regarding his or her impressions of the technique practiced, being sure to identify positive impressions as well as any difficulties the youth had in completing the technique. If necessary, the therapist can modify the procedure to address these challenges. After discussing the youth's impressions of the technique(s), the therapist instructs the youth to practice the technique(s) on a regular basis (e.g., practice deep breathing for 5 minutes twice a day, practice PMR two separate times over the course of the week). Although practicing relaxation techniques outside of the session is important for generalization, adherence can be difficult to achieve. Motivation can be improved by discussing the importance of practicing at home with the youth and his or her parents. The therapist might consider analogizing the challenge to practicing a skill with which the youth is familiar (e.g., shooting a free throw, playing the piano). One strategy for facilitating practice at home is to instruct the youth to teach the technique(s) to his or her parent(s) and/or siblings and practice the skills as a family. Parents may also be provided with relaxation scripts to read to their children to help guide home practice. Additionally, the therapist can provide the child with a CD or digital recording of the session and/or a handout that includes the scripts used during the session to help the child complete practice of the skill at home. While it may be helpful for the therapist to record the specific script that is utilized in the session, relaxation audio files are widely available through online or mobile applications (e.g., at *http://relax.practicewise.com*, or through the "Relax Me" app). Finally, helping the youth determine a convenient place and time to practice the skills, such as right before falling asleep at night or prior to getting out of bed in the morning, can aid in adherence.

## Developmental Adaptations

Relaxation training techniques, particularly PMR and deep breathing, have been adapted for use with children and adolescents to account for developmental differences in attention, cognition, gross and fine motor ability, physical and emotional awareness, and behavioral skills. Children often have difficulty attending to adult PMR scripts owing to the length and depth of the descriptions (Koeppen, 1974), especially in combination with symptoms of inattention and hyperactivity (Grover, Hughes, Bergman, & Kingery, 2006). To help deal with the limits of youth attention, Beidas, Benjamin, Puleo, Edmunds, and Kendall (2010) suggest separating relaxation techniques into manageable pieces rather than engaging in the entire activity at once. For example, the therapist can focus on a single muscle group during PMR, followed by a short break. Cautela and Groden (1978) suggest initially focusing on gross motor areas, such as arms and legs, and then fine motor areas, such as facial features, because it is easier for children to learn to control larger areas of their body before attempting to control smaller ones. Additionally, longer sessions can be broken up into multiple short- ened sessions to maintain the child's attention and ensure retention of skills. As mentioned previously with Koeppen's script, cues such as squeezing the juice out of a lemon can help to engage a younger child in the accurate tensing of their muscle groups. Similarly, the "turtle technique" (Schneider, 1974) has been found to help children relax their muscles to cope with strong emotions by having them pretend they are turtles withdrawing into their shells (Robin, Schneider, & Dolnick, 1976). Finally, reinforcers and special apparatus such as squeeze toys can be used to motivate younger children. Specific to deep breathing, pinwheels, balloons, and/or bubbles may help younger children main- tain their attention throughout the exercise (Cautela & Groden, 1987). Youth may be more engaged if relaxation is presented as a "game" with a certain amount of novelty.

While there is some literature that examines developmental adap- tations for PMR and deep breathing, there is only limited study of such adaptations for guided imagery. Though no reference is made to empirical outcomes, Ott (1996) described a developmental adaptation of guided imagery for two young children with chronic illness. Recom- mendations include collecting an initial assessment of the child's favor- ite things, which may direct the content of the imagery, adequately pacing the guided imagery, and using age-appropriate word choice. The clinician may need to lead the exercise and refocus when neces- sary while allowing the child to participate in the experience by adding details and sensory descriptions.

Some children are not physically capable of performing all tech- niques related to relaxation training, particularly PMR. Cautela and Groden (1978) advise conducting a readiness assessment with younger children, children with special needs, and children with serious illness before engaging them in relaxation training. The assessment is conducted to evaluate the child's gross and fine motor abilities as well as to gauge his or her ability to follow simple instructions. If relevant, consultation with a child's medical, physical, and/or occupational therapists regarding his or her ability to engage in and benefit from relaxation may help guide treatment.

Approaches for relaxation training adapted for adolescents focus more on the "here and now" and utilize briefer methods, such as deep breathing, as opposed to lengthier methods such as PMR (Curry et al., 2000). When PMR is implemented with adolescents, more direct, to-the-point descriptions are used (e.g., press your fingers into your palms and pull up on your wrists, pull your shoulders up and try to touch your ears with them; Ollendick & Cerny, 1981). Relaxation training with older adolescents can be similar to that with adults because older adolescents are capable of understanding instructions and engaging in advanced techniques (King, Hamilton, & Ollendick, 1988). PMR scripts utilized with adults are potentially beneficial for use with older adolescents, and so it is important to know the developmental level of the adolescent with whom you are working (Bernstein & Borkovec, 1973; Cormier et al., 2013).

Kendall and colleagues have created two manualized treatments for children and adolescents with generalized anxiety disorder, social phobia, and/or separation anxiety disorder. Within these manuals, the authors have specifically adapted the use of relaxation techniques according to the developmental level of the client. The Coping Cat program and the C.A.T. Project are typically used with youth ages 7–13 and 13–17 years, respectively (Kendall et al., 2002; Kendall & Hedtke, 2006). Both manuals explicitly link the somatic feelings that produce muscle tension with anxiety; however, the C.A.T. Project provides greater detail about how stress affects the body (Kendall et al., 2002). In Coping Cat, the child is asked to imagine feeling both relaxed and tense and mentally compare those feelings. The manual provides examples that may help children to understand the difference between muscle tension and relaxation (e.g., walking like a robot vs. a rag doll, uncooked vs. limp spaghetti). This is followed by shortened deep breathing and PMR exercises, following either the Koeppen (1974) or Ollendick and Cerny (1981) scripts previously discussed. These exercises are then reinforced through role play and practiced with parents at the end of the session. The C.A.T. Project progresses similarly through deep breathing and PMR, though the script included in the manual provides direct descriptions of the tensing and relaxing of specific muscle groups. The C.A.T. Project focuses on nine different muscle groups, while Coping Cat recommends practicing only two to three basic muscle groups. Adolescents are encouraged to practice these relaxation skills on their own at home, while children are provided with a CD to facilitate skill acquisition (Beidas et al., 2010).

## Diversity Considerations

Given the similarity in physical symptoms of internalizing disorders across cultures, it has been theorized that the core components of CBT presented in a culturally competent fashion will likely be effective for diverse groups (Muñoz & Mendelson, 2005). In a review of evidence-based treatments for anxiety disorders and depression, Huey and Polo (2008) found group CBT that includes relaxation training to be efficacious for Hispanic/Latino and African American populations (e.g., Ginsburg & Drake, 2002; Roselló et al., 2008; Silverman et al., 1999). Generally, however, there are limited evaluations of relaxation skills training in diverse populations, particularly for use with children or adolescents.

In an example of a cross-cultural adaptation, La Roche, Batista, and D'Angelo (2011) developed the culturally competent relaxation intervention (CCRI) for Hispanic individuals. CCRI includes diaphragmatic breathing, PMR, and guided imagery. The authors state that Latino/a cultural values such as relationalism/allocentrism, spiritualism, and familism lead to a mismatch with the traditionally European American medical model. Individuals with allocentric values tend to rely on social support for coping, while those with idiocentric values more frequently engage in self-soothing behaviors (La Roche et al., 2011). Guided imagery was adapted for CCRI to include allocentric imagery exercises (e.g., imagine yourself surrounded by loved ones), compared to the more traditional idiographic imagery exercises (e.g., imagine yourself on a beach) to better reflect the cultural values reported by the participants. The authors examined the effects of the allocentric CCRI on anxiety symptoms among individuals engaged in a group treatment for anxiety and depression. Participants were provided with a tape of the allocentric imagery script and instructed to practice as frequently as possible (La Roche et al., 2011). Results indicated a significant relationship between the individual's allocentric values and his or her adherence to the allocentric imagery exercises. Furthermore, increased levels of adherence to the imagery exercises was related to greater reductions in both anxiety and depressive symptoms, with greater effects found for anxiety than depression (La Roche et al., 2011). Although this study was conducted with adults, adapting relaxation training to specifically address cultural beliefs seems a promising avenue to explore with youth as well.

Several investigations examining the presentation of symptoms in both Western and non-Western cultures have discovered that most non-Western cultures express negative affect such as depression and anxiety in terms of somatic symptoms (e.g., Farooq, Gahir, Okyere, Sheik, & Oyebode, 1995; Thakker, Ward, & Strongman, 1999; Weiss, Raguram, & Channabasavanna, 1995). For example, a person who experiences extreme anxiety may complain of headaches or shortness of breath, whereas a person who experiences depression may complain of stomachaches or fatigue, attributing their discomfort to physical symptoms rather than emotional difficulties. Farooq et al. (1995) suggest that this is attributable in part to the fact that ethnically diverse minorities may lack the terminology to express depression and anxiety in psychological terms common to the majority culture. Thakker et al. (1999) also suggest that the expression of psychological symptoms through somatic complaints is the result of the stigmatization of mental illness in certain cultures and the social disapproval of strong emotional expression.

Because ethnically diverse individuals may experience stigmatization related to mental illness and be discouraged from expressing certain emotions, relaxation training may have potential benefits in treatment with people whose cultural context supports somatic symptoms. More specifically, the primary purpose of relaxation training is to address the physiological symptoms related to internalizing disorders. Thus, even if a client is hesitant or unable to adequately express his or her emotions owing to social disapproval of standard psychological treatment, relaxation training can be used to address the somatic symptoms he or she is experiencing.

Physical disability status is another form of diversity that is important when considering relaxation. Among children with disabilities (e.g., brain injuries, psychomotor deficits), tension and anxiety can be both physiological and psychological (Zipkin, 1985). Relaxation techniques provide the child with the opportunity to directly control his or her own behaviors, which has been found to be more beneficial than other externally implemented forms of treatment (Zipkin, 1985). PMR and guided imagery are the most commonly used relaxation techniques in disabled populations, as they allow for greater flexibility in structure and implementation (Walker, 1979). Additionally, new developments in the technology of treatment implementation, such as multimedia relaxation training, may be beneficial for children with limited mobility (Weersing, Gonzalez, Campo, & Lucas, 2008).

In sum, there is a paucity of research examining specific modifications for relaxation among diverse populations. While the general elements of relaxation skills training may be useful across cultures, ethnicities, and disability status, the specific implementation may require adaptations in order to be most effective. The American Psychological Association (2003) recommends that treatments be specifically tailored to the needs of diverse clients, as miscommunications or value conflicts may lead to treatment failure. For example, treatment manuals for children typically describe deep breathing as "blowing up a balloon," or "blowing bubbles," which may not be relevant to the experiences of all populations (e.g., Kendall & Hedtke, 2006). Culturally appropriate images, metaphors, and stories should be included to illustrate key concepts (Muñoz & Mendelson, 2005). Providing culturally relevant training on relaxation skills is important for treatment, because stress can interfere with the ability to utilize additional coping skills, potentially inhibiting effective treatment.

## CONCLUSIONS

Relaxation training has been present in various forms for centuries and is used to reduce physiological symptoms associated with depression and anxiety in children and adolescents. The relaxation response provides children and adolescents with coping skills that may promote engagement in other components of the treatment process such as exposures or discussions of trauma. Despite the limited use of relaxation alone, there is evidence supporting the use of CBT treatment programs that rely on relaxation training as a core component; however, further research is needed to continue to explore the use and impact of these skills in various treatments. The guidelines for use of relaxation training provided in this chapter can be clinically beneficial, particularly in consideration of the clinical needs, developmental level, and diversity status of the youth.

## BOX 6.2. Illustrative Case Example

Tony was a 10-year-old Latino male whose family was referred for brief outpatient psychological services through the local child advocacy center following the sexual abuse of Tony's sibling by a family friend. Each family member received individual CBT for a total of four sessions to provide support and psychoeducation and to assess the need for additional services.

Tony, in particular, reported experiencing a number of distressing physiological and emotional symptoms that were challenging for him to manage. Tony described experiencing anxiety whenever he encountered the perpetrator, which occurred on a regular basis in their small rural community. In particular, he reported experiencing a racing heart, shallow, rapid breathing, and tension throughout his body. Tony reported feelings of guilt because he believed he could have done something to prevent the abuse. He also talked about feelings of extreme disappointment in the perpetrator and sadness over the loss of this relationship. Tony indicated intense feelings of anger toward the perpetrator, which led to frequent aggressive thoughts of harming that individual to defend his sibling, though he had never acted on these thoughts or angry feelings. When engaged in these thoughts, Tony explained that he could feel his body become warm and sweaty and he would start shaking uncontrollably. His physiological and emotional symptoms were discussed during the initial session.

The second treatment session focused on psychoeducation regarding understanding and coping with feelings. Tony engaged in activities to learn about different emotions and to identify his specific thoughts and behaviors related to the emotions he was experiencing. The concept of positive coping through relaxation was introduced to Tony, and he learned about and engaged in one relaxation technique, deep breathing.

First, Tony was taught that deep breathing would help steady his breath whenever it was short and rapid and would help calm the physical sensations such as shaking and heart racing. Tony was instructed to practice by sitting comfortably in his chair, closing his eyes, and placing one hand on his chest and one hand on his stomach. He was then told to try to make the hand on his stomach move out by taking in one deep, steady breath. After Tony understood this concept and had demonstrated several deep breaths, he was instructed to mentally count each breath in and out. The therapist explained that counting each breath in and out helps to focus thoughts on the relaxation exercise, providing a temporary distraction from other, more distressing, thoughts. For homework, Tony was instructed to practice deep breathing for 5 minutes each day. The therapist recommended he try this when waking up in the morning or right before falling asleep at night. Tony invited his parents to join in at the end of the session and demonstrated the deep breathing skills so that they could practice together at home.

At the beginning of the third session, the homework assignment from the preceding session was discussed. Tony reported practicing and utilizing the deep breathing techniques to manage some of the uncomfortable symptoms he experienced when he was plagued by the thoughts of and/or encountered the perpetrator.

Tony stated that he used deep breathing when he felt his heart start to race and when he noticed his breath speeding up, and he reported that he felt calmer after using the technique. He also stated that when he noticed that he was having distressing thoughts he would mentally count to himself as he was breathing.

The remainder of the third session focused on engaging Tony in PMR and positive imagery. Tony was provided with a rationale for utilizing these techniques. For progressive muscle relaxation, he was told that muscle relaxation helps to release tension that builds up in his body when he experiences stress. Regarding positive imagery, Tony learned that picturing a safe, calm place can be a temporary distraction and may help him feel better when he is experiencing an uncomfortable situation or having a negative thought. After being provided with the rationale, Tony engaged in both PMR and positive imagery.

For PMR, Tony and the therapist sat on the floor with their backs against the wall for support. Tony was informed that he could close his eyes at any time during the exercise if he felt comfortable doing so. He was instructed to listen carefully to the script and, when asked, to tighten his muscles as much as possible without hurting himself. The therapist then read the relaxation script from Koeppen (1974) and observed him tensing and relaxing each muscle group. Tony was somewhat distracted by the fantasy of the script at times, becoming energetic and laughing, which made it difficult to complete the remaining tasks. The therapist began to instruct Tony in a more direct manner for the remainder of the script, omitting the fantasy portion to help him become more focused and relaxed. Following the exercise, Tony noted that his body felt more "like jello" and that this feeling was more relaxing and comfortable than when his body was tense. He was given a handout that included basic descriptions of each step as well as the full script to use at home.

Next, Tony engaged in positive imagery. He was reminded to sit comfortably with his eyes closed and was instructed to picture in his mind a time or place where he felt calm and safe. He identified driving down a country road in his dad's classic convertible. The therapist asked Tony to continue picturing himself driving down this country road while describing it to his therapist using his five senses. Tony described seeing the dirt road, country houses zooming by, his dog in the passenger seat, and cows and horses grazing in the field. He described hearing the car radio, his dog barking at the animals, and the wind swooshing by as he drove with the top of the car down. He described smelling the crisp air, the strong scent of the cows and horses, and smoke from the chimneys of the houses. He described tasting bubblegum in his mouth and feeling the wind on his face, the dog's slobber as it licked him, and the squishy leather seats of the car. At the end of the session, Tony taught his parents about the relaxation techniques he had learned that session. Again, it was recommended that he practice both relaxation techniques when he woke up in the morning or right before falling asleep at night throughout the next week.

During the fourth and final session, Tony reported he was able to use all three techniques to manage the distressing feelings he had been experiencing. He

(continued)

## BOX 6.2 (*continued*)

stated that he liked being able to use these techniques right away without anyone knowing that he was doing them. He said that he was able to picture the country road any time he had aggressive thoughts of harming the perpetrator and that he used deep breathing and muscle relaxation to help address his physiological reactions. Tony indicated that he still felt anger toward the perpetrator but could better manage his emotions whenever he was around the perpetrator or when having negative thoughts.

# 7

# Psychoeducation

with Matthew W. Kirkhart and Jason M. Prenoveau

## BACKGROUND OF THE ELEMENT

Psychoeducation, typically the first component presented in treatments for internalizing disorders in youth, refers to the process of providing information about the prevalence, symptoms, course, and treatments of a disorder. The purpose of psychoeducation is to normalize symptoms, empower youth and families, and instill hope (Fristad, Goldberg Arnold, & Leffler, 2011; Piacentini, Langley, & Roblek, 2007). In addition, knowledge of the theory, rationale, and efficacy of the specific intervention is shared with the youth and family to help increase motivation and commitment to the treatment (Lukens & McFarlane, 2004; March & Mulle, 1998). This chapter first presents the historical context of psychoeducation along with empirical support for its use in practice. Next, step-by-step instructions for the implementation of psychoeducation are discussed, followed by adaptations for youth of different developmental levels and diverse backgrounds. The chapter closes with a case example.

### Brief History

The development of psychoeducation as an intervention component was influenced by sociopolitical and mental health policy factors that occurred during the middle of the 20th century, as well as changes in the understanding of the course and treatment of mental illness. One of the most important of these historical events was the development of chlorpromazine (more commonly known as Thorazine), which is often considered to be the first effective antipsychotic medication (Torrey, 1997). The drug's effectiveness in the management of psychotic symptoms was one of the contributing factors in the deinstitutionalization movement of the 1950s (Lukens & McFarlane, 2004; Torrey, 1997). This movement resulted in the emptying out and eventual closing of many state institutions, with as many as 66% of individuals moving from living in an institution to living with their families (Solomon, Gordon, & Davis, 1984). Both the rise of more effective medications and the decreased reliance on hospitalization led to a shift in treatment philosophy that included more active patient involvement and responsibility for mental illness management, a move toward a recovery model of mental illness, and patient empowerment in terms of choice regarding treatment options. At its core, psychoeducation is designed to prepare the client (youth or adult) and the client's family for more active involvement, or a partnership, with the treating professional (Lukens & McFarlane, 2004).

The acceptance of a biopsychosocial approach to the treatment of mental illness was also growing during this time period. The combination of genetic and biological predispositions and family, social, and psychological vulnerabilities or stressors was viewed in a more holistic way in both understanding the development of mental illness and undertaking its treatment (McFarlane, Dixon, Lukens, & Lucksted, 2003). Two important aspects of the biopsychosocial model relate to the historical development of psychoeducation. First, while effective, medications alone were not adequate to treat all individuals with chronic mental illnesses. Second, family dynamics and psychological functioning were viewed as important protective factors against both developing and relapsing into mental illness (Anderson, Hogarty, & Reiss, 1980). Therefore, it became necessary to provide some type of skills and knowledge-based intervention if the chronic mental illness was to be effectively managed (McFarlane et al., 2003). Thus, this shift to a more comprehensive biopsychosocial model of mental illness also contributed to the development and use of psychoeducation interventions.

The term *psychoeducation*, as we know it, stems in large part, from the work of C. M. Anderson et al. (1980). In their seminal article, Anderson and colleagues described a family-based psychoeducation intervention model for use with individuals with schizophrenia that was specifically aimed at reducing relapse rates. Indeed, the content and goals of their recommended family intervention are similar to current psychoeducation components. The original intervention included information about the etiology, onset, course, treatment, and outcome in clear, easy-to-understand language. In addition, knowledge regarding family management of symptoms was conveyed. Within this discussion, the point was made that the family does not "cause" schizophrenia. Sharing knowledge about the treatment, course, and contributing factors (specifically, expressed emotion) of schizophrenia was intended to reduce family anxiety and increase self-confidence. In this way, it was hoped that the family and patient could make more constructive decisions about care.

The history of psychoeducation also has roots in the rise of cognitive therapy and behaviorally focused therapies. For example, the seminal book *Cognitive Therapy of Depression* encourages therapists to share an educational booklet about depression with the patient and to present the rationale for cognitive therapy during the first session (Beck et al., 1979). Similarly, an early missive on using behavior therapy to treat individuals with anxiety disorders encourages providing information regarding the psychological and physical symptoms of anxiety to reduce fears that the patient is "going crazy" or "going to have a heart attack" (Hanrahan, Gitlin, Martin, Leavy, & Francis, 1984). Hanharan et al. (1984) also wrote that sharing information about the diagnosis with family members may help counteract assumptions that anxiety is incurable or that the client is being manipulative, thus removing obstacles to effective treatment.

Today, this information-sharing element is encouraged in EBT for youth with internalizing disorders to help build collaboration between the therapist and youth and to normalize the experience of the youth and family (e.g., March & Mulle, 1998). These therapy approaches often require a great deal of effort on behalf of the youth and family (e.g., mood tracking, thought monitoring, exposures, homework); therefore, psychoeducation is also considered a way of establishing partnership and motivating the youth and family to fully engage in the therapy. Indeed, basic information on disorder symptoms, prevalence, and an overview of the current treatment are commonplace in most evidence-based interventions for youth with internalizing disorders. For example, TF-CBT uses books and games to teach youth about typical responses to trauma (Cohen, Mannarino, & Deblinger, 2006), and IPT-A includes a description of IPT and other treatments in the first session (Mufson et al., 2011). Although psychoeducation is often addressed

at the start of therapy, many treatments contain aspects of psychoeducation throughout therapy. For instance, in their manual for the treatment of youth with OCD, Piacentini and colleagues (2007) recommend
presenting the rationale behind ERP in the first session as well as in the
third session, when the youth starts engaging in ERP. Similarly, other
treatments may introduce the cognitive-behavioral model in the first
session and then revisit that model many times to help youth understand the connections among thoughts, behaviors, and feelings (e.g.,
Kendall & Hedtke, 2006).

## Theory Base

The main premise of psychoeducation is that simply sharing information with the client and family about the etiology, course, symptoms,
and treatment options is, in and of itself, somehow therapeutic. This
premise rests on multiple schools of thought. In fact, family systems,
cognitive, rational-emotive, and behavior therapy theories all help
explain why psychoeducation is considered part of an effective treatment. This section aims to explore the theoretical foundation of psychoeducation through these multiple lenses.

Many associate psychoeducation with a family systems perspective,
which assumes that mental illness is caused by an interaction between
a biological predisposition and environmental (including family) stress.
Thus, one of the main functions of psychoeducation is to transfer knowledge to empower the family, therefore reducing stress and facilitating
treatment (Anderson et al., 1980). Family stress is reduced by helping
family members to develop an understanding of the symptoms (thus
reducing blaming and conflict), the course of the disorder (thus reducing unrealistic expectations), and treatment options (thus increasing
hope). In addition, current family systems approaches see the family as
an important resource for the client and utilize psychoeducation with
the goal of helping the family to become better equipped to support
positive growth (Schwoeri & Sholevar, 2003). Aspects of this approach
are easily identified in Fristad and colleagues' (2011) psychoeducational psychotherapy for youth with mood disorders. For example, in
addition to information on symptoms, course, and treatments, Fristad
et al. also encourage families to learn how to support healthy sleeping
and eating habits and how to advocate for their child in the school and
mental health system. Overall, this perspective is strengths-based, as
psychoeducation transfers knowledge to the individual and family so
that they can become agents of positive change.

Psychoeducation also has roots in cognitive therapy. Cognitive therapy operates on the assumption that distorted or irrational beliefs are at the root of disordered behavior and emotions (Sharf, 2012). In this framework, psychoeducation could be considered the presentation of accurate information to potentially counter inaccurate assumptions. For example, the sharing of information about the prevalence of mood disorders may challenge an adolescent's belief that he or she is the "only one who ever felt this way." Similarly, data on treatment effectiveness and options for anxiety may help to refute the belief that a child "will always have trouble in social situations." In addition, psychoeducation is used to prevent future negative attributions that might affect early termination (Beck et al., 1979). Specifically, Beck and colleagues encourage the therapist to discuss the "ups and downs" of depression so that the client will interpret setbacks as a natural part of depression instead of a failure of the treatment. Related to cognitive therapy, rational-emotive therapy posits that emotional responses are more influenced by a person's interpretation of a situation rather than the situation itself (Ellis & Bernard, 1985). Therefore, psychoeducation may be understood as an attempt to help the client relabel his or her potential mislabeling of the distress (e.g., "My OCD makes me irritable" instead of "I am an irritable person"; March & Mulle, 1998).

Even behavior therapy, which focuses primarily on external determinants of learning and behavior (like rewards and punishments), recognizes the influence of cognitive mediators of learning. In fact, in their influential book on clinical behavior therapy, Goldfried and Davison (1976) discuss several possible mediators of learning related to psychoeducation that may affect behavioral processes. They recommend sharing the rationale for a behavioral orientation along with a detailed description of what will happen in the treatment at the beginning of therapy. This sharing of information likely increases the client's motivation and commitment to therapy by affecting expectations, which in turn influence his or her behavior. Advance information on therapy content is thought to help the client organize new information presented in therapy and thus facilitate learning. For example, an early discussion of the cognitive-behavioral triad in a treatment for child anxiety may help the youth more readily learn to label cognitive distortions later in treatment. In addition, Goldfried and Davison stress the importance of discussing the effectiveness of behavior therapy in order to engender positive expectations of behavior change, which are thought to potentially increase client engagement both during and between therapy sessions. A discussion of treatment options and effectiveness might also reduce "psychological reactance," a negative feeling caused by the perception that one does not have a choice in a situation, thereby facilitating youth openness and commitment to therapy.

In sum, psychoeducation has its roots in multiple theoretical perspectives. The fact that it contains elements of multiple theories may help explain its presence in most of the empirically based treatments for youth with internalizing disorders. This next section moves on from the philosophy of psychoeducation, examining the empirical evidence for the effectiveness of psychoeducation in the treatment of youth with internalizing disorders.

## Evidence Base

Empirical evidence for the effectiveness of psychoeducation in the treatment of youth with internalizing disorders derives from three sources: research on interventions that use a psychoeducational approach (i.e., psychoeducational psychotherapy; Fristad et al., 2011), a small body of research that evaluates psychoeducation as a sole treatment ingredient, and research on multicomponent treatments that incorporate psychoeducation (e.g., CBT, IPT). See Table 7.1 for an overview of psychoeducation in several representative empirically supported treatments for depression and anxiety in youth.

Although no studies have examined psychoeducation alone in the treatment of youth mood disorders, multicomponent treatments that include psychoeducation suggest that it may be an active treatment ingredient. One such treatment, psychoeducational psychotherapy (PEP; Fristad et al., 2011), is a psychosocial intervention that blends extensive psychoeducation with cognitive-behavioral strategies (e.g., problem solving, communication skills) and is considered a "probably efficacious" treatment for bipolar spectrum disorders (BSDs) when using the American Psychological Association's (Division 12) criteria for empirically supported treatments (Fristad & MacPherson, 2014). Through the psychoeducation components, youth and their parents learn about mood disorders (e.g., symptoms, course, comorbid conditions), treatment (e.g., options, mechanisms, outcomes), healthy habits for mood stability, and navigating mental health and school resources (parents only). Results from waitlist RCTs have demonstrated the efficacy of a multifamily format of this treatment (MF-PEP) for treating depression and BSD in children ages 8–12 years (Fristad, Goldberg Arnold, & Gavazzi, 2002, 2003; Fristad et al., 2009; Mendenhall, Fristad, & Early, 2009). Gains for MF-PEP as compared to waitlist control have been observed at 1-year follow-up (Fristad et al., 2009), are not

**TABLE 7.1. The Psychoeducation Element in Representative EBT Manuals**

| | |
|---|---|
| *Coping Cat* (Kendall & Hedtke, 2006) | • Psychoeducation is used primarily during the first couple of sessions, when information is provided about the nature of anxiety, the presentation and identification of anxiety symptoms, and the treatment of anxiety. |
| *C.A.T. Project* (Kendall, Choudhury, Hudson, & Webb, 2002) | • Psychoeducation is used primarily during the first two sessions, when information is provided about the nature of anxiety, the presentation and identification of anxiety symptoms, and the treatment of anxiety. |
| *Family-Based Treatment for Young Children with OCD* (Freeman & Garcia, 2008) | • Psychoeducation is covered explicitly during the first parent session (Session 1) and the first child session (Session 3) and includes information about OCD as a neurobehavioral disorder as well its course, symptoms, common comorbid disorders, and an overview of treatment. |
| *OCD in Children and Adolescents* (March & Mulle, 1998) | • Psychoeducation is utilized explicitly in the first session and involves both the child and the parent(s).<br><br>• Psychoeducation includes information about the etiology of OCD, deliberately placing it in a neurobehavioral context, as well as information about its prevalence, symptoms, treatment rationale and process, and potential impact of OCD on families. |
| *CBT of Childhood OCD: It's Only a False Alarm* (Piacentini, Langley, & Roblek, 2007) | • Psychoeducation is discussed explicitly during the first two child sessions and the first parent session.<br><br>• Psychoeducation includes information about the prevalence, etiology, treatment rationale, and potential impact of OCD on families. |
| *CBT for Social Phobia: Stand Up, Speak Out* (Albano & DiBartolo, 2007) | • Psychoeducation is utilized explicitly in the first session and reviewed in the second session. Parents may be included in the first two sessions, or a separate parent-only session may be held to discuss the psychoeducational content.<br><br>• Psychoeducation includes information on symptoms, the role of avoidance in the maintenance of anxiety, and the treatment rationale. |
| *When Children Refuse School: A CBT Approach* (Kearney & Albano, 2007): Chapters 4 and 5 on internalizing symptoms | • Psychoeducation is addressed explicitly in the first session and involves a description of the physical, cognitive, and behavioral aspects of anxiety.<br><br>• Psychoeducation also includes an introduction to the rationale underlying the treatment components of relaxation, cognitive restructuring, and exposure. |
| *Treating Trauma and Traumatic Grief in Children and Adolescents* (Cohen, Mannarino, & Deblinger, 2006) | • Psychoeducation is used explicitly in the first session as a way to share information regarding typical responses to trauma or to discuss treatment and to model nonavoidance of the discussion of trauma. The importance of caregiver involvement and the effectiveness of the treatment are also discussed. |

*(continued)*

**TABLE 7.1.** (continued)

| | |
|---|---|
| *Adolescent Coping with Depression* (Clarke, Lewinsohn, & Hops, 1990) | • In this group therapy, psychoeducation is provided during the first session, including discussion of the cognitive-behavioral conceptualization and treatment of depression. |
| *Interpersonal Psychotherapy for Depressed Adolescents,* 2nd edition (Mufson, Pollack, Dorta, Moreau, & Weissman, 2011) | • Providing psychoeducation about depression and therapy is an explicit goal for the first phase of treatment and is implemented with both the adolescent and the parent(s).<br>• Psychoeducation includes the presentation of treatment options for depression, the link between depression and interpersonal functioning, depression as a sickness, and the structure of the treatment program.<br>• Psychoeducation is also recognized as a behavior change technique that may be used as needed throughout treatment. |
| *Treating Depressed Children: Therapist Manual for "Taking Action"* (Stark & Kendall, 1996) | • Psychoeducation about the general process of therapy is provided during the first child session. |
| *Treating Depressed Youth: Therapist Manual for "Action"* (Stark et al., 2007) | • Early sessions provide information—though not explicitly referred to as psychoeducation—about depression, the aims and process of therapy, emotions and how to recognize them, and how mood can be affected by situations. |
| *Psychotherapy for Children with Bipolar and Depressive Disorders* (Fristad, Arnold, & Leffler, 2011) | • Psychoeducation is mentioned explicitly and is a large part of this treatment; being implemented with both the youth and the parent(s).<br>• Psychoeducation includes information about the symptoms, diagnosis, comorbid conditions, and course of the disorder as well as treatment options, how treatments work, healthy habits, mental health, and school services. |

*Note.* Some book titles are shortened to conserve space. See the References at the back of the book for full titles.

significantly different for those with depression as compared to BSD (Fristad et al., 2002), and appear to be attributable in part to parents becoming better consumers of the mental health system and accessing higher-quality services (Mendenhall et al., 2009). Also, at least one RCT has demonstrated the efficacy of an individualized version of this treatment (IF-PEP) for children with BSD (Fristad, 2006).

In addition, CBT treatment manuals, which include psychoeducation, are considered a "well-established" treatment for adolescent depression (David-Ferdon & Kaslow, 2008). One such manual is the CWD-A course (Clarke et al., 1990). As with many CBT therapies, the focus of CWD-A is on developing and practicing skills for overcoming depression (e.g., cognitive strategies, social skills training, problem solving, and self-monitoring). CWD-A also uses psychoeducation, mainly at the beginning of treatment, to teach participants about the presentation of depression (e.g., "depression as a problem in living," discussion of the downward spiral and upward spiral), the CBT model of depression (e.g., there are three aspects to personality: thoughts, actions, and feelings), and the rationale for treatment strategies (e.g., you can change feelings by changing thoughts and actions). Two RCTs found that depressed adolescents, ages 14–18 years, who received CWD-A treatment showed significantly greater reductions in depressive symptoms than those in a waitlist condition, and these gains were maintained at 2-year posttreatment (Clarke et al., 1999; Lewinsohn et al., 1990). Additionally, when depressed 12- to 18-year-olds were treated with CWD-A plus a selective serotonin reuptake inhibitor (SSRI), they improved significantly more than those treated with an SSRI plus primary care treatment as usual at 1-year follow-up on general health, outpatient visits, and medication use (Clarke et al., 2005); differences in depressive symptoms did not quite reach significance ($p = .07$).

IPT-A is also considered a "well-established" treatment for adolescent depression (David-Ferdon & Kaslow, 2008). Objectives of the initial phase of IPT-A are to "complete psychoeducation about depression and the therapy process" and to "explain the theory and goals of interpersonal therapy" (Mufson et al., 2011, p. 40). Within this process, therapists are encouraged to let clients know that their symptoms are part of a known syndrome, give them hope that it can be effectively treated, provide a rationale for IPT-A, and provide information about alternative treatment options. Two RCTs have demonstrated the effectiveness of IPT-A for treating depression in adolescents ages 12–18 years (Mufson et al., 1999, 2011). Compared to those in a clinical monitoring condition that included supportive listening, those who received IPT-A showed significantly more improvement in depression scores, social functioning, and problem-solving skills; additionally, significantly more teens in the IPT-A condition met recovery from depression criteria (Mufson et al., 1999). Those who received IPT-A also showed greater improvement on self- and clinician-reported depression symptoms and self-reported global and social functioning than those who received treatment as usual at a school-based clinic (Mufson et al., 2011).

Few studies have examined the efficacy of psychoeducation as a sole component of treatment for child or adolescent anxiety disorders. However, at least one study attempted to evaluate specific components of panic control treatment for adolescents (PCT-A) by examining changes in panic-relevant symptoms week by week throughout treatment (Micco, Choate-Summers, Ehrenreich, Pincus, & Mattis, 2007). PCT-A is a CBT for panic disorder that has been modified for use with adolescents (Hoffman & Mattis, 2000). The psychoeducation component includes information on the affective, behavioral, and cognitive components of anxiety, the physiology of panic, and the rationale for CBT treatment of panic disorder. In their component analysis, Micco and colleagues (2007) found that, after receiving psychoeducation, the average number of panic attacks per week as reported by adolescents dropped from almost 3 to less than 1.5. Because the PCT-A treatment components were not randomized and psychoeducation occurred at the beginning of treatment for all the adolescents, the authors indicated that the drop in panic attacks could have been related to relief from initiating treatment. However, they also speculated that psychoeducation may have played a role in symptom reduction by increasing adolescents' sense of control.

Interestingly, psychoeducation is often used as a control condition in RCTs examining the effectiveness of other therapies (e.g., exposure-based therapies) for the treatment of anxiety disorders in youth, thereby unintentionally also evaluating the effectiveness of psychoeducation. For example, youth ages 6–16 years with a primary diagnosis of a phobic disorder (specific phobia, social phobia, or agoraphobia) were randomly assigned to a psychoeducation support condition or one of two different exposure-based conditions: contingency management or cognitive self-control (Silverman et al., 1999). Psychoeducation support consisted of providing therapeutic support (e.g., active listening) and information to youth and their parents about the nature, course, etiology, and treatment of phobias in youth. Although various theories and treatments of phobias were discussed, no specific therapeutic strategies were discussed or practiced, unlike the exposure-based conditions in which exposure was taught, practiced in session, and assigned for homework. All three conditions resulted in substantial improvements on child-, parent-, and clinician-rated measures at posttreatment as well as at 3-, 6-, and 12-month follow-ups, and the improvements in the psychoeducation support condition were not significantly different from those in the other two conditions (Silverman et al., 1999).

Similar results were observed for youth ages 7–17 years with a primary diagnosis of specific phobia in an RCT comparing a wait-list condition, an exposure condition, and a psychoeducation support condition (Flatt & King, 2010). Both treatment conditions resulted in significantly larger improvements in behavioral approach tests and self-efficacy ratings than the waitlist condition, and these gains were maintained at 1-year follow-up. Additionally, there were no differences found between the exposure and psychoeducation support conditions at posttest or 1-year follow-up (Flatt & King, 2010). Another RCT compared CBT to psychoeducation support in the treatment of school phobia in youth ages 6–17 years (Last, Hansen, & Franco, 1998). There were no significant differences between the conditions, and both treatments significantly reduced children's anxiety and depressive symptoms, were effective in returning youth to school, and resulted in continued school attendance the following school year. Both of these studies used a psychoeducation support condition based on that of Silverman and colleagues (1999). Although it is tempting to conclude that psychoeducation alone may be as effective as CBT, the results may instead reflect an unintentional overlap in active ingredients between the two conditions. In fact, in one study independent raters indicated that 65% of a psychoeducation control condition (also based on Silverman et al., 1999) unintentionally included CBT content (Kendall et al., 2008).

Regarding multicomponent treatments that include psychoeducation, CBT is considered a "probably efficacious" treatment for child anxiety (Silverman et al., 2008), in large part owing to waitlist RCTs with treatments based on the Coping Cat manual (e.g., Kendall & Hedtke, 2006) and an Australian adaptation of this manual called Coping Koala (Barrett, Dadds, & Rapee, 1991). Although not explicitly referred to as psychoeducation, both Coping Cat and Coping Koala provide information about the nature of anxiety (e.g., fear is normal and beneficial in some situations), the presentation and identification of anxiety symptoms (e.g., somatic symptoms and anxious thoughts), and the treatment of anxiety using CBT. Results from several waitlist RCTs provide evidence for the effectiveness of these programs for children ages 9–13 years (Kendall, 1994; Kendall et al., 1997) and 7–14 years (P. M. Barrett, 1998; Barrett et al., 1996). Children receiving CBT had better outcomes, as indicated by child and parent reports (Kendall, 1994; Kendall et al., 1997) as well as by clinician report (P. M. Barrett, 1998; Barrett et al., 1996). Several studies have demonstrated the maintenance of treatment gains at 1, 2, 5, and even 19 years (P. M. Barrett, 1998; Barrett, Duffy, et al., 2001; Benjamin et al., 2013; Kendall et al., 1997; Kendall, Safford, Flannery-Schroeder, & Webb, 2004; Kendall & Southam-Gerow, 1996).

CBT is also used to effectively treat OCD in youth (Freeman, Garcia, et al., 2014). CBT treatment packages for OCD typically include psychoeducation, cognitive restructuring, and exposure with response prevention (e.g., Freeman & Garcia, 2009; March & Mulle, 1998). The psychoeducation component is considered essential and focuses on framing OCD as a neurological disorder, with analogies to other medical disorders (e.g., asthma, diabetes) often also used. In addition, families are encouraged to "externalize" OCD by creating a name for it (e.g., Worry Monster). Families are also introduced to the theory and rationale behind ERP to help build commitment to and compliance with the intervention. A recent review concluded that both individual and family-based CBT treatment manuals are considered to be "probably efficacious" by APA standards in the treatment of pediatric OCD (Freeman, Garcia, et al., 2014). In addition to posttreatment effects, treatment gains were maintained at follow-up assessments of up to 6 months (Freeman, Garcia, et al., 2014).

## THE ELEMENT IN PRACTICE

The second half of this chapter is devoted to the practical implementation of psychoeducation (see Box 7.1 for a step-by-step task analysis). In addition to the task analysis, possible adaptations for youth of varying developmental levels and diverse backgrounds are discussed. The chapter closes with a case example of psychoeducation applied in the treatment of an 8 year-old Asian American girl diagnosed with OCD (see Box 7.2).

### "Core of the Core" Element

Clear instructions on how to deliver psychoeducation are difficult to find. In many treatment manuals, the psychoeducation element is implied or very briefly described (e.g., Kearney & Albano, 2007). Psychoeducation is a relatively small component in some interventions, often comprising only a portion of the first session (e.g., as in Coping Cat, Kendall & Hedtke, 2006; "ACTION", Stark et al., 2007), while it plays a comparatively much larger role in other treatments (e.g., PEP, Fristad et al., 2011; OCD in Children and Adolescents, March & Mulle, 1998; IPT-A, Mufson et al., 2011). In addition, psychoeducation is sometimes a dyadic exchange between the clinician and youth and other times is a larger family or group therapy process. Yet, in looking across several treatments, common themes and sequences occur in its delivery (see Box 7.1).

Psychoeducation is typically one of the first components of

## BOX 7.1. Task Analysis of Psychoeducation

1. Assess the current level of understanding of the youth (or youth and family) regarding the disorder and treatment.
   a. Assess knowledge regarding causes (e.g., "What do you think causes kids to worry a lot?").
   b. Assess knowledge regarding symptoms (e.g., "How can you tell when someone is depressed?").
   c. Assess knowledge regarding treatment (e.g., "What have you heard about therapy?").

2. Add to existing knowledge with information on symptoms and prevalence.
   a. Discuss the prevalence of the condition to help normalize the youth's experience.
   b. Discuss the continuum of emotion, from adaptive to maladaptive (for example, fear as adaptive vs. fear as a "false alarm").
   c. Emphasize that the symptoms of the disorder are separate from the youth. It may help to externalize the disorder by giving it a name (e.g., Mood Monster).

3. Discuss the etiology of the disorder.
   a. Review current research and theories.
   b. Reduce blame or guilt; emphasize that the disorder is not the fault of the youth or anyone in the family.

4. Present information on treatments.
   a. Describe the current treatment.
   b. Instill hope and increase compliance by presenting information regarding the effectiveness of the current treatment.
   c. Discuss other potential treatment options for the youth's particular disorder.

5. Assess understanding and retention of new information.
   a. Encourage the youth and family to ask questions.
   b. Encourage the youth to summarize the information to better assess understanding.

interventions used to treat youth with internalizing disorders. Perhaps owing to its nature as an initial treatment ingredient, establishing rapport with the youth is often cited as a necessary precursor to starting psychoeducation. To this end, a neutral, nonthreatening conversation that enables the therapist and youth to get to know each other is recommended. Asking about hobbies, likes, and dislikes and gathering information about potential rewards for therapy assignments may be useful in building rapport. Kendall and Hedtke (2006) suggest playing a Personal Facts game that involves asking and supplying answers to simple questions like the number of siblings and favorite TV shows. In their group treatment for depressed children, Stark and Kendall (1996) include a fact-gathering exercise to be completed in pairs and then shared with the group. Similarly, Stark and colleagues (2007) detail a team building activity for their group treatment of depressed girls. In the Connections Game, the therapist ties the end of a ball of yarn around his (or her) wrist, says his name and something he likes to do for fun, and then throws the ball of yarn to one of the group members. The group member then wraps the yarn around her (or his) wrist, repeats the information from the therapist, shares her name and something she likes to do for fun, and then throws the ball of yarn to another group member, whereupon the process is repeated. Once all members have participated, the therapist and youth take turns completing the sentence "I'm happiest when . . . " At the end of the activity, the resulting web of yarn can be discussed as a symbol of the connections among the group members.

Once rapport is established, the first step of psychoeducation involves assessing the youth's and family's current knowledge and understanding of the disorder and treatment (Box 7.1, Step 1). The clinician can begin this process by asking the child why the family is coming to therapy and whether the child has any questions. Prompts like "Tell me about anxiety," "What do you think causes kids to get depressed?", "What do you think therapy will be like?", and "Have you ever heard of cognitive-behavioral therapy?" may also be helpful. As youth respond, the clinician can reinforce correct information (e.g., "You are exactly right that worries can be helpful in some situations and unhelpful in others"), and correct misinformation (e.g., "Not you nor anyone else is to blame for your OCD"). During this phase, it is important to assess the level of knowledge regarding prevalence, symptoms, etiology, and treatment and to take note of areas that are well understood as well as topics where the youth and/or family needs additional information.

The next step begins the imparting of information about the disorder that characterizes psychoeducation (Step 2). Utilizing the framework of knowledge provided by the youth, the therapist adds to the child's existing understanding with additional facts about symptoms and prevalence. One of the goals of this step is to normalize the experience. Knowing how common internalizing disorders are may reinforce the message that the youth is not alone in his or her experience. Information about symptoms may allow youth to place their symptoms on a continuum from adaptive to maladaptive. For example, Kendall and colleagues (2002) recommend discussing fear as a normal and beneficial emotion that at times is unhelpful. They add that "sometimes we feel more fear than we need to in some situations" (p. 4). Piacentini et al. (2007) use the analogy of a fire alarm to help normalize the anxiety associated with OCD. In many cases, a fire alarm warns about a real danger and serves to keep people safe; however, fire alarms can misfire and ring when there is no fire. In this way, OCD is explained as similar to a "false alarm."

Understanding the symptoms of the disorder can also help externalize the illness and separate the identity of the youth from the symptoms of the disorder. In their manual for interpersonal therapy for depressed adolescents, Mufson and colleagues (2011) direct the therapist to clearly communicate that the symptoms the teen is exhibiting are linked to the depression. The teen and the family are urged to think of the teen as having an "illness" and to make allowances for the symptoms of the illness. March and Mulle (1998) also encourage families to separate the symptoms of OCD from the affected child by thinking of OCD as a medical illness much like asthma or diabetes. To underscore this separation of child and illness, they suggest that the youth give their OCD a name (e.g., Worry Monster, Bad OCD) to further externalize the disorder. Similarly, Fristad and colleagues (2011), in their treatment for youth with bipolar and depressive disorders, include a session focused on helping youth separate their symptoms from who they are. In this process, youth participate in an activity called "Naming the Enemy" in which they make a list of their own positive personality characteristics and a list of symptoms, thus serving to remind the youth and family that the symptoms are not fixed attributes of the child.

The next step is to present the etiology of the disorder, with the goal being to dispel myths and to reduce blame or guilt experienced by the youth and/or the family (Step 3). March and Mulle's (1998) treatment contains a detailed account of OCD as a neurobehavioral illness and encourages the therapist to present up-to-date research on the etiology of OCD to the parents and youth. In their treatment for OCD, Piacentini and colleagues (2007) present OCD as multidetermined and include a discussion of possible neurochemical, environmental, behavioral, and hereditary contributors. Mood disorder interventions often include information on the genetics and biology of mood disorders (e.g., Fristad et al., 2011) and how thoughts, feelings, and behaviors contribute to depression (e.g., Clarke et al., 1990). Fristad and colleagues (2011) direct parents to conceptualize mood disorders as "no-fault brain disorders" (p. 90). Indeed, throughout the discussion of etiology, it is important to underscore that the disorder is not the fault of the parent or the youth and that any frustration should be focused on the disorder and not toward family members (e.g., Piacentini et al., 2007).

The fourth step of psychoeducation is to discuss treatment of the disorder, thereby helping to instill hope and increase treatment engagement (Step 4). Information on treatment typically includes an overview of the variety of interventions that currently exist, specifics about the current treatment, and the overall effectiveness of treatment. Psychoeducation regarding the range of available treatments may include a discussion of types of therapy, different medications, and the potential combination of therapy and medication. Fristad et al. (2011) stress that youth with mood disorders often get help from several different sources; hence, the discussion of possible treatments may include a description of a "treatment team" that consists of the school, a therapist, and a psychiatrist. Most EBTs then present an overview of the current treatment and its rationale. For example, many CBTs begin by describing how thoughts, feelings, and behaviors are linked together. For example, Kearney and Albano (2000) recommend drawing three circles connected by arrows and labeled "What I feel," "What I think," and "What I do." The therapist can then help the youth fill in somatic, cognitive, and behavioral symptoms to underscore potential areas of intervention. Finally, presenting information about the effectiveness of therapy serves to increase hope. For example, in their group treatment for youth with depressed mood, Stark and Kendall (1996) include a story about a girl who felt sad at the beginning of the group but felt much better by the end of treatment. At the same time, it is important to communicate that there are other options if the current therapy fails. Mufson et al. (2011) are careful to present IPT-A as one of several options, stating, "If IPT-A doesn't seem to be helping enough, there are other therapies that can be tried, including medication. Let's see how you do with this treatment first" (p. 48).

Finally, the information presented during psychoeducation is reviewed and understanding should be assessed (Step 5). This review can be completed at the close of the treatment element or at the start of the next session, to better assess retention of the material. The therapist can ask the youth to summarize the information or can enlist the youth's help in presenting the information to the parent(s) or other family members. As a homework review, the youth could prepare an information sheet that could be given to newly diagnosed youth.

## Developmental Adaptations

The goal of psychoeducation is to impart knowledge regarding the illness and the treatment in question to aid in reducing distress and instilling hope. In this section, we discuss how to tailor that message to youth of different ages and developmental levels. The EBTs discussed above are designed for use with a range of ages. For example, March and Mulle (1998) note that they have used their manual, *OCD in Children and Adolescents,* to treat children as young as age 4, and yet it is also used with adolescents. Within this age range, a therapist may be presented with a variety of developmental levels. For example, youth will vary in their working memory, abstract thinking, metacognition, and emotional regulation abilities (Berger, 2012). Luckily, psychoeducation is easily adapted to the needs of each individual child.

Young children are likely to rely on their parents to facilitate new learning (Berger, 2012), so it may be best to begin by delivering psychoeducation to parents alone. In their adaptation of CBT for young children with OCD, Freeman and Garcia (2009) recommend this approach so that parents can act as treatment "coaches," reduce their inadvertent accommodation of compulsive behaviors, and be adequately prepared for the ERP aspect of treatment. Moreover, as it is unlikely that very young children will understand and/or remember all the information presented, parents may continue the process of psychoeducation outside of the treatment session.

Psychoeducation with the young child should include simple language, concrete examples, and descriptive imagery and metaphors. To assess the child's understanding of the disorder, a therapist might play an interview game, taking turns passing a microphone back and forth to ask questions about sadness or worry. When presenting prevalence rates, it may be helpful to focus on how many children in a classroom or school are likely to have depression or anxiety. Within this explanation, therapists can encourage the young child to help glue colored dots on a piece of paper or to draw different colored stick figures to demonstrate prevalence (e.g., blue for a child with depression, red for one without). In discussing adaptive versus maladaptive emotions, specific examples of helpful worry (e.g., when crossing a busy street) and unhelpful worry (e.g., when Mom goes upstairs) may be used. Making the distinction between the child and the disorder may be done by encouraging the younger child to draw a picture of OCD, for example, and give it a name, thus helping prepare the child to "boss back" OCD (March & Mulle, 1998). In addition, there are several simple books about worries or sadness that are appropriate for young children (see Magination Press at *www.apa.org/pubs/magination*).

Similarly, the discussion of both etiology and treatment may be simplified for younger youth. For example, it may be more appropriate to discuss OCD as a "brain problem" or "brain hiccup" instead of detailing the neurochemistry of the disorder. In preparing the young child for treatment, it may be helpful to give specific examples of what therapy will look like (e.g., "We will talk, play games, and learn about feelings and how things you think and do affect how you feel") or to draw a cartoon about the things you will do together during treatment. The exposure component of anxiety treatment may be presented as slowly learning to face your fears. Freeman and Garcia (2009) recommend working with the child to identify personal examples of other fears the child has overcome. Kendall and Hedtke (2006) suggest having the therapist share a personal story of a fear that was conquered through exposure (e.g., fear of giving a speech that disappeared with practice). Exposures can also be presented by using the metaphor of getting into a swimming pool on a hot day: At first, the water feels cold and you want to get out, but if you stay in your body gets used to the water and the water starts to feel good.

The basic structure of psychoeducation will likely differ for adolescents or more cognitively advanced youth. More developmentally mature youth tend to rely less on their parents and desire higher levels of independence (Santrock, 2010), and so it may be beneficial to present psychoeducational content to the youth first. As it remains important to share information about the disorder and treatment with the parents, having the youth present the material in a family meeting serves the purpose of educating the family while giving the youth the opportunity to demonstrate competence.

The content of psychoeducation can also be adapted for older youth. Older youth are more likely to understand percentages in discussing prevalence, and the therapist can quiz older youth regarding what the rates mean (e.g., "So, 2% would mean how many in your school? How many in your neighborhood? What do you think the chances are that you know someone else who is also depressed?"). Similarly, more cognitively advanced youth will be able to take a larger role in the discussion of emotions. For example, older youth may be able to volunteer personal examples of situations in which feelings of sadness have been appropriate/adaptive and times when the emotion has been less adaptive. In discussing symptoms of the disorder, older youth may benefit from collaboratively reviewing the diagnostic criteria for the disorder. Older youth may also be able to readily externalize the disorder by identifying thoughts and behaviors that are a reflection of their "true selves" versus symptoms of the disorder.

Psychoeducation about etiology and treatment can also occur at a more advanced level for some youth. Different theories of etiology may be presented while encouraging the youth to ask questions. One of the goals in discussing etiology is to dispel mystery and potential guilt and to increase empowerment through understanding (Cohen, Mannarino, & Deblinger, 2012). Therefore, being open to questions and being prepared with informational handouts or brief videos is useful. Discussion of current and alternative treatments should be similarly interactive and informative. In their manual for treatment of OCD, March and Mulle (1998) have a helpful handout titled "Your CBT Program" that outlines session and treatment structure as well as lists specific skills the youth will learn. This handout could be easily adapted for other disorders. In discussing treatment, it is important to communicate to the youth that the current treatment has a good chance of working (Mufson et al., 2011). Older youth may be curious about research supporting the effectiveness of the treatment. Depending on the treatment plan, older adolescents may also benefit from a conversation about how medications may complement the current intervention. Finally, it is important to facilitate hope by letting the youth know that, if the current treatment does not work, there are other possible treatments (Mufson et al., 2011).

## Diversity Considerations

The American Psychological Association (2003) encourages psychologists to utilize a "cultural lens" in all aspects of the profession of psychology, including training, research, and practice. This focus on the cultural context of the individual is also echoed in the Association's recommendations for evidence-based practice (American Psychological Association, 2006). Research supports these directives, suggesting that these contextual variables "influence almost every aspect of the diagnostic and treatment process" (Bernal, Jiménez-Chafey, & Domenech Rodríguez, 2009, p. 361). Cultural sensitivity in delivering empirically supported interventions has taken two forms: delivering manualized treatments in a flexible manner that stays true to the fundamental components of the treatment (i.e., the flexibility within fidelity approach; Kendall & Beidas, 2007) and creating new culturally enhanced versions of existing manualized treatments (e.g., BigFoot & Schmidt, 2012). Treatments that include psychoeducation as a core component for youth with internalizing problems fall into both of these categories.

Interventions for internalizing disorders that incorporate psychoeducation as a treatment module have been shown to be effective with diverse youth. Specifically, manualized treatments for anxiety are effective with African American teens (Ginsburg & Drake, 2002) and Hispanic/Latino youth (Pina et al., 2003) and have been successfully adapted for use in other countries (e.g., Coping Koala; Barrett et al., 1991). Research supports the use of manualized treatments for depression that include psychoeducation with Puerto Rican youth (e.g., Rosselló et al., 2008) and incarcerated Hispanic youth (Sanchez-Barker, 2003), with preliminary evidence for effectiveness with Haitian American adolescents (e.g., Nicolas, Arntz, Hirsch, & Schmiedigen, 2009). Moreover, a meta-analysis of controlled trials of treatment effectiveness concluded that there are treatments for both anxiety and depression that are "probably" or "possibly efficacious" for use with minority youth (Huey & Polo, 2008).

Interestingly, in cultural adaptations of trauma-focused CBT, psychoeducation is considered one of the crucial components of treatment. De Arellano and colleagues (De Arellano, Danielson, & Felton, 2012) designed a culturally adapted form of TF-CBT for Latino youth based on a thorough review of the literature on working with Latino clients and their clinical experience working with TF-CBT in this population. In this process, they identified common cultural themes (e.g., spirituality, involvement of family, traditional parenting style), held focus groups with caregivers and health providers, and integrated the collected information into a treatment, culturally modified TF-CBT (CM-TF-CBT). In response to parents identifying several questions about mental health treatment during the focus group sessions, de Arellano et al. (2012) increased the range of information discussed within the psychoeducation module of the treatment. For example, they recommend assessing the family's understanding of what a therapist is, what therapy is, and the role that each member of the family may play in the course of therapy. De Arellano and colleagues encourage cultural sensitivity in the psychoeducation process by considering Latino values and integrating metaphors common in Latino culture. For instance, the cultural value of *respeto*, or respect for authority, may prevent family members from asking questions, and so it may be more effective for the therapist to ask specific questions (e.g., "What does a therapist do?"; "Who comes to therapy?") rather than open-ended questions (e.g., "What questions do you have?"). The use of a short proverb may aid in imparting information regarding psychoeducation and also help to communicate respect for and integration of the culture. For instance, de Arellano et al. recommend the proverb *"Despues de la tormenta, sale el sol entre las nubes"* ("After the storm, the sun shines through the clouds") to instill hope. As with all minority groups, there is significant within-group variability, so it is important to remember that each client will come to therapy with a different level of understanding as well as a different level of acculturation, and psychoeducation should be modified to match the needs of the client.

Psychoeducation plays a similarly central role in the cultural modification of TF-CBT for Native American youth called Honoring Children—Mending the Circle (HC-MC; BigFoot & Schmidt, 2012). The authors describe HC-MC as TF-CBT integrated with complementary elements of indigenous culture (e.g., the consideration of extended family connections, interconnections between spirituality and healing, use of the sacred symbol of the circle to represent connectedness). Within this framework, psychoeducation is considered a critical treatment component, as "it is here that the therapist begins to learn about the family and join with them in the healing process" (BigFoot & Schmidt, 2012, p. 290). The authors stress that, given the historical context of discrimination toward indigenous peoples, the client and family should be encouraged to share with the clinician details regarding their values, perspectives, traditions, and family relationships, thereby establishing a more collaborative approach to healing. To enhance the psychoeducation element of treatment, BigFoot and Schmidt (2012) recommend sharing facts and statistics on trauma in American Indian and Alaska native populations, discussing well-being as an interconnected circle (an elaboration of the traditional CBT triangle) and utilizing culturally congruent analogies and stories. For example, beading could be used as a useful metaphor for treatment. The beading process has a common structure of steps and necessary tools (much like manualized treatment), but is also made unique by each individual's approach and style (in much the same way that treatment will be adapted to the needs of the individual).

## CONCLUSIONS

Psychoeducation involves the process of sharing relevant information regarding the prevalence, symptoms, etiology, and specifics of treatment with the youth and their families. The common use of psychoeducation is grounded in sociopolitical and psychological movements that historically valued clients' knowledge and, thereby, their increased empowerment in the treatment process. Evidence for the efficacy of psychoeducation as a core element in the treatment of youth with internalizing disorders has been bolstered by multiple RCTs that evaluated multicomponent treatment packages as well as RCTs that included a psychoeducation-only comparison group. Psychoeducation is typically implemented at the beginning of the treatment process, as its goal is to normalize symptoms, demystify treatment, provide hope, and empower the youth. Additional research is needed to further evaluate adaptations of psychoeducation for youth of diverse backgrounds.

## BOX 7.2. Illustrative Case Example

Sophie was an 8-year-old Asian American girl referred to therapy by her pediatrician for treatment for OCD. She was brought to therapy by her parents and her maternal grandmother, who also lived in the home. According to her parents, Sophie became very concerned about germs and getting sick at the start of second grade. Mr. and Mrs. C. stated that Sophie frequently talked about her fear of getting sick and began washing her hands and using hand sanitizer many times a day. Her family began to get really concerned when she started getting out of bed at bedtime to wash her hands—even though she had just washed them a few minutes earlier. In addition, Sophie's teacher called her parents with concerns about her frequent trips to the bathroom and repeated in-classroom use of hand sanitizer. Her parents, grandmother, school nurse, and pediatrician all reported noticing that Sophie's hands were red and cracked owing to the excessive washing. Mr. and Mrs. C. also reported that Sophie protested and had tantrums when she was prevented from washing her hands. Sophie's pediatrician recommended a trial of CBT prior to considering medication. A diagnosis of OCD was confirmed through a clinical interview paired with use of the Children's Yale–Brown Obsessive Compulsive Scale.

Treatment followed the *It's Only a False Alarm* manual (Piacentini, Langley, & Roblek, 2007). This manual begins with two sessions of psychoeducation involving the child and parents (siblings or additional caregivers may also be involved). Sophie, both parents, and her maternal grandmother attended the first two sessions. While chatting with the family about Sophie's hobbies to facilitate rapport, the therapist took note of interests that might be helpful to integrate into later examples or activities (e.g., Sophie swims, makes bracelets, enjoys reading). The therapist then helped the family to transition to a discussion of Sophie's history (e.g., developmental, social, academic) and current symptoms. The therapist also asked questions regarding how the current symptoms were affecting her schoolwork, friendships, and family life.

Next, the therapist assessed the child's and family's knowledge of OCD, providing information and correcting misinformation as needed. The therapist asked Sophie if she had ever heard of OCD and, if so, whether she could describe the disorder. Sophie stated that her doctor said that she had OCD, and that she knew that OCD was making her worry about germs and wash her hands but that she didn't understand how that happened or what she could do to stop it. Sophie added that she was embarrassed and thought she might be the only kid "in the whole world" with this problem. Mr. and Mrs. C. reported that they read some information online but still had many questions about what caused Sophie's symptoms. In response, the therapist defined obsessions and compulsions, using Sophie's specific worries and behaviors to provide relatable examples. The therapist then discussed the prevalence of OCD to help Sophie understand that she was not alone and to reduce any feelings of stigma. Specifically, the therapist pointed out that one or two kids of every 100 have OCD. Mr. and Mrs. C. were able to report that there were about 300 children in Sophie's elementary school, which meant that between 3 and 6 children in her school likely had OCD. To further normalize Sophie's experience, the therapist talked about how everyone has worries, but OCD makes kids worry and act on those worries when it is not needed (like a false alarm). Together, the therapist, Sophie, and her extended family generated examples of helpful and unhelpful worries that children may have (e.g., about nightmares, burglars, tests).

Next, the therapist discussed the family's current understanding of the causes of OCD. The therapist started by explaining that OCD is likely a brain and behavior disorder. To help keep Sophie engaged, the therapist used a large sheet of drawing paper and had Sophie help draw a picture of the brain. The therapist explained that OCD is similar to asthma or diabetes, all of which are medical problems that need treatment and ongoing management. Together, the therapist and Sophie also drew a diagram of the obsession, worry, hand washing, and relief cycle to demonstrate how hand washing is contributing to the problem. Finally, the therapist discussed how OCD often runs in families but that Sophie's OCD was not anyone's fault.

Finally, the therapist talked to Sophie and her parents about treatment, first asking what they knew of treatment options and then supplementing their existing knowledge. Both Sophie and her parents had heard about the possibility of medication from the pediatrician and had many questions about how therapy might also help. Sophie's understanding of therapy was "a place you go to talk about your feelings"; so, the therapist validated her statement and added that this specific therapy involved talking about feelings, helpful and unhelpful thoughts, and helpful and unhelpful behaviors—and that this approach was called "cognitive-behavioral therapy," or CBT. In addition, the therapist explained the concept of exposure with response prevention by drawing a series of graphs with Sophie. First, Sophie and the therapist drew a graph of Sophie's worries increasing and then decreasing in response to hand washing. Then, the therapist and Sophie drew a new graph (similar to the first, with the worries perhaps going a little higher and lasting a little longer) to demonstrate what would happen if Sophie did not wash her hands. Finally, the therapist added more lines to the graph to demonstrate how habituation through practice would result in fewer worries that lasted for a shorter period of time. Sophie, her parents, and her grandmother were given the opportunity to ask questions about this process. Toward the end of the session, the therapist stressed the effectiveness of the treatment and briefly summarized other treatment options (e.g., medication) if the current approach didn't prove effective for Sophie. The psychoeducational content was reviewed briefly during the second session. Although the formal psychoeducation unit was thus completed, the content was revisited during therapy as needed.

# 8

## Social Skills Training

### BACKGROUND OF THE ELEMENT

Social skills training (SST) is a widely used procedure for increasing competence in interpersonal situations. SST is based on behavioral and social learning theory and commonly includes providing instructions and rationales, modeling of the skills being taught, opportunities for rehearsal, positive and corrective feedback, and praise and reinforcement (Smith, Jordan, Flood, & Hansen, 2010). SST may target a variety of interrelated social skills, such as those needed for social initiation, conversation, and assertiveness. Given the importance of interpersonal interactions in daily functioning and the fact that many clinical presenting problems have associated social skills deficits, SST is a widely applicable treatment and a common element of EBTs for internalizing disorders in youth. For example, a youth with social anxiety disorder may receive systematic desensitization for anxiety reduction and SST to address skills deficits that contribute to experiencing anxiety. Similarly, a depressed youth may participate in treatment that includes cognitive strategies to address maladaptive thinking and SST to increase social reinforcement and support. This chapter provides a brief overview of the historical and theoretical foundations of SST and the evidence base for using this technique in the treatment of youth experiencing internalizing problems. Specific procedures for implementing SST are described, including a step-by-step task analysis, discussion of developmental and diversity considerations, and a case example using SST with a 13-year-old adolescent experiencing interpersonal problems and depressive symptoms.

## Brief History

A brief review of the history of SST provides a valuable context for examining its current use. The foundations of SST can be traced to early work in behavioral models of psychotherapy that included assertion training, for example, Andrew Salter's (1949) conditioned reflex therapy, Joseph Wolpe's (1958) reciprocal inhibition, and Arnold Lazarus's (1971, 1973) multimodal behavior therapy. Deffenbacher (2000) noted that "the focus on teaching of effective coping skills stood in marked contrast to the psychodynamic models of the day, which viewed social interpersonal problems as a result of developmental difficulties, intrapsychic conflicts and traumas, ineffective defenses, and underlying personality structure" (p. 371). Although the original focus of assertion training was to inhibit anxiety in social situations, its overall value for interpersonal functioning was recognized and expanded to training in additional social skills. This broadened focus also expanded the range of problems addressed by SST, including serious clinical concerns. In particular, research on individuals with depression (e.g., Lewinsohn & Graf, 1973) and schizophrenia (e.g., Hersen & Bellack, 1976; Zigler & Phillips, 1961) was very influential in the development and expansion of SST. The use of SST by clinicians and researchers was also aided by books detailing its procedures (e.g., Galassi & Galassi, 1977; Kelly, 1982).

Much of the initial SST work was with adults, but there were also early developments with children (Van Hasselt, Hersen, Whitehill, & Bellack, 1979). Early applications focused on problems of aggressive behavior (e.g., Bornstein, Bellack, & Hersen, 1980; Gittelman, 1965) and social isolation and withdrawal (e.g., Oden & Asher, 1977; Walker & Hops, 1973). As the field developed, researchers examined SST with children in different contexts, including school (Oden & Asher, 1977), outpatient (Michelson et al., 1983), and inpatient settings (Hansen, St. Lawrence, & Christoff, 1989). Single-case experimental designs were widely used in the development and evaluation of SST with youth, including research documenting efficacy with a variety of clinical samples, such as "emotionally disturbed" inpatient children (Matson, Ollendick, & Adkins, 1980), adolescents diagnosed with mental retardation (Bradlyn et al., 1983), and "emotionally disordered" adolescents (Plienis et al., 1987). Across this work, interventions were often described as broadly addressing "social skills," though in some cases specific skills were the focus, including assertiveness (e.g., Bornstein, Bellack, & Hersen, 1977) and conversation skills (Hansen et al., 1989). The use of SST to help youth with internalizing problems, such as social anxiety, grew from work with youth identified as "shy" or "withdrawn" (e.g., Christoff et al., 1985; Walker & Hops, 1973).

Decades of research documenting social skill deficits in emotional (e.g., anxiety, depression) and behavioral problems (e.g., oppositionality/aggression) led to the inclusion of SST in many multicomponent treatment programs for youth (Chorpita & Daleiden, 2009). As discussed in a later section, research on the effectiveness of SST for addressing emotional and behavioral problems has been somewhat mixed, including limited generalization and maintenance in real-world settings. This has led to "a shift from excitement about the potential of social skills training (SST) as a panacea for many different psychological disorders to a gradual recognition that SST represents a valuable therapeutic approach but only as an integrated component of more complex cognitive-behavioral interventions" (Spence, 2003, p. 84).

## Theory Base

Social skills deficits and interpersonal problems have long been documented as contributing to the development and exacerbation of symptoms of depression (Segrin, 2000) and social anxiety (Rapee & Spence, 2004) in children and adults. A variety of research has also shown that poor peer relations and peer rejection in childhood predict later maladjustment, including internalizing symptoms (Hawker & Boulton, 2000; Kupersmidt, Coie, & Dodge, 1990). Emotional problems may in turn contribute to further development of interpersonal problems and social skills deficits by increasing social withdrawal or rejection and limiting opportunities for naturally occurring social learning and development. For example, children who report feeling anxious are perceived as anxious and less likable by their peers (Verduin & Kendall, 2008), and depressed youth are perceived as less popular, less likable, and less desirable as friends (Connolly, Geller, Marton, & Kutcher, 1992). Trower, Bryant, and Argyle (1978) proposed two ways that the development and severity of psychological disorders may be influenced by social skill deficits: (1) social incompetence leads to social isolation and/ or rejection, which causes problems such as depression or anxiety; and (2) psychological disturbance may cause a range of problems, including social difficulties, and the ensuing isolation and rejection lead to further stress and deterioration. The need for social skills interventions for youth with internalizing disorders derives from the complex bidirectional relationship of social skills deficits to these clinical problems.

The major theoretical basis for the developing SST procedures stems directly from social learning theory (SLT). Building on the work of Neal Miller and John Dollard (1941) and others, Albert Bandura (1977c) pioneered the development of SLT. He outlined a four-step process of observational learning that includes *attention* to an action in the environment, *retention* of what was observed, *reproduction* of that action, and *motivation* via consequences for the action (i.e., reinforcement or punishment). While based primarily on the operant principles of reinforcement and punishment, SLT also emphasizes the role of cognitive processes and the social context. It integrates behavioral and cognitive therapy approaches to learning via modeling, imitation, and consequences, and it is central to the development of many treatment procedures.

The development of SST corresponded closely with the development of SLT. Both saw a progression of theory development from emphases on basic operant conditioning principles to models that incorporate observational learning and cognitive processes (Nangle, Erdley, Adrian, & Fales, 2010). Jeffrey Kelly (1982) summarized the active ingredients of SST as including the following: (1) instructions and rationales provided to the client; (2) exposure to modeling of skills being taught; (3) overt practice or behavior rehearsal; and (4) reinforcement and feedback to shape behavioral practice. Thus, SST utilizes the same mechanisms by which most youth learn social skills in their natural environment as they are growing up, including direct reinforcement of social behaviors, observational or vicarious learning experiences, receiving interpersonal feedback, and cognitive experiences organized around interpersonal situations (Kelly, 1982).

Modeling is an essential part of SLT and SST (see Chapter 5). This may include live modeling, symbolic modeling (through such media as movies, books, and the Internet), and verbal instruction. Bandura (1977c) identified vicarious learning as that which occurs when individuals modify their own behavior based on observations of the consequences that others receive for the same behavior. Bandura (1978) also described the concept of *reciprocal determinism* as a critical part of how we learn; this involves the relationships among an individual (including his or her personal characteristics and cognitions), that person's behavior, and the environment. Each of these elements influences the other in a reciprocal fashion. For example, a shy child (personal/cognitive component) who enters a playground for the first time and sees other children interacting (environment) is inclined to go off to a quiet area and sit on a swing (behavioral component). However, a friendly child who is happy to see someone new on the playground asks him or her to join her or him in the sandbox and as a result changes the shy child's behavior.

Also important to the development of SST was the distinction between acquisition and performance deficits (Gresham, 1981). Acquisition deficits reflect an absence of the knowledge or ability to perform the needed social skill, while performance deficits occur when the skill is in the person's behavioral repertoire but he or she fails to exhibit it in social situations. These are sometimes referred to as "can't do" and "won't do" deficits. For instance, a socially isolated and anxious youth who doesn't know what topics his or her peers find interesting to talk about could benefit from SST to acquire the skill, while a depressed youth who knows what topics to talk about but can't find the energy or opportunity to use the social skill may need alternative interventions (e.g., reinforcement and activity scheduling). For SST to be effective, it must address the development of skills acquisition, enhance skills performance, and facilitate generalization in use of the skills in the natural environment (Ladd & Mize, 1983; Smith et al., 2010). The focus on performance and generalization of SST also focuses attention on the need to address interfering or competing problem behaviors (Gresham, 2002), such as internalizing (e.g., anxiety, depression, social withdrawal) or externalizing problems (e.g., aggression, impulsivity).

## Evidence Base

The evidence base for the value of SST interventions with youth includes decades of research across a variety of interpersonal difficulties (Gresham, 2002; Spence, 2003). The problems addressed range from students with poor peer relations in school (e.g., Bornstein et al., 1977; Oden & Asher, 1977) to "emotional problems" and extreme shyness in clinical samples (e.g., Christoff et al., 1985; Plienis et al., 1987). As the promise of SST grew from research using individual subject designs, group comparison studies increased, including RCTs for youth with social adjustment problems and poor peer acceptance (e.g., Bierman & Furman, 1984; Ladd, 1981; Michelson et al., 1983). While not specifically focused on internalizing disorders, this foundational work often addressed closely related problems, such as shyness and withdrawal. The research overall supports the efficacy of SST, but a commonly expressed concern is the need for further demonstration of lasting effects that have an impact on real-world interactions (Gresham, 2002; Spence, 2003).

A number of meta-analyses have been conducted to examine the broad research literature on the impact of SST with youth (e.g., Beelman, Pfingsten, & Losel, 1994; Mathur, Kavale, Quinn, Forness, & Rutherford, 1998; Schneider, 1992). Overall, these meta-analyses document moderate effect sizes, with significant outcomes primarily noted for specific social behaviors versus broad indices of adjustment. For example, in a meta-analytic review of 79 controlled studies with children, Schneider (1992) concluded that the short-term overall effectiveness of SST was moderate. Efforts to explore variation in effect sizes showed that withdrawn youth were more responsive to SST than aggressive youth and youth without a diagnosis (i.e., "normal" ones). Effects were stronger on measures related to social competence (e.g., observation of social interaction, peer and self-report) than more peripheral variables (e.g., academic achievement). Effects continued, though lessened somewhat, through follow-ups that were generally 3 months or less.

Similarly, in a meta-analysis of 49 studies of social competence training with youth that included at least one control group, Beelman et al. (1994) concluded that intervention was overall moderately effective across a variety of samples, including youth identified as internalizing (i.e., exhibiting social withdrawal, depression, childhood neglect), externalizing (i.e., aggression, conduct disorder, rejection), and at-risk (i.e., social deprivation, facing critical life events). Effects varied somewhat across groups and types of outcome measures. For example, all groups showed a moderate-to-strong effect for social-cognitive skills (e.g., problem solving, perspective taking). Social interaction skills (ratings of actual social behavior) showed low-to-moderate effects for the internalizing and externalizing groups, but no significant effects for the at-risk group. Measures of social adjustment (e.g., general adjustment or problem scores; ratings of aggressiveness or popularity) revealed a moderate effect for only the internalizing and externalizing groups. There were no significant effects across the groups for self-related cognition/affect (e.g., social anxiety, depression, self-concept, and control beliefs). This analysis also provided evidence for the superiority of multimodal SST approaches over mono-modal interventions that used modeling, coaching, or reinforcement in isolation. Though there were encouraging findings, there were also concerns. Significant effect sizes were found only on the most direct measures of social skills targets (e.g., social interaction skills) with limited effects on broader constructs (e.g., adjustment). It was also noted that long-term effects were weak overall and that the research does not allow drawing firm conclusions about generalization of behavior change in real-world social interactions.

After decades of research on SST, the field has recognized that SST is generally not sufficient as a sole treatment for internalizing disorders of youth, but it is a valuable element in more comprehensive interventions (Spence, 2003). As a result, research on use of SST on its own has become much less common, and SST is more likely to be included as part of a larger treatment package. As documented by Chorpita and Daleiden (2009) in a review of randomized trials of EBTs for children and adolescents, SST is a relatively widely utilized component of interventions for internalizing problems.

A number of EBT programs for youth with anxiety disorders include SST as an important element (e.g., Albano & DiBartolo, 2007; Kendall et al., 2002; see Table 8.1 for examples). These are typically cognitive-behavioral interventions that also use a combination of elements, including psychoeducation, cognitive restructuring, exposure, relaxation, problem solving, and contingency management. For example, cognitive-behavioral group treatment for social phobic adolescents (CBGT-A; Albano & DiBartolo, 2007) incorporates psychoeducation, problem solving, social skills, cognitive restructuring, and exposure to anxiety-provoking social situations. The SST portion of CBGT-A includes the identification of the skills to be taught (e.g., assertive behaviors), imaginary practice of the skill, the examination of difficulties that may interfere with *in vivo* practice and coping strategies to address these difficulties, practice in real-world social interactions, and self-reinforcement following practice. In an RCT with 35 adolescent girls, Hayward et al. (2000) found a moderate short-term effect of CBGT-A as compared to a waitlist control condition, including a decrease in social phobia diagnoses. Differences between subjects receiving CBGT-A and those in the control condition were not present 1 year later, when social phobia was the primary outcome. However, the treatment of social phobia likely lowered the risk for relapse of major depression for those youth with a history of depression.

Social effectiveness therapy for children (SET-C; Beidel, Turner, & Morris, 2004) is a multielement behavioral treatment program for youth with social anxiety. It combines SST, peer generalization experiences (i.e., social activities with outgoing but unfamiliar peers), and individualized *in vivo* exposure. SET-C includes training on a number of interpersonal skills, including conversation skills, assertiveness, joining groups, establishing and maintaining friendships, and giving

**TABLE 8.1. The Social Skills Training Element in Representative EBT Manuals**

| | |
|---|---|
| *C.A.T. Project* (Kendall, Choudhury, Hudson, & Webb, 2002) | • The clinician explicitly discusses communication skills during the eighth session. The clinician leads the youth through practice conversations during the session. |
| *CBT for Social Phobia: Stand Up, Speak Out* (Albano & DiBartolo, 2007) | • The clinician explicitly teaches social skills, using a five-step model for improving social skills during the fifth session. The youth engage in imaginary practice of the skills, participate in role plays related to verbal and nonverbal skills, create a self-assessment of their social skills difficulties, and learn basic assertiveness skills. |
| *When Children Refuse School: A CBT Approach* (Kearney & Albano, 2007) | • The clinician explicitly teaches communication skills and peer refusal skills during the initial phase of treatment. The youth participate in role plays and feedback with family members. |
| *Treating Trauma and Traumatic Grief in Children & Adolescents* (Cohen, Mannarino, & Deblinger, 2006) | • Social skills training is included in a supplemental section of Component 4 of the initial, trauma-focused, phase. The clinician can elect to provide information about, model, and practice social skills in the context of problem solving. |
| *Adolescent Coping with Depression* (Clarke, Lewinsohn, & Hops, 1990) | • The clinician explicitly teaches social skills throughout the course of treatment. Initial sessions teach the youth about positive peer interactions, starting conversations, meeting new people, introducing oneself to a stranger, and skills for joining and leaving conversation groups. Later sessions focus on improving these "friendly" skills as well as listening and making appropriate responses within conversations, and interpersonal negotiation. Youth participate in role plays and activities to demonstrate these skills. |
| *Interpersonal Therapy for Depressed Adolescents,* 2nd edition (Mufson, Pollack Dorta, Moreau, & Weissman, 2011) | • The clinician explicitly teaches communication skills and analysis to those youth experiencing negative and ineffective communication. The clinician leads the youth through the analysis of significant social interactions and teaches alternative strategies for communicating feelings, opinions, and empathy. |
| *Treating Depressed Youth: Therapist Manual for "Action"* (Stark et al., 2007) | • The clinician explicitly teaches the youth about interpersonal compliments during the fifth session. The youth are encouraged to compliment their peers during the session. Interpersonal communication is also discussed during the ninth session in the context of problem solving. |
| *Psychotherapy for Children with Bipolar and Depressive Disorders* (Fristad, Arnold, & Leffler, 2011) | • The clinician explicitly teaches the youth about verbal communication, nonverbal communication, and conversation skills during the latter part of treatment. The youth are provided a handout on the communication cycle. Social skills that are covered include facial expressions, body gestures, body posture, the tone of one's voice, and personal space. |

*Note.* Some book titles are shortened to conserve space. See the References at the back of the book for full titles.

and receiving compliments. SET-C has been evaluated and compared to both waitlist and attention controls (Beidel et al., 2004). For example, Beidel and colleagues (2000) compared SET-C with a nonspecific active intervention (Testbusters) and found that the SET-C group showed significant improvements in social skills, increases in social interaction, reduced social fear and anxiety, and fewer social phobia diagnoses through a 6-month follow-up. Beidel, Turner, and Young (2006) examined the long-term maintenance of treatment gains for these youth 3, 4, and 5 years later. Using multidimensional assessment including self-report, parent report, clinical ratings, and direct behavioral assessment, they found that SET-C treated youth maintained treatment gains and that their functioning was no different from youth who never had a disorder.

SST is also an integral element in multicomponent treatments for depressed youth (e.g., Clarke et al., 1990; Mufson et al., 2011; see Table 8.1). For example, the CWD-A course, which has been shown to be effective for adolescents across a number of RCTs (e.g., Clarke et al., 1999; Lewinsohn et al., 1990), integrates SST into a larger program along with psychoeducation, relaxation training, cognitive strategies, and problem solving. Using role plays and group activities as well as homework assignments to encourage practice, this program teaches social skills that include approaching others and starting conversations, meeting new people, joining and leaving conversations, listening, and interpersonal negotiation (Clarke et al., 1990). IPT-A, which has been evaluated by Mufson and colleagues (e.g., Mufson et al., 2011; Mufson, Weissman, et al., 1999), also includes efforts to improve social interaction skills. The goals of IPT-A include clarifying problems (such as grief, interpersonal conflict), identifying and implementing strategies to address the subject's problems, and improving interpersonal functioning and communication. With the goal of eliminating negative and ineffective communication, the therapist uses communication analysis to help the youth examine difficult social interactions and teach alternative approaches for expressing feelings, opinions, and empathy. Research demonstrating its effectiveness includes RCTs comparing IPT-A to a clinical monitoring control (Mufson, Weissman, et al., 1999) and to "treatment as usual" in school-based mental health clinics (Mufson, Pollack Dorta, & Wickramaratne, 2004).

## THE ELEMENT IN PRACTICE

With a strong historical and theoretical foundation established, the latter portion of this chapter shifts to a practical discussion of the implementation of SST for anxious and depressed youth. A task analysis of the multiple steps of SST is presented in Box 8.1, and a case study illustrating implementation is elaborated in Box 8.2 at the end of the chapter. The following discussion expands on the task analysis, providing additional details on the many considerations that arise when conducting SST.

## "Core of the Core" Element

An essential first step is conducting an assessment to determine a need for SST (Box 8.1, Step 1; Smith et al., 2010). A critical issue in identifying whether SST is needed is determining whether the youth has not yet acquired the social skills of interest or, rather has acquired the skills but is not exhibiting them because of interfering or competing problem behavior, such as social anxiety or a lack of motivation attributable to depression (Gresham, 2002). A variety of measures are available for use in social skills assessment of youth, including interview, self-report, ratings by others, analogue/role play, and observational measures (see Nangle, Hansen, Erdley, & Norton, 2010, for a review of measures).

If the determination is that there is a skills deficit, the therapist must identify the specific target behaviors that need improvement. For example, if conversation skills are limited, what are the basic conversational components that need improving (e.g., asking questions, making eye contact)? A basic premise of SST is that youth learn a skill area in its entirety by learning its component parts and practicing integrated use of these behaviors. If there is a performance deficit that is accounting for some or all of the failure to use appropriate social skills, the problem behaviors that interfere must be identified and additional treatments provided as needed. For example, if the underlying problem is social anxiety, other core elements described in this book may be needed, such as relaxation training and exposure. If the youth is failing to exhibit social skills because of depression, activity scheduling, contingency management, and cognitive strategies may be valuable.

Once the need for SST has been identified, the focus shifts to skills acquisition. The therapist begins by providing the rationale and instruction for the specific skills to be trained (Step 2). The social skills being targeted must be clearly defined and described, with multiple examples. For example, in conversational skills training, appropriate self-disclosure may be described as providing information about yourself, including sharing about interests, hobbies, background, preferences, and opinions (e.g., "I like to play basketball"). In addition, a rationale for using the skill should be provided. When possible, it is

## BOX 8.1. Task Analysis of Social Skills Training

1. Conduct an assessment of the youth to determine the need for social skills training.
   a. Determine whether there is a social skills acquisition deficit, performance deficit, or both.
   b. If a skills deficit exists, identify the specific target behaviors that need to be improved.
   c. If a performance deficit exists, identify interfering or competing problem behaviors (e.g., anxiety) that inhibit skill acquisition and/or performance, and provide additional treatment as needed to address these concerns.

2. Provide the rationale and instruction for the skill(s) to be inculcated.
   a. Describe each skill, providing examples, and encourage the youth to offer examples.
   b. Describe the purpose and benefits of using the skill.

3. Model the target behavior.
   a. Model the appropriate use of the skill being taught.
   b. In addition to therapist modeling, consider the use of video and/or covert modeling (e.g., the visualization of behavior being exhibited by an admired peer).
   c. Discuss and model the positive consequences associated with the proper use of the skill.

4. Have the youth exhibit and rehearse the skill.
   a. Guide the youth in role playing the use of the skill. Practice may be verbal (with only verbal components), overt (verbal and behavioral components), and/or covert (the visualization of one's self exhibiting the behavior).
   b. As training progresses, have the youth practice integrated use of the skills that have been taught.

5. Provide positive and corrective feedback.
   a. After a rehearsal, provide feedback about the effort and the appropriate behaviors exhibited. Feedback should be specific and constructive, with clear examples and instruction (at the youth's level of understanding).
   b. Provide suggestions to improve performance. Use feedback to refine the behavior in the desired direction.

6. Provide praise and reinforcement.
   a. Provide specific praise to the youth immediately following the desired behavior.
   b. As needed to elicit and maintain participation, provide rewards to the youth. Identify potential reinforcers, with input from the youth and/or significant others (e.g., parents, teachers).

7. Provide homework assignments for practicing the skills.
   a. Choose the assignment in collaboration with the youth. Consider the youth's strengths, ability, and motivation when identifying the assignment.

    b. Discuss and problem-solve potential obstacles that might interfere with the assignment.

    c. For younger children, have the child explain the assignment to his or her parent(s). Elaborate as needed.

8. Repeat Steps 2–7 as needed.

    a. Continue the training cycle until the youth demonstrates successful performance of the skill.

    b. End on a positive note, with the youth having been reinforced for success.

9. Encourage generalization and maintenance.

    a. Enlist significant others, such as parents and teachers, to encourage and reinforce the use of social skills in everyday social situations.

    b. Teach the youth to self-reinforce the use of social skills.

    c. Schedule booster sessions or follow-up contacts as needed following treatment to facilitate continued progress in real-world interactions.

---

valuable to elicit this from the client to be sure the youth understands the function and benefits of using the skill before moving forward with training (e.g., "Self-disclosure helps the other person get to know me and helps us have something to talk about").

The therapist then models appropriate use of the target behavior being trained (Step 3; see also Chapter 5). Modeling also provides the opportunity to demonstrate and discuss positive consequences that may occur with the proper use of the skill. The demonstration of multiple exemplars is valuable for providing varied versions of the targeted behavior and facilitating generalization (Stokes & Baer, 1977; Stokes & Osnes, 1989). The typical scenario is that the therapist models the skill being trained for the youth. For example, the therapist might demonstrate multiple examples of talking about an age-appropriate high-interest topic. Video and/or covert modeling may also be helpful. Video modeling can be created (e.g., with peer-age models), purchased from publishing companies (e.g., "Model Me" videos from *www.modelmekids. com*), and increasingly found for free on YouTube. An advantage of video modeling is that it allows for repetition and instills confidence that the skill is clearly and correctly modeled. With covert modeling, a youth can be asked to close his or her eyes and imagine the behavior being exhibited by an admired peer. As discussed in Chapter 5, it is valuable to use models that may be perceived by the youth as similar (e.g., in age, gender, ethnicity, interpersonal context) to increase identification with and imitation of the model (Rosenthal & Bandura, 1978). Modeling often utilizes a mastery model (where the skill is modeled flawlessly), but coping models are also valuable as training progresses (where the model first experiences some difficulties but eventually exhibits the desired behavior).

After modeling the desired behavior, the youth is prompted to exhibit and practice the skill (Step 4). Practice may be verbal (with only verbal components), overt (verbal and behavioral components), and/ or covert (visualization of oneself exhibiting the behavior). The verbal and covert rehearsals are used to improve encoding, retention, and retrieval of skill information (Ladd & Mize, 1983). For example, with verbalization, a youth may be asked to state questions they may ask a peer in order to maintain a conversation. With covert practice, they may be asked to visualize themselves doing so in various social situations. Overt forms of practice (performing the desired behavior) enable the youth to also develop and refine the motor elements of the skill (e.g., maintaining appropriate eye contact; Ladd & Mize, 1983).

Practice situations may range from structured role plays to semi-structured or unstructured interactions. In structured role plays, a scenario is typically described as the background or context for the interaction. Then the therapist (or another role-play partner) acts in a manner intended to give the youth an opportunity to exhibit the desired skills. Practice may also occur in less structured ways and for more extended periods. For example, a socially anxious youth might be asked to carry on a conversation as if he or she is meeting a peer-age youth for the first time. Use of a wide variety of practice scenarios, including those that closely resemble real-world situations for the youth, may encourage generalization to the natural environment (Hansen, Nangle, & Meyer, 1998; Kelly, 1982). As training progresses, rehearsal opportunities should allow for practice of the integrated use of the skills that have been taught. For example, an extended practice session may allow the youth to exhibit a variety of verbal and nonverbal component skills (e.g., appropriate questions, self-disclosure, speech acknowledgers, eye contact, posture).

The youth's engagement in practicing the skill is accompanied by positive and corrective feedback from the therapist regarding the effort and appropriate behaviors exhibited (Step 5). Using specific and constructive feedback, with clear examples, the therapist provides suggestions to improve the youth's performance and refine the behavior in the desired direction. It may be valuable to provide a limited number of suggestions at a time (e.g., one or two) so that the instructions are understandable and the youth does not feel overwhelmed (Kelly, 1982). Reviewing video recordings of the youth practicing the skill can also be useful in providing feedback about both verbal and nonverbal behaviors and may be easier for the youth to attend to and understand than purely verbal feedback (Hansen et al., 1998). This also facilitates teaching the youth to engage in self-evaluation.

Praise and reinforcement are always provided along with practice and feedback (Step 6; see also Chapter 9). Specific praise immediately following the youth exhibiting the desired behaviors encourages continued use of the skill and helps keep the youth engaged in the treatment process. The use of rewards for participation can be particularly valuable for youth whose motivation to engage in treatment is low and/or who are not yet receiving naturally occurring reinforcement via successful social interactions. This may include tangibles (e.g., candy, small toys), activities (e.g., playing a game with a parent), or tokens (e.g., stickers, points) to be exchanged later for desired rewards. Such reinforcement may also be valuable in facilitating homework completion (described below).

Homework assignments are important for having youth practice these newly acquired behaviors outside of the therapy session (Step 7; see Chapter 13). The homework goals for SST can evolve with the motivation and progress of the youth. For example, a youth who is intimidated by an assignment of practicing conversational skills at school might first be tasked with observing peer conversations. It is helpful to have the youth describe and practice the assigned task and make a commitment (verbal and/or written) to carrying it out. For example, if the assignment involves initiating an interaction with a peer at a nearby locker, the youth and therapist could role-play that scenario. For younger children, it is valuable to have the child explain the assignments to parents. It is valuable to discuss and problem-solve potential challenges that might interfere with completing the assignment. For example, if a youth says he or she might "forget," discuss the strategies that might help him or her remember (e.g., a reminder on a school notebook). Finally, during the subsequent session review the homework assignment and praise efforts at completion to demonstrate the importance of the tasks.

Given that SST requires teaching the integrated use of multiple component behaviors involved in successful social interactions, the steps in the skills acquisition phase may be repeated multiple times (Step 8, repeating Steps 2–7 as needed). This skills acquisition training cycle continues until the youth demonstrates successful performance of the desired set of social behaviors.

Once the desired skills have been acquired, the focus shifts to facilitating generalization of the skill's use in the natural environment and maintenance over time (Step 9). Because generalization typically does not occur spontaneously, therapists must make specific efforts to actively program for it (Stokes & Baer, 1977; Stokes & Osnes, 1989). There are many approaches for doing so (see Hansen et al., 1998, for a discussion of strategies specific to SST). For example, youth can be prompted and encouraged by parents, teachers, or other caregivers to use their social skills in naturally occurring social situations. These adults can also praise and reinforce successful use of social skills, as they have the opportunity to observe them in regularly occurring social situations. Youth may also be taught to monitor and self-reinforce their use of appropriate social skills as a means to keep motivation up and progress continuing. These efforts at reinforcement can be valuable because newly acquired social skills are not always responded to positively by peers, in part because of their previous history with the youth (Hymel, Wagner, & Butler, 1990). And finally, it can be helpful as treatment winds down to allow greater time between sessions and to schedule booster sessions or encourage follow-up contacts as needed to facilitate continued progress in real-world social interactions.

## Developmental Adaptations

As children develop, there are many changes in their social context that accompany advances in conceptual understanding, perspective taking, emotional awareness, problem solving, and independence (Berger, 2014). Consideration of these differences in developmental and social contexts is essential when conducting SST for youth with internalizing problems, as they may impact the goals and behaviors targeted by SST (Christopher, Nangle, & Hansen, 1993; Hansen, Christopher, & Nangle, 1992). For example, social interactions typically progress from the parallel play of toddlers to the cooperative play of preschoolers as the children progressively learn how to interact with others, follow rules, ask to join in, and be assertive when needed. During the elementary school years, children further develop conversational skills, including listening and taking turns talking. They also continue to refine their assertiveness skills, including negotiation and their ability to say "no," and giving and receiving compliments. SST for children typically addresses these peer relationship skills in the context of informal prosocial situations, though sometimes specific applications are the focus, such as sports etiquette (e.g., not being a sore loser) and academic success (e.g., ignoring peer distractions while working; Smith et al., 2010).

Adolescence and the high school years bring further changes that impact the focus of SST, including physical maturation, more advanced cognitive abilities, and the increased salience of one's peer group (Berger, 2014). Skills are needed for a variety of social situations as the peer group becomes larger and more complex, more time is spent with peers, and one's interest in dating and sexual interaction increase (Christopher et al., 1993; Hansen et al., 1992). The psychosocial tasks of adolescence can be even more challenging for youth with internalizing problems that may lead to increased avoidance and decreased motivation for social engagement. Involvement in romantic relationships becomes a major focus for many youth that may present both opportunities and challenges (Berger, 2014). In fact, research has shown that romantic break-ups in adolescence are associated with the first onset of major depressive disorder in adolescence (Monroe, Rohde, Seeley, & Lewinsohn, 1999) as well as suicide and suicide attempts (Gould, Greenberg, Velting, & Shaffer, 2003). Because of the social nature of sexual behavior, social skills also play a major role in appropriate sexual interaction and prevention of high-risk sexual behavior, which can present significant difficulties for youth who are unassertive or socially anxious (Nangle & Hansen, 1998). For example, assertiveness skills are needed for initiating and declining sexual contact, including, for example, asking a partner to use a condom. For gay, lesbian, and bisexual youth, the dating and sexual interaction context may be further complicated by peer and adult attitudes toward homosexuality (Smith et al., 2010).

Although the skills targeted in SST will vary with the developmental level, the basic techniques used tend to be the same across all ages (Kelly, 1982; Smith et al., 2010). Additions or modifications to the skills training steps (as outlined in Box 8.1) can be made to adjust for differences in social context and opportunity, interests, cognitive and emotional abilities, and attention capacity. For example, the language used in providing rationales and instructions, or giving feedback, should be adjusted to the individual youth's developmental level, with repetition and clarification as needed. Also, younger children may require exposure to additional modeling as well as additional opportunities for practice. For encouraging generalization of SST with children, it can be relatively easy to enlist others (e.g., parents, teachers) to prompt and reinforce the use of social skills. Given the independence and larger social environment for adolescents, enlisting others may be less practicable for them, and so self-monitoring and self-reinforcement may be needed.

A procedure that can be used in isolation or in combination with standard SST is peer mediation (Hansen et al., 1998). By its very nature of involving peers, this intervention adjusts to the developmental level of the youth. In peer mediation interventions, one or more peer helpers without social skill deficits serve as a positive role model and practice partner for the client in facilitating interaction with other children. While this may be impractical in many clinical situations, this procedure works well in school settings because of the readily available similar-aged peers who interact in a variety of social contexts, such as at recess and lunchtime during elementary school (e.g., Bierman & Furman, 1984; Christopher, Hansen, & MacMillan, 1991). The peer helpers receive brief training on how to engage and interact with the youth with social skills deficits, and at times reinforcement for their efforts (e.g., stickers after a recess period). Although this approach has primarily been used in elementary settings, it has also shown value with high school youth (Hansen, MacMillan, & Shawchuck, 1990). Peer mediation creates opportunities for youth to practice their newly acquired skills in interactions with peers in natural settings and to receive the naturally occurring reinforcement that comes with successful social interaction. Peer-mediated intervention is believed to help overcome the negative views of the youth that might have developed during the youth's prior history in the peer group. This "reputational bias" (Hymel et al., 1990) can reduce the likelihood that improved social skills have a positive impact in social exchanges with youth who have previously rejected or have a negative social opinion of the youth. Positive association with peer mediators can help break that cycle and facilitate entry into the natural "trappings" of interactions with the larger peer group (Christopher et al., 1991).

Another variation in treatment procedure that involves developmental consideration is the use of group interventions. Much SST is conducted individually, but opportunities for group treatment are valuable when peer-age youth also in need of social skills intervention are available. There are no clear guidelines regarding at what ages group work may be most valuable, but SST group interventions have been successfully used across a wide age range, from preschool (e.g., Mize & Ladd, 1990) to elementary (e.g., Bierman & Furman, 1984) and high school youth (e.g., Plienis et al., 1987). Some of the multicomponent treatment packages for internalizing disorders that include SST use a group approach, including SET-C for treating social phobia in youth ages 8–16 years (Beidel et al., 2004) and CWD-A for treating depression in youth ages 14–18 years (Clarke et al., 1990). Group treatment provides increased opportunities for modeling and rehearsal with more individuals as well as exposure to increased stimulus and response exemplars. This opportunity to practice with and observe same-age peers may also increase engagement and motivation to participate, enabling the youth to receive the naturally occurring reinforcement associated with positive peer interactions. Also worthwhile is the inherent social context provided by the group setting, where the treatment session itself is an arena in which newly acquired skills can be readily practiced with same-age peers in both structured and unstructured situations.

As noted earlier, video recordings may be useful in providing instruction, exposure to models, and feedback. Video may have special advantages for younger children and those experiencing difficulties in learning and attending, as the same basic interaction can be paused and replayed as needed to discuss the performance (Kelly, 1982; Smith et al., 2010). In addition to providing the opportunity for repetition, videos may be seen as more interesting and attention-grabbing than a therapist modeling skills of interest or describing the youth's performance during feedback. Video training has progressed to also include opportunities for practice in "virtual reality" (i.e., interactive three-dimensional computer-generated simulations). For example, Sarver and colleagues (2014) did a feasibility study of an "interactive virtual school environment" in the treatment of social anxiety disorder in children (ages 8–12 years). All children were treated with SET-C (Beidel et al., 2004), with the usual *in vivo* peer generalization sessions and homework assignments replaced by practice in a virtual environment. The virtual environment program was well received by the clinicians, children, and parents, and the results support the acceptability, ease of use, and credibility of the technology. As virtual reality technology advances and becomes more available, the contributions to SST will be substantial.

## Diversity Considerations

Evidence-based practice in psychology necessitates consideration of the "context of patient characteristics, culture and preferences" (American Psychological Association, 2006, p. 273). The need for doing so is especially apparent in SST, given the focus on interpersonal skills that are effective in a myriad of naturally occurring social contexts. Individual differences that may impact social interactions and social identities are many, including age, race and ethnicity, physical disability, sexual orientation, socioeconomic status, cultural and ethnic identity, acculturation level, and religious and spiritual orientation. By them-selves, these are heterogeneous and distal variables that tell us very little about the behaviors, beliefs, attitudes, or values of an individual, as there are also many within-group variations (Sue, 1988). Thus, it is essential that a clinician implementing SST gain a detailed understand-ing of the youth, his or her family, and his or her social environment.

Understanding the theoretical basis and basic procedures of SST provides a strong foundation for its proper application with diverse youth. Like other CBTs, SST may be well suited for adapting to the needs of diverse youth, as it is grounded in theories that may have relatively universal application across populations (i.e., social learning, operant conditioning; Hansen, Zamboanga, & Sedlar, 2000). In addi-tion, emphasis on thorough and repeated assessment and functional analysis that examines the conditions and contingencies that influence behavior are valuable for understanding key issues, concerns, and rela-tionships in the youth's sociocultural environment. This helps with understanding the youth's specific social ecology and avoiding appli-cation of simplistic and universal notions about minority populations. SST research and practice also emphasize focusing on socially relevant target behaviors that will be effective in the individual's naturally occurring social interactions and that can be maintained well over time and context. This emphasis on the social validity of intervention goals and on programming for generalization of the effects of treatment is well suited for adapting SST to diverse youth (Hansen et al., 1998).

In a valuable discussion of social skills instruction in school set-tings with "culturally and linguistically different" youth, Cartledge and Loe (2001) made several recommendations for culturally respon-sive SST. They note that diverse youth may be more inclined to have a collectivist orientation that emphasizes the values, goals, and norms of relevant groups, such as peers and their extended family. Those teach-ing social skills must establish a positive connection to the youth and also encourage their sense of responsibility to one another, creating a "community of learners" focused on helping each other. They also emphasize teaching social behaviors that go beyond the immediate peer group, noting that culturally informed SST must help youth have success "within their own subculture as well as the mainstreamed school environment" (p. 41). In addition, Cartledge and Loe recom-mend learning the "generic" model of skills training, versus just fol-lowing a curriculum that teaches a specific set of skills, as that gives the trainer the ability to teach additional specific skills needed by youth in their social context.

Although there is substantial research evaluating SST, relatively little work has been done to specifically examine its application and effectiveness with diverse youth. In a unique effort to examine whether culturally focused SST would be more effective for inner-city youth, Banks, Hogue, Timberlake, and Liddle (1996) compared a group-based "Afrocentric curriculum" to an SST curriculum that was "culturally relevant but not Afrocentric." The Afrocentric curriculum included black history, cultural experiences, values and principles (e.g., purpose, faith), and an examination of the ways in which behaviors may lead to optimal (e.g., unity) or suboptimal (e.g., materialism, self-centeredness) outcomes. Both curricula had similar impact, including reducing anger and increasing assertiveness and self-control. The comparable effects may be attributed to the similarity of the interventions, including being peer-based with culturally relevant elements and language. Despite the lack of differences, Banks et al. (1996) concluded that the Afrocentric approach showed promise as an intervention but needed further study.

In another SST program designed for African American youth, Hammond and Yung (1991) evaluated an intervention for health promotion and risk reduction, positive adolescents choices training (PACT). This group intervention uses role plays and discussion along with a series of videos featuring African American peer role models. The videos were developed to model the targeted behaviors in a more culturally relevant fashion, including language, dress, and situations that would be relatable for minority urban adolescents. The video series, called "Dealing with Anger: A Social Skills Training Program for African-American Youth," is available for purchase (at *www.researchpress.com/books/502/dealing-anger*). The three videos (14–20 minutes long) address: (1) Givin' It—expressing criticism, disappointment, anger, or displeasure calmly in a nonthreatening manner, setting the stage for nonviolent verbal resolution of disputes; (2) Takin' It—listening, understanding, and accepting criticism and anger appropriately; and (3) Workin' It Out—negotiating a solution by listening, identifying problems and solutions, proposing alternatives, and learning to compromise. Results suggest that participation in PACT improves communication, problem solving, and negotiation conflict resolution skills, and it reduces involvement in fighting and juvenile court as compared to untrained youth at the school (Hammond & Yung, 1991).

While not specifically evaluated with minority youth, group interventions can be an effective mode of delivering SST (Smith et al., 2010) that may have some benefits when used with diverse populations. For example, group interventions with peers from similar circumstances (e.g., inner-city youth, Latina youth) increase the cultural relevance of discussions and peer modeling. A group-based format for SST may also provide a valuable alternative for minority youth who have concerns about or who have not responded well in individual-based counseling (Banks et al., 1996). For minority youth with concerns about possible stigma or labels associated with participation, it can be helpful to refer to the treatment group as a "club" (Hammond & Yung, 1991).

Multielement interventions for youth with internalizing disorders that include SST as a component have been demonstrated to be effective for diverse youth. The meta-analysis by Huey and Polo (2008) identified a number of treatments for anxiety and depression in ethnic minority youth as probably or possibly efficacious. For example, Rosselló and colleagues have demonstrated the effectiveness of CBT and IPT in both individual and group formats for treatment of depression in Puerto Rican youth (e.g., Rosselló & Bernal, 1999; Rosselló et al., 2008). Rosselló and Bernal (1996), in a discussion about adapting CBT and IPT for Puerto Rican adolescents, recommended considering several elements or dimensions that have implications for SST. These include language (e.g., culturally appropriate and syntonic), persons (e.g., therapist characteristics, perspective, and relationship), and metaphors (e.g., culturally consonant ideas, sayings, images). Content is also emphasized, including the importance of being consistent with values and traditions, such as *familismo* (e.g., identification and attachment to family), *respeto* (e.g., looking to authority figures for guidance), *simpatia* (e.g., agreement and harmony in relationships), and present-time orientation.

As evidence grows for the effectiveness of various treatment packages with SST elements for internalizing disorders, researchers have begun to examine the utility of the treatments with different populations, including cross-cultural endeavors. For example, Olivares et al. (2002) conducted a quasi-experimental study of adolescents with social phobia who received either CBGT-A, social effectiveness therapy for adolescents—Spanish version (SET-Asv), or *intervención en adolescentes con fobia social*—treatment for adolescents with social phobia (IAFS). Compared to a no-treatment control, all three treatments showed significant reductions in social anxiety as well as improvements in self-esteem and social skills (Olivares et al., 2002). Treatment gains for anxiety symptoms were maintained at a 5-year follow-up (Garcia-Lopez et al., 2006).

The FRIENDS program, a group-based cognitive-behavioral intervention for preventing and treating anxiety and depression, has been examined across a number of different populations, including African American children exposed to community violence who have anxiety problems (Cooley-Quille, Boyd, & Grados, 2004), former Yugoslavian adolescent refugees (Barrett, Moore, & Sonderegger, 2000), and culturally diverse migrant youth with a non-English speaking background (Barrett, Sonderegger, & Sonderegger, 2001). This work has led to a variety of recommendations for the culturally sensitive application of FRIENDS, including consideration of specific cultural needs, such as intergenerational family conflict that accompanies acculturation. Other suggestions include sharing responses verbally instead of writing them down and lessening the number of activities in both sessions and homework, especially when writing was involved, to allow time for completion and not feeling rushed. To make the intervention more culturally relevant and fun, they recommended "incorporation of music, art, and creative stories that are personally relevant" to the youth (Barrett, Sonderegger, & Sonderegger, 2001, p. 89). Cooley-Quille et al. (2004) recommended that examples involving experiences contextually relevant to inner-city children be incorporated into the sessions, including their fears (e.g., death, kidnapping) and challenges (e.g., fights, limited resources). They also recommended that training materials be adapted by using names, pictures, and situations commonly heard or known in the youth's community. Because family structures can be so different, and the concept of family can be very inclusive in some cultures, Cooley-Quille et al. (2004) suggest that questions like "How many people are in your family?" should be changed to "How many people live with you?" (p. 117).

## CONCLUSIONS

Grounded in behavioral and social learning theory, SST has a long history of use for a variety of psychological disorders, including internalizing problems of youth. SST typically involves instructions and rationales, modeling, rehearsal, feedback, praise and reinforcement. It relies heavily on use of other core elements examined in this book, including psychoeducation, modeling, praise and rewards, and homework. Since the 1970s SST has been widely used and extensively researched across many populations and clinical problems. Early research and applications often focused on SST as a sole intervention strategy, although evidence on its effectiveness, including its generalization to real-world interaction and its maintenance over time, was mixed. Presently, it is

most common to find SST for youth with internalizing disorders implemented as an element in multicomponent EBT packages that have been
supported by RCTs. Consideration of the youth's cognitive and social
capabilities, as well as his or her interpersonal context and personal
goals, is important for conducting SST. In addition, efforts to adapt SST
procedures to youth associated with diverse sociocultural backgrounds
and developmental levels are essential.

## BOX 8.2. Illustrative Case Example

Molly R., a 13-year-old Caucasian female, was brought to the clinic by her mother
owing to concerns about her shyness, worry, and depressed mood. Molly was
finishing eighth grade and would be a freshman in a large public high school in a
few months. Her mother, Mrs. R., had noticed that Molly had become increasingly
withdrawn and unhappy during the previous two years of middle school. Mrs. R.
was concerned that high school might be an even more challenging time for Molly
and wanted to help her "get started with more success." Mrs. R. approached Molly
about seeking help from a therapist, and after initially expressing reluctance Molly
came to like the idea and expressed a desire for therapy to help her "be happier
and have friends."

Both Molly and her mother reported that she had often been "shy" and that
this was pervasive from an early age. Through elementary school it was not a concern, as she had several close girl friends whom she hung out with during school
as well as evenings and weekends. During middle school, Molly gradually became
less socially active with friends and lost interest in participating in extracurricular
activities, including the school band. By the end of middle school, girls that were
once close friends were now distant, and Molly had few peer interactions outside of
school. Mrs. R. reported that, even though Molly was a talented musician (playing
both saxophone and piano), she was not enjoying playing music and participating
in the band activities, and so the mother allowed Molly to quit. Eventually, Molly
stopped playing instruments altogether.

Molly's shyness and anxiety in social situations did not meet the criteria for
social anxiety disorder, though features were present, including concerns about
being evaluated negatively by others and some avoidance of social situations.
Depressive symptoms were consistent with mild dysthymia. Molly described herself as becoming increasingly shy and less confident in social situations. She found
daily social situations, like lunchtime in the cafeteria, aversive. As she progressed
through middle school, she found herself sitting more at the fringes of peer discussions and often opening a book to pretend that she were reading while sitting at
the lunch table.

Assessment with Molly focused on determining whether she had not acquired
basic social skills or whether she had the social skills but was not exhibiting them
(e.g., a performance deficit resulting from anxiety and depression). Based on a
variety of information, including interviews with Molly and her mother and informal

role plays with the therapist, it was determined that Molly was lacking in age-appropriate social skills and that her shyness and mild depression interfered with the opportunity and motivation to engage in social interactions. As Molly became less active, less socially confident, and less involved with peers during recent years, she became increasingly unhappy and depressed, which further heightened her withdrawal and isolation. As these problems worsened and Molly's social interactions decreased, she became less confident in and more avoidant of social situations. This resulted in her having less opportunity to socially engage and therefore fewer chances to continue to develop and refine age-appropriate social skills.

Molly agreed to participate in individual CBT that would focus on enhancing her social skills, increasing her successful engagement in social activities, and reducing her depression. Molly's treatment included a number of elements, including (1) psychoeducation on depression, peer relationships, and social skills; (2) activity scheduling to increase engagement in pleasant activities (via setting goals, making plans for behavior change, and self-monitoring and reinforcement); and (3) SST to improve conversational and assertiveness skills. Given this chapter's focus, this illustration primarily details the social skills training aspects of her treatment.

Therapist role plays with Molly indicated that she had basic conversational skills, especially in the nonverbal components (e.g., eye contact, posture, speech volume, etc.). Molly expressed concerns that her challenges were in "knowing what to say," and her awkwardness and lack of confidence regarding conversational content were evident in role plays. Training focused on asking appropriate questions in conversations (e.g., about topics that the other person initiated or about topics that might be of interest to the partner); disclosing appropriate information about one's own interests, hobbies, and background; talking about topics likely to be of interest to peers (e.g., TV, movies, music, school events/activities, food, hobbies); and using speech acknowledgers to convey verbal and nonverbal interest and attention to a partner (e.g., "Yeah," "Really," head nods). The notion that conversational partners should take turns listening and speaking, and spend relatively equal amounts of time talking, was also addressed. Some effort focused on addressing questions and concerns posed by Molly, such as recognizing appropriate times to start a conversation (e.g., the person makes eye contact or says "Hello," vs. looks preoccupied or angry) and how to get started (e.g., good "conversation starter" questions).

In addition to conversation skills, training also focused on basic assertiveness skills. This included reviewing the differences between assertiveness, passiveness, and aggressiveness, and the benefits of being assertive. Attention was focused on situations that required commendatory, refusal, and request assertiveness. Commendatory situations included expressing positive feelings, such as expressing appreciation, and giving and receiving compliments. Refusal situations included saying "No" to others' requests and disagreeing with the opinions or actions of others. Request assertiveness, which may accompany either commendatory or refusal situations, involves asking something of someone to meet a goal or need (e.g., "Will you go to a movie with me?"). This training built on the previous conversational skills taught by addressing different contexts and including the use

(*continued*)

## BOX 8.2 (continued)

of "I statements." Though cooperative, Molly didn't show much interest in the focus on assertiveness except on that for commendatory situations.

The skills training sessions had a common structure that began with identifying the skill being targeted and providing instruction on its importance and use. The therapist then modeled the skill and asked Molly to practice the behavior. For example, the therapist and Molly role-played interactions such as starting up conversations with an unfamiliar peer in the cafeteria and asking an acquaintance to hang out after school. The therapist regularly offered praise, feedback, and suggestions. The sessions concluded with homework assignments to practice the skills Molly was learning. These assignments progressed in complexity and difficulty over the course of treatment as her skills and confidence grew. For example, an early assignment was to ask two conversational questions to familiar peers during the school day, and a later assignment was to ask a peer to hang out after school or a weekend (e.g., a trip to the mall). After assigning homework, the therapist initiated a brief role play to practice the assignment and encourage success. Molly's mother was brought in at the end of sessions periodically to review progress and the goals for the week.

Treatment continued for a total of 18 sessions over 7 months, with the last two sessions scheduled 3 weeks apart to fade treatment and allow time for practice. The efforts to enhance Molly's social skills complemented efforts to increase her engagement in pleasant activities. Molly and her therapist regularly discussed activities that she might enjoy doing and established activity goals for each week. Initially, pleasant activities included practicing the piano, baking with her mother, and journaling. As Molly's social skills and confidence increased, activity goals, included opportunities to interact with peers across a variety of social situations. She was progressively more engaged in school activities, enjoying time with peers, and more active overall. This included participating in a high school "Key Club" (for service and leadership) and a film club. Molly and her mother were both pleased with the progress made, reporting that Molly was more active and engaged with peers, more confident in her social skills, and happier and less depressed.

# 9

## Praise and Rewards

### BACKGROUND OF THE ELEMENT

Praise and rewards are behavioral strategies that use positive rein-forcement, such as social praise, tangible prizes, tokens, and reward-ing activities, to increase or strengthen desired behaviors. Through the use of positive consequences, clinicians, parents, or teachers can help children to develop more adaptive behaviors (King & Ollendick, 1997). More formally defined, a positive reinforcer is "an event, behav-ior, privilege, or material object that will increase the probability of occurrence of any behavior upon which it is contingent" (Masters et al., 1987, p. 189). For example, a socially anxious child who earns a small prize, verbal praise, or special privilege for introducing him- or herself to a new peer will be more likely to repeat that behavior in the future. Similarly, a depressed adolescent may feel more motivated to complete pleasant events scheduling if he or she earns points that can be exchanged for tangible prizes for completing a daily assignment. As both of these examples illustrate, praise and rewards can be used to gradually modify behavior consistent with treatment goals and thereby aid in the alleviation of anxiety or depression. Although other contingency management strategies such as negative reinforcement (i.e., withdrawing an aversive stimulus to increase the rate of perfor-mance) or punishment can also be used to change behavior, it is usu-ally preferable to increase adaptive behaviors through the use of posi-tive reinforcement (Masters et al., 1987). As such, this chapter focuses on the positive reinforcement strategies (i.e., praise and rewards) commonly used in the cognitive-behavioral treatment of internalizing disorders among children and adolescents.

## Brief History

Gaining a broader contextual understanding of praise and rewards begins with a brief review of its history. Edward Thorndike was one of the first individuals to discuss the concept of positive reinforcement when he studied how cats learned to escape from wooden puzzle boxes to reach food that was placed outside of the box. Thorndike (1911) observed that, through a process of trial and error, the cats learned the connection between the action required to escape the box and the food reward. This research led Thorndike to formulate the law of effect, which states that responses to a given stimulus that are rewarding or satisfying to an animal will lead to stronger stimulus-response connections. Consistent with most learning theorists, Thorndike believed that the gradual strengthening effect of rewards was a general law of behavior. As such, this rule applied to humans and animals and across a wide variety of situations. Several decades later, Clark Hull (1943) echoed Thorndike's ideas by asserting that behavior consists of sets of stimulus–response connections that have formed as a result of reinforcement. He expanded upon the law of effect by proposing that there are many factors that can enhance or inhibit the development of stimulus-response connections, including drive (e.g., hunger level), the strength or amount of reinforcement, and the number of times that reinforcement has been presented after a particular stimulus.

With his introduction of the operant conditioning concept, B. F. Skinner (1953a, 1969) made a landmark contribution to principles of reinforcement. Specifically, Skinner posited that any emitted behavior could be considered an "operant" because it is operating on the environment. Once emitted, that operant results in consequences that can be either rewarding (i.e., strengthen a response) or punishing (i.e., weaken a response) through a process called operant conditioning. Skinner also introduced an important variant of operant conditioning referred to as "shaping," which involved rewarding a series of random movements one step at a time until a specific sequence of behavior was learned. In formulating this concept, Skinner conducted research with rats and pigeons using a puzzle box that contained a bar that would dispense pellets of food when pressed (for rats) or a disk that would release a drawer of food when pecked (for pigeons). In addition to having equipment outside of the box that recorded the animal's behavior, the box could be programmed to reinforce behavior after regular or intermittent intervals, which allowed Skinner to study the effects of various schedules of reinforcement on behavior. Based on such laboratory research, Skinner set forth several principles of reinforcement that also applied to human behavior. For instance, intermittent reinforcement delivered at irregular intervals results in behavior that is more difficult to extinguish than intermittent reinforcement delivered at regular intervals (Hunt, 2007). Skinner's methods for operant conditioning and shaping behavior (i.e., rewarding successive approximations of the desired behavior until the desired behavior is achieved) influenced behavior management strategies used in schools and mental hospitals, providing the foundation for all contemporary behavior modification programs.

## Theory Base

The history review provides a solid foundation for understanding the theoretical underpinnings for the use of praise and rewards in the treatment of internalizing problems. Importantly, various reinforcement contingencies can serve to maintain or even exacerbate children's symptoms of anxiety or depression. For example, children's anxious behaviors may be both positively reinforced through attention from parents or teachers and negatively reinforced through avoidance of anxiety-provoking situations (Gosch, Flannery-Schroeder, & Compton, 2006). Similarly, depressed children or adolescents who have withdrawn from previously enjoyable activities and are lacking positive reinforcement may set small goals for increasing their activity level and reward themselves for reaching these goals. Whether the goal is to increase children's ability to face feared situations or their willingness to engage in daily pleasant events and social activities, praise and rewards can be used to positively reinforce and shape more adaptive behavior. An in-depth understanding of several basic theoretical principles related to reinforcement enables one to more effectively implement this core treatment element.

One of the most widely known reinforcement principles is sometimes referred to as "Grandma's rule" but is more technically known as the Premack principle (Premack, 1965). The principle is that more frequently occurring (i.e., higher probability) behaviors can serve as reinforcers for less frequent (i.e., lower probability) behaviors. For example, going out to play can be made contingent on completing homework. Interestingly, this principle holds regardless of whether the higher probability behaviors are considered particularly enjoyable, although those that are aversive are not typically reinforcing. For example, Azrin, Vinas, and Ehle (2007) found that among children with attention-deficit/hyperactivity disorder (ADHD), calm and attentive behavior (lower probability behavior) could be reinforced through opportunities to engage in physical activity (higher probability behavior). Similarly, for a socially anxious child, engagement in social activities (e.g., ordering food at a restaurant, attending a birthday party) could be reinforced with higher probability behavior, such as quiet time to read or work on a hobby.

A closely related principle comes from the response deprivation hypothesis, which states that if an organism is deprived of the opportunity to respond as often as it typically would, that response becomes a reinforcer (Timberlake & Allison, 1974). For example, video game playing will not be reinforcing for a child who typically spends a great deal of time playing video games. However, if the child is deprived of the opportunity to play video games for several days and then told that he or she can play video games after completing one's homework, the child will complete the homework quickly because the video games have become a powerful reinforcer. As these examples highlight, principles related to these response theories of reinforcement could lead to more effective implementation of the praise and rewards treatment element, ensuring the selection and administration of rewards that are particularly reinforcing for a given child.

More recent conceptualizations of the etiology of anxiety and depression also inform our understanding of praise and rewards. According to the approach–withdrawal theory of anxiety (Delprato & McGlynn, 1984), the development of avoidance is conceptualized as "relaxation-approach" behavior. Individuals faced with an aversive stimulus actively approach situations that signal safety. When the safe area is reached, relaxation or relief responses occur, and it is these responses that positively reinforce the avoidance behavior. Therefore, avoidance behavior is maintained through the relationship between avoidance and relaxation. Notably, approach–withdrawal theory is one of the few theoretical perspectives on the etiology of anxiety with positive reinforcement as a key component (Delprato & McGlynn, 1984). Drawing upon this theory, the treatment of phobias and school refusal behavior involves closely examining factors that positively reinforce the avoidance behavior (e.g., positive attention from a parent, participating in enjoyable activities when staying home from school), eliminating these contingencies, and implementing positive reinforcement of more adaptive behavior.

Applying these principles to mood disorders, Lewinsohn (1975) posited that overall low rates of positive reinforcement and high rates of negative reinforcement led to dysphoric mood and ultimately to depression. Lending empirical support to this theory, Lewinsohn and Amenson (1978) found that depressed individuals reported significantly lower frequency and enjoyability of pleasant events and significantly higher frequency and aversiveness of unpleasant events, in comparison to nondepressed individuals. Lewinsohn (1975) also theorized that modifying learned social behaviors (e.g., assertiveness, communicating with others) and increasing pleasant events would lead to more rewarding social interactions and decreased levels of depression. Indeed, Grosscup and Lewinsohn (1980) reported that during the course of treatment, decreases in the frequency of unpleasant events and increased engagement in pleasant events were associated with clinical improvement in depressive symptoms among depressed adults.

Following Lewinsohn's theory, Rehm (1977) emphasized the role of self-control, linking depression with impairments in individuals' abilities to self-monitor, evaluate, and reward their own behavior. Supporting this theory, Fuchs and Rehm (1977) evaluated a behavior therapy program for adults based upon Rehm's self-control theory of depression. The program focused on self-monitoring of daily pleasant events and mood, setting goals, and self-evaluating and self-rewarding by using a point system with reward menu to reinforce progress with goals. In comparison to individuals in nonspecific group therapy, those in self-control therapy demonstrated significantly greater reductions in depressive symptoms, greater improvement in overall distress, and improved self-control skills. Empirical support for self-control training with children and adolescents has also been reported (e.g., Stark et al., 1987) and is discussed in a subsequent section of this chapter. Both Lewinsohn and Rehm emphasized strategies aimed at increasing rates of positive reinforcement, such as rewarding oneself for engaging in pleasant events and implementing ongoing self-evaluation and reward for treatment progress, which are key components of the praise and rewards element in contemporary CBT programs.

## Evidence Base

Several classic anxiety treatment studies provide empirical support for the theories of reinforcement offered by the behaviorists. For example,

Obler and Terwilliger (1970) successfully treated children with phobias (e.g., of using a public bus or seeing a live dog) through gradual exposure to the feared stimulus, followed by verbal encouragement and tangible rewards. Another study targeted fear of the dark among preschool and kindergarten-aged children with a "reinforced practice" approach in which children received reinforcement (e.g., verbal praise, small prizes) for spending increasingly more time in a dark room and were given feedback on their progress (Leitenberg & Callahan, 1973). Children in a treatment group improved significantly relative to a no-treatment control group. Also targeting nighttime fears, Graziano and colleagues (Graziano, Mooney, Huber, & Iginasiak, 1979) implemented a program that included giving "bravery tokens" to children for practicing various skills (e.g., relaxation, positive imagery, brave self-statements) and for sleeping in their rooms alone at night. With eight to nine sessions of training, all seven children reached the criterion of 10 consecutive fearless nights, and gains were maintained through a 1-year follow-up.

There is also ample evidence supporting the effectiveness of praise and rewards as part of multicomponent interventions for internalizing disorders among youth. In addition to briefly reviewing the empirical evidence in this section, readers may refer to Table 9.1 for a description of how the praise and rewards element is incorporated into various treatment manuals. The list is illustrative, not exhaustive, and highlights representative manuals that are evidence-based and commonly used for the treatment of anxiety and depression among youth. For example, Coping Cat is a well-known anxiety treatment manual that utilizes contingent reinforcement (i.e., verbal praise during session, reward system implemented by clinician and/or parent) to reward children's gradual progress toward facing their fears (Kendall & Hedtke, 2006). Children are taught to evaluate their own efforts and use self-reinforcement when appropriate. Results of several waitlist-controlled trials provide evidence for the effectiveness of this program for 9- to 13-year-old children, demonstrating significant treatment effects at posttreatment with gains maintained across 1-year (Kendall, 1994; Kendall et al., 1997), 2- to 5-year (Kendall & Southam-Gerow, 1996), 7.4-year (Kendall et al., 2004), and 16-year follow-up periods (Benjamin et al., 2013).

Similarly, Silverman et al. (1999) found support for the efficacy of a 10-week exposure-based contingency management program for 6- to 16-year-old children and adolescents with phobias. In this program, parents were trained in behavioral principles that included positive reinforcement, shaping, and extinction (i.e., removal of existing

TABLE 9.1. The Praise and Rewards Element in Representative EBT Manuals

| | |
|---|---|
| *Coping Cat* (Kendall & Hedtke, 2006) | • The clinician explicitly teaches the use of praise and rewards as part of the R (results and rewards) step of the FEAR plan. The youth practice this skill during the second half of treatment as they complete exposure tasks, rating their level of success with each task and rewarding themselves accordingly. Rewards for effort (not just total success) are emphasized. |
| *C.A.T. Project* (Kendall, Choudhury, Hudson, & Webb, 2002) | • The clinician explicitly teaches the use of praise and rewards as part of the R (results and rewards) step of the FEAR plan. The youth practice this skill when completing exposure tasks, rating their level of success with facing fears and rewarding themselves accordingly. Rewards for effort are encouraged. |
| *Family-Based Treatment for Young Children with OCD* (Freeman & Garcia, 2009) | • The clinician explicitly discusses praise and rewards, and this skill is utilized throughout treatment. The parents learn about the importance of positive reinforcement and develop a reward program that is discussed with the youth. The parents are taught to provide praise and positive attention when the youth complete their homework tasks. |
| *OCD in Children and Adolescents* (March & Mulle, 1998) | • The clinician explicitly teaches the child and parents about the use of praise and rewards, and this skill is practiced throughout treatment as the child works to "boss back" OCD. The parents are coached in providing specific praise, and the child's accomplishments in resisting OCD are rewarded with verbal praise, prizes, and ceremonies. |
| *CBT of Childhood OCD: It's Only a False Alarm* (Piacentini, Langley, & Roblek, 2007) | • The clinician explicitly teaches the use of praise and rewards to the youth and parents. A behavioral reward program is used to reinforce completion of ERP tasks completed in-session and for homework. Rewards for compliance are negotiated between the child, clinician, and parents throughout treatment. |
| *CBT for Social Phobia: Stand Up, Speak Out* (Albano & DiBartolo, 2007) | • Praise and rewards are briefly mentioned in the context of other skills being taught during treatment. For example, the youth learn to administer praise or self-reinforcement for successfully changing automatic thoughts during cognitive restructuring, and they reward themselves for the effective use of problem solving. |
| *When Children Refuse School (Treatments That Work): A Cognitive-Behavioral Approach* (Kearney & Albano, 2007): Chapters 4 and 5 on internalizing symptoms | • Praise is mentioned briefly in the context of using problem solving to identify and change negative thoughts related to social situations (i.e., "Praise yourself for using these steps"). Other chapters in this manual mention implementing rewards for school attendance (Chapter 6—refusing school for attention) and designing a treatment contract that incorporates rewards (Chapter 7—refusing school for tangible rewards outside of school). |

*(continued)*

**TABLE 9.1.** (*continued*)

| | |
|---|---|
| *Treating Trauma and Traumatic Grief in Children and Adolescents* (Cohen, Mannarino & Deblinger, 2006) | • The use of praise and rewards is discussed within the parenting skills component of treatment. The parents are taught to effectively praise positive behavior while ignoring negative behavior and to use behavior charts with rewards to increase appropriate behavior. |
| *Adolescent Coping with Depression* (Clarke, Lewinsohn, & Hops, 1990) | • Praise and rewards are explicitly introduced and practiced during treatment. The youth are taught to notice and praise group members' positive behavior, and the group leader provides specific praise for the completion of pleasant events scheduling, relaxation skills, and role-play exercises. The youth also create a treatment contract that includes rewards for accomplishing treatment goals. |
| *Treating Depressed Children: Therapist Manual for "Taking Action"* (Stark & Kendall, 1996) | • Praise and rewards are explicitly taught and practiced throughout the treatment. At the beginning of treatment, clinicians help the children establish a reward system to be used during group sessions and work with the parents to establish rewards that their children can earn for completing daily workbook assignments at home. |
| *Treating Depressed Youth: Therapist Manual for "Action"* (Stark et al., 2007) | • The use of praise and rewards is explicitly taught and practiced on a weekly basis during treatment. A within-group reward system is used in which the youth earn prizes for attending sessions and completing homework assignments. They are also taught to notice and record positive things that happen each week by using a Catch the Positive Diary and to compliment other group members for positive behavior during each session. |
| *Psychotherapy for Children with Bipolar and Depressive Disorders* (Fristad, Arnold, & Leffler, 2011) | • The use of praise and rewards is briefly mentioned as a general therapeutic issue that relates to individual and multifamily versions of this treatment. The clinicians are encouraged to establish basic rules for the children and a reward system for behavior management during sessions that incorporates points or tokens that can be exchanged for prizes. |

*Note.* Some book titles are shortened to conserve space. See the References at the back of the book for full titles.

rewards for nondesired behavior to hopefully eliminate those behaviors). Parents and children created a contingency contract that outlined the rewards children would receive for completing exposure tasks listed on their fear hierarchies. Participants in the exposure-based contingency management program improved significantly, and these gains were maintained across 3-, 6-, and 12-month follow-up assessments. There was not a significant difference in terms of treatment outcomes between the exposure-based contingency management and the other two groups (i.e., exposure-based cognitive self-control, education support) in this study. Notably, however, praise and rewards were incorporated in the exposure-based cognitive self-control condition, as children were taught to use self-evaluation and self-reward when practicing in-session and out-of-session exposure tasks. Children and parents in the education support condition were not taught about praise and rewards or any other therapeutic strategies, but did learn about behavioral theory related to the maintenance of anxiety disorders (e.g., that phobias may be maintained owing to positive consequences).

Regarding the use of praise and rewards for depression, several studies have evaluated self-control training, which includes coaching in self-reinforcement strategies. As depressed individuals tend to engage in high levels of self-punishment and low levels of reinforcement, training in self-reinforcement (i.e., self-reward for performance of desired behaviors) helps youth increase their activity level and learn other skills for coping with depression (Reynolds & Stark, 1987). In evaluating self-control training, Stark et al. (1987) randomly assigned 9- to 12-year-old children with moderate to severe levels of depressive symptoms to either a 12-session (5-week) self-control (SC) or behavioral problem-solving (BPS) intervention, or a waitlist control group. Both treatment groups were trained in self-monitoring to track involvement in pleasant activities and received rewards and praise for completing self-monitoring log sheets. Participants in the self-control group were also taught to hold more realistic standards for their performance, adopt a more adaptive attributional style, and monitor and self-reward their performance and cognitions across a variety of situations. Both intervention groups evidenced significant improvement in both self-reported and clinician-assessed symptoms of depression as compared to the waitlist control group at posttreatment, and gains were maintained through an 8-week follow-up (Stark et al., 1987). There is also empirical support for self-control training for depressed adolescents, with those enrolled in self-control or relaxation training with use of rewards showing significantly greater improvement in depressive symptoms (as well as anxiety and academic self-concept) than those in a waitlist control group, both at posttreatment and at a 5-week follow-up assessment (Reynolds & Coats, 1986).

Several studies have evaluated the efficacy of CWD-A, a group treatment program for depressed adolescents that includes various skill modules, including cognitive restructuring, increasing activity level and social interactions, problem solving and communication, relaxation training, and goal setting (Clarke & DeBar, 2010). Self-reward is incorporated at various points in the program. Adolescents are taught to set small goals for increasing particular skills (e.g., activity level, positive thinking), make a written contract that specifies rewards they will receive for accomplishing these goals, and then reward themselves accordingly. Lewinsohn and colleagues (1990) assessed the efficacy of CWD-A with a sample of 14- to 18-year-old adolescents. Participants were randomly assigned to an adolescent-only treatment group, adolescent-and-parent treatment group, or the waitlist condition. Both treatment groups had significantly more improvement in depressive symptoms relative to the waitlist group at posttreatment, and gains were maintained a 1-, 6-, 12-, and 24-month follow-up assessments for the two treatment groups (Lewinsohn et al., 1990). A recent meta-analysis also provides support for the efficacy of CWD-A in preventing a reoccurrence of major depressive disorder (MDD) in adolescents (Cuijpers, Muñoz, Clarke, & Lewinsohn, 2009). Results showed that teens previously diagnosed with MDD (but not currently) have a 38% lower chance of developing a new case of a major depression compared to nonparticipants.

## THE ELEMENT IN PRACTICE

This section of the chapter focuses on the "nuts and bolts" of implementing the praise and rewards element with anxious and depressed youth. A step-by-step description is summarized in the task analysis format in  Box 9.1 and supplemented by a narrative below offering several basic principles to consider when implementing praise and rewards. Suggestions for tailoring this element to particular diagnoses are provided, along with a case example at the end of the chapter illustrating what the praise and rewards element would look like in practice when implemented with an 8-year-old male with separation anxiety disorder (see Box 9.2). Finally, possible adaptations for use with youth of different developmental levels and diverse racial and ethnic backgrounds are discussed.

### "Core of the Core" Element

Across the various treatment manuals for anxiety and depression, praise and rewards are implemented in different ways. All, however, aim to teach children the basic principles of praise and rewards and how to monitor their progress and self-reward. Therapists work together with the youth to develop a list of possible rewards for accomplishing

## BOX 9.1. Task Analysis of Praise and Rewards

1. The clinician conducts a functional analysis of stimuli that are positively or negatively reinforcing the youth's target behavior.

2. The clinician introduces the concepts of self-rating and reward to the youth during a session:
   a. Provide the definition of a reward, using concrete and age-appropriate examples.
   b. Introduce the idea of evaluating one's performance in particular situations by using self-ratings, employing cartoon strips and clinician modeling.
   c. Emphasize the importance of rewarding one's effort and partial success rather than perfect performance.

3. The clinician and youth collaboratively brainstorm a list of potential reinforcers to increase target behavior, using the following strategies:
   a. The clinician develops a list of possible rewards with the child during treatment sessions.
   b. The clinician obtains input from parents, particularly for younger children.
   c. The clinician may observe the child in his or her natural environment or informally in the waiting room before or after therapy sessions.
   d. Consider diverse types of rewards, including tangible (prizes), social (praise), activities, or tokens/points that can be redeemed for tangible or activity rewards.

4. The clinician trains the child to assess and record his or her target behavior and administer appropriate reinforcement. Have the child practice this sequence in session first, then at home:
   a. Choose a specific target behavior to focus on.
   b. Decide on a reward that will be earned for completing the target behavior.
   c. For homework, ask the child to perform the target behavior a specific number of times during the week or to choose specific days or times or situations in which it would be appropriate to practice the behavior.
   d. The child records his or her progress and whether the goal is accomplished; if so, the appropriate reward is administered by the child or parent.

5. Depending upon the youth's age, the clinician may need to train the parents in the basic principles of praise and rewards and to give them guidelines for helping the child to administer reinforcement for assignments completed outside of therapy sessions.

6. The basic principles for clinicians to keep in mind when implementing praise and rewards are:
   a. Reinforcement should immediately follow the desired behavior.
   b. Reinforcement should be administered in a consistent manner.
   c. The relationship between the target behavior and the reward should be made explicit to the child.
   d. Use continuous reinforcement initially, followed by intermittent reinforcement once a target behavior is established.
   e. Modify the list of rewards if they appear to be losing their effectiveness over time.

treatment goals and engage the parents by discussing the basic principles of praise and rewards with them. The extent to which parents are involved depends on the child's developmental level.

Step-by-step procedures for implementing praise and rewards with anxious and depressed youth are listed in Box 9.1. During the assessment and continuing through the early weeks of treatment, the therapist initiates praise and rewards (Step 1) by conducting a functional analysis to determine events or situations that are positively or negatively reinforcing the child's target behavior (e.g., avoidance of anxiety-provoking situations). To assist in this process, children complete daily diaries to track their mood related to particular events as well as the antecedents and consequences of target behaviors. This information is used to better understand the ways that the child's maladaptive behaviors are being maintained and to alter these contingencies by establishing a reward system for more adaptive behaviors. Therapists typically discuss goals for more adaptive behaviors when reviewing the treatment plan with the children and their parents and revisit these goals to assess progress throughout treatment.

After the functional analysis has been conducted, the concepts of self-rating and reward are introduced (Step 2). The skill of self-evaluation is often practiced by using cartoon strips that show individuals completing an activity such as facing an anxiety-provoking situation and then rating their performance and giving themselves a reward. The cartoon strips include blank thought bubbles that the child fills in to describe the situation. Therapists can also model self-ratings for performance by discussing with the child real-life situations that he or she has faced. Next, the therapist collaboratively brainstorms a list of rewards with the child (Step 3). This process may continue across several sessions, with the clinician asking the child direct questions to determine which rewards will serve as the most powerful reinforcers. Rewards should closely match each child's developmental level and individual preferences. Inventories such as the Children's Reinforcement Survey Schedule (CRSS; Phillips, Fischer, & Singh, 1977) can be used as a tool to help children select effective rewards. This measure includes 89 commonly used reinforcers listed in 12 categories, such as food, toys, sports and games, and excursions. Each category also includes blank spaces in which children can write rewards that are not already listed. Children rate each item on a 1 ("not at all") to 5 ("very much") scale to indicate how appealing the item is to them. Reviewing the CRSS with the child can help determine which items to use as rewards during treatment.

After collaboratively generating a list of possible rewards, the child is taught to record his or her progress in completing the target behavior and then to administer the predetermined reward (Step 4). For younger children, this process may begin with the therapist or parent administering rewards, with a gradual shift to self-administered rewards (Step 5), and is facilitated by helping the child choose a behavior to focus on (e.g., from the treatment plan, fear hierarchy, pleasant events scheduling list) along with a corresponding reward to be earned for completing that behavior. After performing the behavior, the child records his or her progress, and if progress is made the reward is either self-administered or given by the parent.

There are several basic principles to keep in mind when implementing praise and rewards (see Step 6). Reinforcement should immediately follow the desired behavior and be administered as consistently as possible (Spiegler, 2016). In addition, the relationship between the target behavior and reward should be made explicit to the child. Initially, rewards may need to be provided for successive approximations, or small steps made toward the behavior, consistent with treatment goals (Kendall & Hedtke, 2006). It is also important to determine whether the rewards are effectively reinforcing the desired behavior. If not, the rewards may need to be adjusted accordingly. Similarly, the list of rewards may need to be modified during the course of treatment if they seem to lose their effectiveness.

An understanding of such concepts as reinforcement schedules and differential reinforcement is also crucial when implementing praise and rewards. Reinforcement schedules determine how often a target behavior will be reinforced. With continuous reinforcement, target behaviors are rewarded every time they occur. When using intermittent schedules of reinforcement, target behaviors are reinforced after a particular interval of time has passed (i.e., on an interval schedule) or after a particular number of times that the behavior has occurred (i.e., a ratio schedule; Houston, 1991). Although continuous reinforcement is more effective when a new behavior is being established, intermittent schedules are less costly and better for maintaining a behavior over the long term, and the latter also more closely mimic what occurs in a child's natural environment (Spiegler, 2016). In the treatment of anxiety and depression, it is common to use continuous reinforcement at first, followed by intermittent reinforcement once a target behavior is established. Differential reinforcement is also utilized in the treatment of anxiety and depression. Often referred to as *differential reinforcement of other behaviors*, this process involves ignoring maladaptive behaviors (e.g., fear, withdrawal, avoidance) and rewarding target behaviors that are not compatible with the maladaptive behavior (e.g., facing feared situations, engaging in pleasant activities) every time they occur.

In addition to varying the frequency with which rewards are administered, the therapist can employ a variety of different *types* of rewards, including tangible prizes and activities (Kingery et al., 2006). Tangible rewards include material objects such as snacks, toys, and other small prizes. If a reward chart is being used, token reinforcers (e.g., stickers, points) can be exchanged for tangible items. Activities such as special one-on-one time with a parent (e.g., cooking, playing a board game) or inviting a friend to play are social activities that often serve as effective forms of positive reinforcement. Social reinforcement, such as positive attention and praise from other people, can be administered verbally (e.g., "Great job facing your fear!"), in writing (e.g., a note or certificate of accomplishment), or through physical gestures (e.g., pat on the back, smiling). Although therapists or parents may assume that certain events or objects positively reinforce a particular child's behavior, they cannot know for sure whether a potential reinforcer is effective until they observe increases in the desired behavior after that reinforcer is administered (Masters et al., 1987). When administering praise and rewards, it can also be useful to work collaboratively with the youth and their families to create contingency contracts that outline specific behaviors and the reward that a child or adolescent will earn upon completion of those behaviors (Masters et al., 1987).

Although manualized treatments share common principles for implementing praise and rewards, the procedures for administering this treatment element are often tailored to particular diagnoses. In treatment programs that target generalized anxiety disorder, social phobia, and separation anxiety disorder, such as Coping Cat (Kendall & Hedtke, 2006), the youth learn to evaluate their efforts for coping with anxiety and self-administer rewards as they accomplish steps on the fear hierarchy. Emphasis is placed on rewards for effort rather than actual performance. The extent of parental involvement varies, depending upon such factors as the child's age and particular diagnosis. For an example of how the praise and rewards element of Coping Cat and similar programs would be implemented with a young child with separation anxiety disorder, see Box 9.2 at the end of the chapter. In treatment programs for OCD, parents are more directly involved, learning how to provide specific praise and administer tangible rewards such as small prizes and mini-certificates (March & Benton, 2007; March &

Mulle, 1998). Throughout treatment, the clinician, child, and parents collaboratively identify behavioral goals that will be celebrated with particular rewards, ceremonies (e.g., an ice cream party with a friend to celebrate a new stage in treatment), and notifications (e.g., letting others know about children's progress in treatment). Similar to the treatment of other anxiety disorders, obsessions and compulsions are ranked and placed on a stimulus hierarchy. The child utilizes ERP tasks to work his or her way up the hierarchy, with praise and rewards administered as the child completes these tasks successfully by "bossing back" OCD (March & Mulle, 1998).

The use of praise and rewards in the treatment of depression has a slightly different focus. The CWD-A course emphasizes reinforcement during the behavioral activation portion of treatment (Clarke & DeBar, 2010). Teens are taught basic principles related to rewards (e.g., immediately available, something that they really enjoy). They are also asked to create a list of rewards as well as a written contract that specifies rewards that they can earn for meeting daily goals related to engaging in pleasant activities. The youth are taught similar self-evaluation and reward skills during the cognitive restructuring portion of treatment. They set goals related to changing negative thoughts to more positive ones and reward themselves accordingly. One of the group rules of the CWD-A is to be supportive and encouraging of other group members, focusing on the positive things that others are doing and offering praise when appropriate. Similar to CWD-A, the ACTION program for depressed youth incorporates praise and rewards, with the clinician providing verbal praise for group members during each session and the children learning to compliment one another and themselves for exhibiting prosocial behavior. In-session rewards (via a prize bag) are provided for attendance and homework completion, and progress toward individual treatment goals is documented with stickers or points (Stark et al., 2006).

## Developmental Adaptations

To maximize the effectiveness of a reward system, it is crucial to select rewards that match a child's developmental level and individual preferences. Reward lists should be generated collaboratively, as this process helps to ensure that the rewards are valuable for each child and increases the motivation to comply with treatment (Kingery et al., 2006). The types of tangible and activity rewards that appeal to younger children are likely to differ from those that are motivating for older children. Younger children gravitate toward tangible rewards such as candy, school supplies, Matchbox cars, movie rental coupons, and other small prizes. Regarding activities, younger youth might appreciate spending special one-on-one time with a parent or the clinician (e.g., reading a book, playing a board game), choosing a favorite restaurant for a family outing, or having a play date with a friend. In contrast, older children and adolescents may prefer such rewards as gift cards for clothing stores or MP3 downloads, video games, additional computer or phone time, or the privilege of staying up later. Although they may also enjoy special activities with a parent or clinician, adolescents tend to prefer peer-oriented activities, such as inviting a friend over, earning the privilege to stay out later, or engaging in special activities with friends (e.g., at an amusement park or sporting event). Keep in mind that rewards need not be monetary, which could be stressful for some families. Many of the rewards noted above are social and cost the family little if anything.

Praise and rewards administered during treatment sessions also need to be developmentally appropriate. For example, the ACTION program for depressed girls uses individual charts to track progress toward treatment goals during each session, with stickers utilized for younger children and check marks for older children and adolescents (Stark, Hargrove, et al., 2006). During the course of treatment, reward lists may need to be updated to reflect a child's current interests and to ensure that rewards are maintaining their potency. Regardless of a child's age, praise from therapists and parents and a child's own feelings of pride in his or her accomplishments often serve as one of the most powerful motivators, allowing tangible rewards to be faded out gradually over the course of time (Kendall & Suveg, 2006).

In addition to matching the *types* of rewards to a child's age or developmental level, the *frequency* and *timing* of rewards may need to be modified, particularly when working with younger children. With respect to the treatment of OCD, Freeman and Garcia (2009) emphasize that rewards can be administered to older children over longer periods of time (e.g., resisting checking or counting behavior for a whole day), whereas younger children need more frequent feedback (e.g., rewards given for resisting hand washing every few hours or before each meal). Relatedly, older children usually respond to reward systems that involve earning points, stickers, or tokens that can be saved and exchanged for tangible prizes at a later point in time. Given their limitations with abstract reasoning, younger children often require tangible reinforcers (e.g., small prizes) that are given immediately after a desired behavior. With older children, it may be possible to connect a reward to several related behaviors (e.g., a series of steps in an exposure task), whereas younger children may need the task to be broken down into smaller steps with a reward provided after each step that is successfully accomplished.

The extent of parental involvement is another important developmental consideration. For younger and less developmentally advanced children, parents often need to provide direct assistance with executing exposure exercises, coaching children in coping skills learned during treatment, and keeping track of rewards earned for treatment progress (Kingery et al., 2006). Older children and adolescents are likely to implement the self-evaluation and reward skills learned in treatment with more autonomy, relying on parents to provide subtle reminders about the reward system or verbal praise for completing homework assignments outside of therapy sessions. Manualized treatment programs vary in terms of the extent to which parents are formally incorporated into treatment. For example, the Coping Cat program (Kendall & Hedtke, 2006) includes just two formal parent sessions, but parents are involved in a supportive role throughout treatment. With respect to praise and rewards, parents are encouraged to praise children's progress, offer input on the rewards list, and assist with administering rewards earned for exposure tasks (particularly for younger children). Other manuals, such as the FRIENDS program, involve parents more directly in treatment. This program incorporates four 1½-hour group parent sessions in addition to weekly group sessions for children (Barrett & Shortt, 2003). In this program, one of the parent sessions is focused on contingency management strategies, including the use of tangible rewards, specific praise, and planned ignoring. After learning the basic principles, parents practice the contingency management strategies through group role-play exercises and then implement them with their child outside of treatment sessions.

Regardless of the specific treatment manual being used, Suveg, Roblek, and colleagues (2006) emphasize the importance of training parents of anxious children in effective contingency management strategies, including parental reinforcement for "brave" (i.e., approach) behavior and ignoring inappropriate behavior. Parents can also be taught the importance of removing unintentional reinforcers, such as parental attention for anxious and avoidant behaviors. According to Suveg et al., written contingency contracts that outline the exposure task to be completed and the corresponding reward are an effective way to reduce parents' tendency to "rescue" their child from anxiety-provoking situations (e.g., not leaving the child with a babysitter, allowing the child to stay home from school or social events).

Another approach, proposed by Ginsburg, Silverman, and Kurtines (1995), is a transfer of control model. This model proposes that effective treatment of child anxiety involves a gradual transfer of treatment strategies from clinician to parent to child. With respect to praise and rewards, clinicians can coach parents in generating a reward system, who then implement the system at home. Children gradually gain more autonomy as they learn to use self-control strategies such as cognitive restructuring, self-evaluation, and self-reward. Khanna and Kendall (2009) evaluated associations between specific parent training techniques for the treatment of childhood anxiety, including transfer of control and parent anxiety management training, on child outcomes. Results indicated that the transfer-of-control component of treatment contributed significantly to improvements in global functioning for 7- to 14-year-old children who were involved in a CBT program with a family component.

In summary, many of the developmental modifications discussed in this section rely on parents' ability to understand and implement reward systems effectively outside of the therapy sessions. As Freeman and Garcia (2009) emphasize, it is important to develop reward systems in collaboration with parents so that they understand what is expected of them and feel that it is feasible for them to implement the program in a consistent manner. Similarly, it is crucial for parents to understand the treatment rationale and importance of daily practice so that they can reinforce skills learned in therapy with their child at home.

## Diversity Considerations

Sensitivity to cultural and ethnic background is another important consideration. Unfortunately, however, research evaluating the effectiveness of cognitive-behavioral interventions in general and examining the praise and rewards component specifically across youth from diverse ethnic backgrounds is fairly limited. Nonetheless, there is robust support for the notion that reinforcement is a powerful motivator for all individuals. In fact, positive and negative reinforcement are considered to be "laws of behavior" that are universal and therefore not limited to a particular situation or species (Skinner, 1969; Thorndike, 1911).

Several studies evaluating CBT programs that include a praise and rewards component have reported similar levels of improvement across ethnic groups. For example, Treadwell, Flannery-Schroeder, and Kendall (1995) reported that African American and Caucasian children (ages 9–13 years) experienced similar improvements in anxiety symptoms and diagnoses in response to a 16-session CBT program. Similarly, Southam-Gerow, Kendall, and Weersing (2001) found that child ethnicity was not a predictor of response to cognitive-behavioral treatment of anxiety, either at posttreatment or 1-year follow-up. Notably, these two studies involved *primarily* Caucasian participants, limiting the ability to draw firm conclusions about differential outcome by ethnicity from these findings.

Several studies also have examined the effectiveness of CBT for particular ethnic groups, yielding promising results. For example, Ginsburg and Drake (2002) evaluated the feasibility and effectiveness of school-based CBT for a small sample of anxious African American adolescents ($N = 12$), in which participants were randomly assigned to CBT or an attention-support control condition. Participants in this study were recruited from an urban high school, where 35% of the students were living below the poverty level and 75% were from single-parent households. The CBT program utilized in this study included psychoeducation, relaxation skills, cognitive restructuring, and exposure tasks using a fear hierarchy, contingency contracts, and self-administered rewards. According to the researchers, examples from the treatment manual were modified to include situations that participants encountered in their daily lives, including neighborhood violence, drug use, and financial hardship. Results revealed significantly greater diagnostic and symptom-level improvement for adolescents in the CBT group. Ginsburg and Drake indicated that the response rates for this study were similar to those in studies involving predominantly Caucasian samples and concluded that CBT can be used successfully with adolescents from diverse backgrounds.

In another study, Pina and associates (2003) evaluated data from two randomized clinical trials for anxiety disorders to examine response rates of Hispanic/Latino and European American youths to an exposure-based cognitive-behavioral anxiety treatment. Across the two trials, 60% of the participants were European American, and 40% were Hispanic/Latino. The intervention being evaluated included contingency management procedures such as positive reinforcement, shaping, and contingency contracting. Results indicated that the two groups had similar response rates (in terms of diagnosis and symptoms), comparable effect sizes, and similar maintenance of treatment gains across 3-, 6-, and 12-month follow-up periods. Pina and colleagues point to the importance of additional treatment research with Hispanic/Latino youth to examine the role of immigration and acculturation stressors, evaluate treatments administered to youth from particular Hispanic/ Latino subcultures, and examine the effectiveness of treatments that are administered in Spanish. Although the role of a Spanish-speaking cotherapist has been discussed in a case study for the behavioral treatment involving exposure and contingency management for a 10-year-old Hispanic female with selective mutism (Vecchio & Kearney, 2007), very few studies have addressed this topic and further research is needed.

Harmon, Langley, and Ginsburg (2006) emphasize the importance of taking the time to understand differences in beliefs and norms when working with children and adolescents from diverse backgrounds. Specifically relevant to the use of praise and rewards, it may be important to involve grandparents or other extended family members in implementing reward systems. To show sensitivity to a family's socioeconomic situation, it may be necessary to incorporate activity-based and tangible rewards that are low in cost. For families in which parents have multiple jobs and very little time to spend with their children, the expectations for implementing reward systems also need to be feasible. Regardless of a family's cultural or socioeconomic background, parents or other adult family members may hold particular beliefs about praise and rewards. For example, some parents believe that children should not receive rewards for behaviors that they should be exhibiting on a regular basis (e.g., attending school or social events, completing other tasks assigned during therapy sessions). They may believe that they are "bribing" their children. When working with such parents, it can be helpful to spend more time explaining the rationale and strategies behind the praise and rewards aspect of treatment. Making a distinction between a bribe and reward may also be useful. Whereas a bribe reinforces *undesirable* behavior, a reward reinforces *desirable* behavior. Emphasizing that the ultimate goal is for children to reap the intangible rewards associated with engaging in target behaviors (e.g., feeling proud for facing their fears, having fun when engaging in a pleasant event) so that tangible rewards can be faded out gradually over the course of time is important as well.

## CONCLUSIONS

The praise and rewards treatment element is grounded in a rich history as well as core behavioral principles and theory. Furthermore, the evidence base supporting the effective use of this treatment element includes studies evaluating the praise and rewards element alone and multicomponent CBT programs that include praise and rewards. To implement this core treatment element effectively, it is essential to understand the basic theories and principles related to reinforcement. The step-by-step procedures outlined in this chapter can serve as a helpful and practical resource. Modifications may be needed for various diagnoses, developmental levels, and children and adolescents from diverse backgrounds. As with other components of manualized treatment programs, the strategies related to praise and rewards must be continually adapted to meet the needs of each individual child and family.

## BOX 9.2. Illustrative Case Example

Sam was an 8-year-old Caucasian male who met the criteria for separation anxiety disorder and was seen for 12 sessions of individual CBT. He was in the third grade and lived with his mother, father, and 12-year-old sister. Regarding the symptoms of separation anxiety, Sam slept in his parents' bed every night because he was afraid to sleep alone. During the day, he followed his mother and/or father around the house and was afraid to spend time in a room by himself at home. He became very upset when his mother or father needed to go somewhere without him, because he worried that something bad would happen to them. Although he invited friends to play at his home, Sam avoided going over to friends' houses to play unless his mother or father could stay with him. He did not attend events such as birthday parties or sleepovers and refused to stay at home with a babysitter. When faced with potential separation from his parents (e.g., before school in the morning), Sam cried and begged his parents to let him stay home. During school hours, he visited the nurse frequently with stomachaches and headaches and often called his parents for reassurance that they were safe. In terms of strengths, Sam had several friends whom he invited to his house to play on a regular basis. He participated in swimming lessons each week but was not involved in any other structured group activities outside of school. Sam and his parents were both motivated to participate in treatment; they attended weekly sessions regularly and practiced CBT skills outside of the therapy sessions each week.

During the assessment phase and first several weeks of treatment, Sam was reluctant to separate from his parents and became tearful when he was asked to do so. Owing to Sam's separation anxiety symptoms and his young age, the clinician encouraged him to participate by incorporating fun and engaging activities into each treatment session. In addition, the clinician promised Sam that if he separated from his parents while participating in treatment he could choose a small prize from a prize box (containing stickers, candy, pretend tattoos, rubber balls, bubbles, and small dinosaur toys) or play a fun game with the clinician at the end of each session (e.g., Guess Who?, Go Fish, Hangman, Pictionary, checkers). Sam responded well to these small tangible and activity rewards provided by the clinician.

Using information gathered during the assessment and through further conversation with Sam and his parents during the early weeks of treatment, the clinician developed an anxiety hierarchy that included a list of exposure tasks to help Sam gradually face his fears. After brainstorming the list of exposure tasks, Sam and his parents helped the clinician put the tasks in order from least to most difficult. For example, Sam first practiced staying in a room alone at home, using a timer to gradually increase the amount of time. Eventually, Sam worked his way up to attending playdates without his parents, staying home while his parents visited a next-door neighbor, staying home with a babysitter, and sleeping alone. To address Sam's difficulties with sleeping alone, the clinician helped his parents to establish a bedtime routine and incorporated sleep-related tasks into the anxiety hierarchy.

With respect to the praise and rewards component of treatment, each separation-related task on the hierarchy was broken down into small, manageable steps, and Sam could earn various rewards when he practiced facing his fears. The clinician worked with Sam and his parents to develop a menu of rewards. The reward list included both tangible and activity rewards that Sam was motivated to earn. The clinician made sure that the list included small rewards that could be administered immediately as well as larger, more long-term rewards that Sam could work toward. Initially, Sam responded best to rewards given immediately after completing a particular exposure task, such as a small prize given by parents or the clinician (e.g., a Matchbox car, a board game with parents, staying up a few minutes later) or a privilege such as choosing a special dessert or television program. After Sam successfully completed several initial exposure tasks, the clinician initiated a token system in which he could earn a certain number of stickers for completing subsequent tasks on his hierarchy. After completing a particular task, he could choose to redeem the stickers immediately for a small prize or activity, or he could choose to "save up" his stickers for a larger reward, such as a special toy (e.g., LEGO kit, superhero action figure) or a more substantial activity with his family or a friend (e.g., movie, bowling, miniature golfing, family game night, meal at favorite restaurant or favorite food cooked at home, ice cream outing). The clinician created a sticker chart for Sam, which he kept on the family's refrigerator and brought to the treatment session each week so that the clinician could assess his progress. During weekly check-ins at the beginning of each session, the clinician discussed the reward system with Sam and his parents and made adjustments as needed. Notably, the clinician made sure that Sam understood that he could earn rewards for effort (e.g., a partial number of stickers for attempting a task), given that perfect performance was not expected.

In addition to weekly check-ins with Sam's parents, there were a few parent-only sessions, when the clinician discussed how Sam's parents' tendency to "rescue" him from anxiety-provoking situations played a role in the maintenance of his anxiety symptoms. The clinician also explained ways in which Sam's parents could ignore his fearful behaviors and selectively attend to "brave" behaviors by providing encouragement, verbal praise, and rewards for his efforts. During the parent sessions, the clinician also helped Sam's parents understand basic principles related to praise and rewards (e.g., the importance of immediate feedback) as well as their role in tracking Sam's progress and implementing rewards outside of the session each week. Toward the end of treatment, the reward system was gradually faded as Sam's engagement in the exposure tasks became inherently rewarding. For example, at the end Sam felt proud of himself for becoming more independent and had fun while participating in various activities without his parents.

# 10

## Activity Scheduling

### BACKGROUND OF THE ELEMENT

Activity scheduling is the process of working with a client to generate a list of enjoyable activities along with a plan to engage in those activities. Unlike the majority of the other elements described in this book that are applied to a variety of internalizing disorders, activity scheduling is found almost exclusively in treatments for depression. Based on evidence that supports a link between engagement in pleasant activities and mood, activity scheduling encourages the child or adolescent to increase involvement in activities that are likely to be positive experiences. For example, a depressed adolescent who has dropped out of the high school orchestra and is spending much of her spare time alone may be encouraged to schedule times to play her violin and socialize with friends. After presenting an overview of the historical and theoretical foundations of activity scheduling, this chapter reviews the empirical evidence supporting the element and provides detailed suggestions for its implementation in interventions for depressed youth. Also included are a discussion of the use of activity scheduling with diverse youth and a case example highlighting the application of activity scheduling in the treatment of a depressed African American adolescent.

### Brief History

A brief review of the history of activity scheduling helps fit its current use in the treatment of depressed youth into a broader context. Activity scheduling, or pleasant events scheduling as it is sometimes called, is rooted in the behavioral principle of reinforcement, which states that behavior is learned and maintained through rewards that are awarded contingent on occurrence of the behavior (Glaser, 1971; Skinner, 1953b). In other words, behaviors that result in some sort of reward are more likely to be repeated. Positive reinforcers (or rewards) increase or maintain the behavior. Positive reinforcers can be tangible (e.g., an ice cream cone, an allowance) or intangible (e.g., feelings of connection, satisfaction, accomplishment; Thorndike, 1935). Positive reinforcement can be used to increase desired behavior. For example, if a child completes his or her homework inconsistently, a system of rewards may be instituted to increase the frequency of homework completion. In contrast, the absence of positive reinforcement leads to a reduction in behavior, and less frequent behavior then results in lower levels of reinforcement. Therefore, if the reward frequency is decreased in our example, the child will likely decrease his or her homework completion. This consequent decrease in homework behavior then means less chance of the homework behavior being rewarded, simply because the behavior occurs so infrequently.

Beginning in the 1930s, early discussions of positive reinforcement included debates regarding the optimal timing of rewards to increase behavior, investigations of the differential effectiveness of various types of reinforcement, and theories as to how rewarding certain behaviors could result in complex cognitive operations like problem solving or reasoning (Glaser, 1971). Within this early context, Thorndike (1935) noted an association between repeated participation in an activity and a subsequent increase in mood. Interestingly, Thorndike (1935) observed that this relation occurred even when an individual did not cognitively appraise the activity as inherently positive. Thus, even if an individual does not expect to enjoy a party, but attends anyway, it is likely that the individual will feel happier. Thorndike (1935) stated that the increase in mood likely results from unexpected positive results/rewards from participating in the activity. Early clinical applications of positive reinforcement included behavioral modification programs primarily in educational settings with youth and influenced later behavioral conceptualizations of mental illness, including depression (Ferster, 1973).

The use of activity scheduling emerged from the observed association between positive reinforcement and mood, and early theories of depression considered a lack of reinforcement as a potential cause of the disorder and an increase in activities that engender reinforcing experiences as central to treatment. Early theorists viewed withdrawal from social interactions, low rate of activity, and feelings of dysphoria as key symptoms of depression and suggested that they were interrelated (Lewinsohn, Sullivan, & Grosscup, 1980). Increased social isolation and reduced activity likely lead to lower levels of positive reinforcement and thus lower levels of positive mood. Activity scheduling became a component in behavioral treatments for depression in an attempt to facilitate awareness of the link between reinforcement and mood and to actively increase positive mood through the planning and participation in activities that had a high likelihood of engendering rewards (Lewinsohn et al., 1980).

## Theory Base

An understanding of the theory underlying the use of activity scheduling assists in its clinical application. Early evidence that positive reinforcement could increase human behavior influenced behavioral theories of the etiology and treatment of depression. For example, Ferster (1973) theorized that the initial depressed state likely occurs in the context of a dramatic change in the individual's environment that results in a reduction of available positive reinforcers. For example, the illness of a parent could be a precipitating factor for a child, as the parent may be physically unable to provide many of the usual rewards in the child's life (e.g., smiles, hugs, praise, and play). As there are fewer reinforcers available in the context of this life event, contingent behaviors begin to decline through a process of extinction. Thus, the depressed child may stop trying to engage with the parent, which further reduces the chances of being rewarded by the parent.

As Ferster (1973) further theorized, the increased dysphoria that occurs in response to low levels of positive reinforcement leads the depressed individual to engage in increased levels of escape behaviors (e.g., crying, complaining) in an attempt to end the negative emotional state. Although these behaviors may have been rewarded in the past (e.g., a complaint may have resulted in a parent's aid), in the current situation the escape behaviors fail to alleviate the depressed feelings. In fact, the increase in these behaviors has the unintended effect of reducing the behaviors that could garner positive reinforcement. For example, if there is an increase in time spent crying, then there is a consequent decrease in the engagement of alternative enjoyable behaviors, such as playing a board game with a sibling or enjoying a laugh with a parent. This reduction in enjoyable behaviors then leads to even lower levels of positive reinforcement and increased dysphoria. Compounding the situation, symptoms of depression (e.g., fatigue, hopelessness) may further decrease interaction with the environment and maintain the low levels of reinforcement.

In Ferster's conceptualization, the goal of therapeutic intervention is to increase the rate of behaviors that will likely lead to positive reinforcement. The byproduct of the increased positive reinforcement will be an increase in positive mood and a decrease in depressed mood. Indeed, there is empirical evidence to support the view that engagement in behaviors that elicit positive reinforcement is associated with improved mood. Using the Pleasant Events Schedule (PES; MacPhillamy & Lewinsohn, 1982), a measure created to assess the type, frequency, and degree of enjoyment of an extensive variety of pleasant events, Lewinsohn and Libet (1972) found that positive mood and engagement in pleasant activities were highly correlated. The content of the specific pleasant activities linked with mood fell into three broad categories, including those that resulted in a mood state that was incompatible with depression (e.g., laughing), those that involved social interaction (e.g., seeing old friends), and finally those that engendered a feeling of competence (e.g., learning to do something new). In a follow-up study, depressed participants reported engaging in a significantly lower rate of pleasant activities as well as a smaller range of activities over a 1-month period as compared to psychiatric and normal control groups (Lewinsohn & Libet, 1972). In one of the earliest studies to test the possible treatment effects of activity scheduling, Grosscup and Lewinsohn (1980) found that increasing the rate of pleasant events was associated with improvements in mood in a depressed adult sample over a 42-day treatment period and 1-month follow-up assessment.

Although Lewinsohn's work provided empirical evidence of the theorized link between rates of contingent positive reinforcement and depressed mood, the behavioral assumption that a reduction in positive reinforcement *precedes* the onset of depressed mood has yet to be empirically established. In fact, Lewinsohn found stronger associations between engagement in pleasant events and mood in concurrent assessments, when mood and activity level were assessed in the same day, than when mood was assessed either prior to or following engagement in activity (Lewinsohn & Libet, 1972). Interestingly, Lewinsohn documented high levels of individual differences in the timing and strength of association between activity level and mood, thus suggesting that an activity scheduling-based intervention for depression may be differentially effective, depending on the individual's vulnerability to the effects of pleasant and unpleasant events (Lewinsohn, 1975).

The association between engagement in pleasant events and mood appears to hold true for children and adolescents as well. Wierzbicki and Sayler (1991) gave children ages 8–14 years and their parents rating scales of pleasant/unpleasant events and depressive symptoms over the latest 2 weeks. Both the child and parent reports indicated a positive relation between engagement in unpleasant activities and depressed mood, whereas the parent reports of child behavior yielded a negative correlation between engagement in pleasant activities and depressed mood. Also looking at ratings that considered the prior 2-week period, Carey, Kelley, Buss, and Scott (1986) documented a positive correlation between engagement in unpleasant activities (e.g., having an argument, taking a test) and depressed mood in adolescents.

Lewinsohn's original activity scheduling intervention, although multifaceted, focused on increasing pleasant events in the daily experience of depressed adults (Grosscup & Lewinsohn, 1980). During the early sessions of treatment, therapists encouraged clients to keep a daily record of events and mood to facilitate their understanding of the association between the two. Therapists used these daily logs to point out mood increases that were concurrent and/or subsequent to engaging in a pleasant activity. Once the link between activity and mood was understood by the client, the therapist and client collaboratively engaged in activity scheduling by planning the type and frequency of activities for the upcoming week. The intervention also included components of social skills and time management training; however, both were used to support the activity scheduling intervention. For example, a client may indicate that spending time with friends would be a pleasant activity but lack the social skills to arrange a social event and/or to ensure that the social interaction would be rewarding to both the client and the friends. Similarly, for the client who reports feeling overwhelmed by demands, the therapist might introduce time management skills to facilitate the planning and execution of planned activities. Later, Clarke et al. (1990) adapted Lewinsohn's adult-focused treatment for an adolescent population by increasing the number of role plays and interactive activities, reducing and simplifying homework assignments, and adding parent sessions and supplemental skills training (e.g., communication, conflict negotiation).

Building on Lewinsohn's work, activity scheduling continued on as a central component of behavioral interventions for depression. The broad scope of pleasant events scheduling was narrowed by subsequent theorists to focus on the scheduling of events that increased the frequency of mastery experiences (Jacobson et al., 1996), reflected client values (Lejuez, Hopko, & Hopko, 2001), or replaced targeted avoidance behaviors (e.g., staying in bed; Jacobson, Martell, & Dimidjian, 2001). As another variant, some interventions suggest the grading of activities from easiest to most difficult and include rehearsal and role-play practice to prepare the client for engagement in the activity (Lejuez et al., 2001; Martell, Addis, & Jacobson, 2001). Regardless of the specific approaches, all activity scheduling interventions focus on increasing the amount of positive reinforcement garnered from the environment by increasing the amount of contact the client has with situations that are likely to provide positive reinforcement.

## Evidence Base

This section describes the research evidence for activity scheduling as an effective treatment component in interventions for youth with depression (see Table 10.1 for an overview of activity scheduling in representative empirically supported manuals). Although the effectiveness of activity scheduling as a sole component in the treatment of child and adolescent depression has not been evaluated, studies with adults and those evaluating multicomponent treatment packages with youth suggest that it is likely an active ingredient (Clarke et al., 1990; Gaynor & Harris, 2008; Ruggiero, Morris, Hopko, & Lejuez, 2007; Stark & Kendall, 1996). In addition, results of recent trials (e.g., Bilek & Ehrenreich-May, 2012) suggest that unified or transdiagnostic treatments that include activity scheduling may be effective in the treatment of youth with depression and/or anxiety.

A landmark dismantling study in the adult literature provides strong support for activity scheduling as an effective component in the treatment of depression. In a randomized controlled study, Neal Jacobson and colleagues (1996) found that a purely behavioral intervention was effective in the treatment of adult depression, and the addition of cognitive therapy elements (e.g., testing of automatic thoughts, testing of cognitive schemas) did not enhance effectiveness. Since the behavioral intervention in Jacobson et al. (1996) consisted of activity scheduling, behavioral techniques for sleep problems, and social skills training, the results of the study suggested that activity scheduling may be an agent of change in behavioral treatments of depression. These results inspired researchers to renew their focus on solely behavioral treatments of depression. For example, behavioral activation treatment for depression (BATD; Lejuez et al., 2001) emerged in this context and has garnered empirical support as an effective treatment for depression in adults.

TABLE 10.1. The Activity Scheduling Element in Representative EBT Manuals

| | |
|---|---|
| *Adolescent Coping with Depression Course* (Clarke, Lewinsohn, & Hops, 1990) | • Activity scheduling is explicitly taught, and the youth engage in activity scheduling throughout the treatment. The youth learn to target specific behaviors, obtain a baseline, create realistic goals for behavior change, and develop a contract for changing their behavior. |
| *Treating Depressed Children: Therapist Manual for "Taking Action"* (Stark & Kendall, 1996) | • Activity scheduling is explicitly taught early in the treatment. It is considered one of the core treatment elements, the "A" in Action standing for "Always do something that makes yourself feel better." The youth keep ongoing daily diaries of mood and activities and are encouraged to make the connection between doing something fun and feeling better. |
| *Treating Depressed Youth: Therapist Manual for "Action"* (Stark et al., 2007) | • Activity scheduling is explicitly taught in the context of "Taking Action" and includes creating a list of fun things to do as well as keeping logs of activities and mood. Therapists help the youth make the connection between doing something fun and feeling better. Activity scheduling extends over several sessions of treatment. |
| *Psychotherapy for Children with Bipolar and Depressive Disorders* (Fristad, Arnold, & Leffler, 2011) | • The manual includes the importance of scheduling exercise but does not discuss the broader context of activity scheduling. |

*Note.* Some book titles are shortened to conserve space. See the References at the back of the book for full titles.

BATD is a highly individualized treatment that involves a functional analysis of depression symptoms and centers on decreasing reinforcement of depressive symptoms and increasing reinforcement of healthy behaviors. Activity monitoring and scheduling are central aspects of this approach; however, the treatment may also include additional behavioral components as needed (e.g., relaxation, skills training).

At present, evidence for the effectiveness of behavioral activation therapy in youth has been documented in some initial small-sample studies. Gaynor and Harris (2008) followed four depressed adolescents being treated with BATD to determine whether an increase in the rate of potentially reinforcing activities mediates the reduction of depression symptoms. All four teens reported reduced depression symptoms following the therapy. In addition, for half of the participants, the pattern of symptom change suggested that increasing pleasant events may be an active mediator. For those two teens, the decrease in depression symptoms occurred directly following a reported increase in engagement in potentially reinforcing events. In another small-sample study, Ruggiero and colleagues (2007) utilized BATD in the treatment of a 17-year-old adolescent with depression. The functional analysis completed at the beginning of treatment revealed that recent changes in the teen's foster family had greatly reduced her opportunities for social activities with friends and positive interactions with her foster mother (reduced pleasant events) and had increased her household responsibilities and negative interactions with her foster mother (increased negative events). Therefore, the treatment focused on restructuring the adolescent's household duties and increasing pleasant events (e.g., social activities with friends, taking photographs). At the end of the 8-week treatment, the adolescent reported lower levels of depression and less conflict with her foster mother. Clearly, behavioral interventions with activity scheduling as one of the primary components have shown promise in the treatment for adolescent depression; future research will need to examine efficacy further by using RCTs.

Activity scheduling is considered an active treatment component in several manualized treatments for children and adolescents with depression. Perhaps two of the most well known are the Taking Action (Stark & Kendall, 1996) treatment manual for depressed children and the CWD-A course (Clarke et al., 1990). The Taking Action intervention (Stark, 1990; Stark & Kendall, 1996) is a school-based group CBT package for children with depression. Although the original treatment manual was designed for youth ages 9–13 years, Stark and Kendall (1996) state that the procedures could be appropriate for additional ages with some developmentally appropriate modifications. Stark, Brookman, and Frazier (1990) explain that activity scheduling is included in the treatment to decrease social withdrawal and increase enjoyment in previously enjoyed activities. They also note that engagement in pleasant activities may increase mastery experiences and self-esteem. Activity scheduling is introduced early (Session 3 out of 18 child sessions) with the individual identification of pleasant events. Further identification of pleasant events along with tracking of engagement in pleasant events occurs in several subsequent sessions. Later sessions reinforce the link between pleasant events and mood and support continued mood monitoring and activity scheduling.

Although Taking Action is one of the more researched interventions for children with depression, the research base is small, and most of the results are presented in chapters and not in empirical articles. Therefore, although the results thus far are promising, additional effectiveness and/or efficacy research is needed. In the first study to evaluate the treatment (in 1990), the Stark group compared Taking Action to a nonspecific supportive therapy (as described in Stark, Swearer, Kurowski, Sommer, & Bowen, 1996). A small sample of 24 children (fourth to seventh graders) were randomly assigned to one of the two conditions and assessed at pre- and posttreatment and at 7-month follow-up. Youth in the Taking Action condition reported significantly fewer depression symptoms and higher levels of self-esteem than those in the control group. The two groups were equivalent at the 7-month assessment; however, high attrition rates across conditions yielded very small sample sizes, resulting in inadequate power to detect differences between groups. More recently, Taking Action has been utilized to reduce depressive symptoms in children (ages 10–12 years) at risk for depression (defined as elevated scores on a parent-report depression survey and at least one criterion of major depressive disorder). Initial results in this population were promising, as children in the treatment group exhibited improvement on measures of depression symptoms and self-worth while children in a waitlist control did not (De Cuyper, Timbremont, Braet, De Backer, & Wullaert, 2004).

One of the first manualized treatments for adolescents with depression emerged out of Lewinsohn's work and manualized treatment for depressed adults. Clarke et al. (1990) adapted Lewinsohn's adult-focused Coping with Depression to create the CWD-A treatment manual. CWD-A is a group (typically school-based) multicomponent treatment that consists of 16 2-hour sessions over 8 weeks (Clarke & DeBar, 2010). The treatment is composed of both cognitive and behavioral elements, and the manual highlights six core treatment components that include the scheduling and monitoring of pleasant events, which is taught and/or discussed in 13 of the 16 sessions. RCTs provide support that CWD-A is more effective in reducing self-reported depression symptoms in depressed adolescents than a waitlist control, and these treatment effects are maintained over a 2-year period (Clarke et al., 1999; Lewinsohn et al., 1990). Empirical studies have also demonstrated a trend toward increased effectiveness with the addition of a brief parent component, compared to treatment without the parent component (Lewinsohn et al., 1990), and the incremental benefit of monthly booster sessions during a 2-year follow-up. Booster sessions appeared to accelerate recovery for those participants who remained depressed at the end of the initial treatment phase (Clarke et al., 1999). In an RCT that included adolescents with both depression and conduct disorder diagnoses, CWD-A proved to be more effective at posttreatment than the alternative life skills intervention (Rohde et al., 2004), though treatment differences were nonsignificant at 12-month follow-up.

Depression and anxiety often co-occur in youth (Costello, Mustillo, Erkanil, Keeler, & Angold, 2003), and thus treatments that target both disorders may be beneficial. The Unified Protocol for the Treatment of Emotional Disorders in Children: Emotion Detectives (UP-C:ED; Ehrenreich-May & Bilek, 2009) and the adolescent version (UP-A; Ehrenreich et al., 2008) contain treatment components aimed at reducing the symptoms of both depression and anxiety. The connection between activities and mood is made early in the treatment. For example, in the UP-C:ED intervention, the therapist throws a brief surprise "dance party" during the first session and then has the youth compare their ratings of mood before and after the dance party. Ehrenreich-May, Bilek, Queen, and Rodriguez (2012) recommend assigning behavioral activation homework throughout the treatment to those youth with depression symptoms. In addition, increasing activity levels may also facilitate exposures that help ameliorate anxiety symptoms. In a recent study, Bilek and Ehrenreich-May (2012) found that youth with an anxiety disorder and comorbid depression symptoms enrolled in UP-C:ED ($N$ = 22, ages 7–12 years) exhibited lower levels of both anxiety and depression symptoms at posttreatment.

In sum, although no existing studies have evaluated the effectiveness of activity scheduling alone in the treatment of depressed youth, several treatment packages that include activity scheduling as a primary treatment element have drawn empirical support. Research on activity scheduling utilizing adult samples suggests that it is an active ingredient in depression treatments (see Kanter et al., 2010, for a further review). Future research needs to examine more closely whether activity scheduling is an active ingredient in the context of existing treatments for children and adolescents with depression.

## THE ELEMENT IN PRACTICE

This section of the chapter presents the practical aspects of applying activity scheduling in treatment. A step-by-step task analysis is provided in Box 10.1 to aid in its implementation. In addition, later in the chapter, possible adaptations by developmental level and for diverse youth are presented, along with (at the end) a case example of activity scheduling implemented with an African American adolescent with depression (see Box 10.2).

## BOX 10.1. Task Analysis of Activity Scheduling

1. Obtain baseline measurements of the client's activities and mood.
   a. The youth keeps a diary of activity engagement and daily mood.
   b. The clinician uses these initial diaries to help the youth make the connection between activity levels and mood.

2. Assess potential reinforcing events.
   a. Events may include those that are currently enjoyed or those that used to elicit enjoyment, those that elicit feelings of mastery or accomplishment, and/or those that align with the child or adolescent's values.
   b. Collaboratively (the therapist and youth, perhaps with help and approval from the parents) make a list of potentially reinforcing events.

3. Schedule activities.
   a. Utilizing the youth's unique list of events, create a goal for the upcoming week (or time period to the next session).
   b. The goal should include the number and types of activities. The goal may also include specific days and times for the events to occur.
   c. The activity schedule should be collaborative and agreed on by both the clinician and the youth.

4. Monitor engagement in the activities and mood.
   a. The youth keeps a log of both activities and mood. Adaptations include ratings of mastery and/or pleasure in addition to, or in place of, mood.
   b. The log entry may be made directly after each activity or at the end of each day.
   c. The log should include all scheduled activities but allow additional space for unscheduled pleasant activities.

5. Increase the client's engagement in activities.
   a. Work on developing small and realistic goals for increasing the youth's engagement in activities.
   b. Activity scheduling goals should increase over time and reflect the current interests and goals of the child/adolescent.

6. Troubleshoot activity scheduling.
   a. Remove or amend activities that are no longer enjoyable or feasible.
   b. Teach any skills that are requisite for completing the scheduled activities.
   c. Consider gradual exposure to potentially reinforcing events that may elicit some anxiety in the youth.

## "Core of the Core" Element

Overall, activity scheduling can be thought of as unfolding across three phases: assessment, implementation, and follow-up. The assessment phase consists of the first two steps of the task analysis (i.e., obtaining baseline measurement of the client's activity level and mood, and assessing potentially reinforcing events). In the majority of treatment packages for depressed youth, assessment of pleasant events and current activity engagement occurs within the first couple of treatment sessions. Regarding Step 1 (Box 10.1), to obtain an initial picture of current activity engagement and mood, the youth is encouraged to keep a daily log. Typically, this log is kept on a chart with time intervals plotted down the left-hand side and the days of the week printed across the top. The youth can then fill in the activities that occurred at different times during each day. Next to the activity, they may also rate their mood during their engagement in that activity (see Chapter 11). In some variations, the youth may also rate the pleasantness of the activity or the sense of accomplishment the youth felt in completing the activity (for sample logs, see J. S. Beck, 2011, and Stark, Kendall, et al., 1996). The resulting information can be utilized to determine the baseline rate of positive (e.g., spending pleasurable time with family or friends) and negative activities (e.g., watching TV alone for hours, skipping school). In addition, review of these initial ratings may help the youth understand the relationship between engagement in pleasurable activities and mood. Socratic questioning may help to make this connection: "What activities were most enjoyable for you over the past week? Let's look at your ratings . . . how did you feel when you were doing that activity? What activities were not fun? Let's see what happened to your mood when you were doing the not-fun activities."

Moving on to Step 2, a full assessment of activities that have the potential to be rewarding to the youth is useful. Pleasant events may be identified through an interview with the youth and family or with the assistance of a formal assessment measure like the Pleasant Events Schedule, Adolescent Version (PES-A; available in the CWD-A student workbook). The PES-A is particularly useful if the youth has trouble verbalizing activities, as it presents a list of 320 activities (e.g., reading a book; playing with pets) and asks the youth to, first, rate whether the event has occurred during the past 30 days and, second, rate how pleasant he or she found the event to be. Stark (1990) developed a similar scale for fourth, fifth, and sixth graders. It is important to assess for activities that are currently enjoyed as well as those that the youth previously enjoyed but may be currently avoiding owing to a lack of energy, motivation, or desire to participate because of the depressive episode. It is also helpful to assess for mastery activities, that is, those that have the potential for eliciting feelings of accomplishment (e.g., working on a hobby or a school project) and for those activities that reflect the values of the youth (e.g., participating in a fund-raiser for the local animal shelter). The assessment should also include a list of necessary activities (e.g., doing homework, taking care of a pet). Although engagement in these types of activities may not be as positively reinforcing as pleasant activities, they have the potential to greatly reduce negative experiences (e.g., family conflict, feelings of stress over schoolwork or bad grades). The resulting list of activities becomes a useful resource for scheduling activities during the next phase.

The next section is the main implementation phase, in which activity scheduling actually occurs (Steps 3–5). Once the link between engagement in pleasant activities and mood is established, the rationale for increasing engagement in pleasant activities to decrease depressed mood can then be explained. Utilizing the list of events created during the first phase, the youth and therapist collaboratively determine the exact content (e.g., walk the dog) and frequency (e.g., every day) of activities to be scheduled for the coming week (or until the next therapy session). When possible, a specific schedule of the days and times that activity will take place (e.g., go to the playground on Saturday afternoon, walk the dog every day) helps to increase compliance with the activity schedule. Compliance can also be facilitated by the use of a "contract," or agreement signed by the youth. Some activities need family financial (e.g., taking karate lessons) or scheduling (e.g., having a sleepover) support, and in these cases the therapist may need to act as a liaison between the youth and the family to help determine what is feasible. Throughout this first week, the youth continues to keep the log of activities and mood to track the relation between the increase in engagement in activities and the expected decrease in depressed mood. The number of scheduled activities occurring between therapy sessions should gradually increase over time. The "optimal" number of activities is indicated when the youth's depressed mood adequately decreases, and/or when additional activities are no longer feasible (i.e., the youth is at risk of being "overbooked").

The process of monitoring (Step 4) and increasing engagement in pleasant activities (Step 5) typically takes place alongside additional skill training. For example, a session may include work on problemsolving skills followed by a check in on activity scheduling. Activity scheduling may also be used as a platform to work on other skills, such as when a discussion of initial reluctance to engage in an activity is used as a vehicle for identifying negative automatic thoughts or core beliefs (e.g., "What is the use? Nothing is fun anymore!"). Activity scheduling may also be used to test automatic thoughts. For instance, a child can be encouraged to add "asking a friend to play" to the activity schedule to test the assumption that no one wants to play with him or her. Similarly, an adolescent client may be encouraged to practice problem solving in response to a desired activity that seems overwhelming (e.g., saving up for a ticket and obtaining a ride to a concert).

The final phase of pleasant activity scheduling involves following up on the ongoing process and troubleshooting any difficulties that may arise (Step 6). For example, preferred activities may change over time and as a child matures; activities that once were pleasurable may no longer be experienced as such (regardless of the depression). A child that may have found jigsaw puzzles pleasurable in the past but no longer enjoys them may end up replacing that activity with a different one. Thus, the list of activities originally drawn from to create the weekly schedule may need to be routinely evaluated and amended. In addition, the content or frequency of some activities may need to be altered for feasibility. For instance, parents may not have time to drive their adolescent to a friend's house every day but might be able to commit to three times per week. Finally, noncompliance in activity scheduling may reflect skills deficits (e.g., a child may not know how to join a game of tag during recess) or anxiety. In either case, adjunctive elements may need to be added to the treatment. If the noncompliance is related to a skills deficit, the therapist will need to assess related skills (e.g., social, time management) and add targeted skills training to therapy. In an anxiety framework, activity scheduling may be easily meshed with exposure by breaking down desired activities into smaller parts and scheduling them in a graded approach; a child could first role-play calling a friend for a play date with the therapist before making the actual call. In addition, establishment of a reward system for completion of activity scheduling homework tasks may increase compliance (see Chapter 9).

## Developmental Adaptations

Just as the content of an activity schedule is highly individualized, the process of activity scheduling is also easily adapted to the unique developmental needs of the youth. For instance, to set the groundwork for activity scheduling, an assessment of potentially reinforcing events is needed. Some youth may be readily able to list activities they currently, or used to, enjoy. For younger children or those who have more difficulty generating ideas, this process may involve incorporating the family's input by supplementing the child's list of activities with information from the parents or other youth in a therapy group.

For example, the Taking Action workbook has a page for brainstorming "fun things to do," which could be used to gather ideas from the
group (Stark, Kendall, et al., 1996). In addition, youth may be prompted
through such questions as "Can you tell me what you used to do during the day last summer?" If needed, examples of commonly enjoyed
activities in picture books, oral stories, or comics may be presented to
garner additional ideas. For adolescent clients, the PES-A may be helpful in identifying potentially pleasant events.

Similarly, the process of keeping a log of activities and corresponding ratings of pleasure in engagement and mood may be adapted for
youth at different developmental levels. More advanced adolescents
will likely be able to complete a log that includes the time of day, the
activity engaged in (e.g., called a friend, washed the dishes, took a
nap), and ratings of mood and other potential supplemental ratings
(e.g., pleasantness, feelings of mastery). This log may also be simplified as needed. For example, youth can be given larger blocks of time
(e.g., morning, afternoon, evening) to record activities and ratings, thus
greatly reducing the amount of potential ratings. The Taking Action
workbook includes sample weekly log sheets for activities and mood
(Stark, Kendall, et al., 1996). In addition, rating scales may be reduced
from the 7-point scale used in the adolescent interventions (e.g., Clarke
et al., 1990) to a 3- or 4-point scale or may include pictures instead
of numbers to represent emotions and their intensity. Helping facilitate an understanding of the link between mood and engagement in
activities may take different forms, as well. More advanced youth may
be able to graph their ratings of pleasant events and mood to see the
connection (see Clarke et al., 1990). Other children may be guided by
actively engaging in a fun activity during the session (e.g., hula hoop-
ing is recommended in Stark, Kendall, et al., 1996) and then discussing
how they currently feel and how this feeling is different from when
they are thinking negative thoughts.

The scheduling of activities may also vary depending on the
developmental level of the child or adolescent. For younger children,
engagement in activities is likely to be parent-mediated, as parents may
need to provide transportation (e.g., drive to karate lessons) or arrange
the activities (e.g., obtain craft supplies, arrange time with a friend). In
addition, it is likely that for younger children a greater percentage of
activities will actually involve parents (e.g., having a family game night,
talking a walk with a parent; Ruggiero et al., 2007). For all youth, it is
important to consider the developmental appropriateness of selected
activities. For example, youth with few friends should be encouraged to

add social activities onto the activity schedule. Similarly, an adolescent may be encouraged to engage in activities with an appropriate level of independence. Ruggiero and colleagues (2007) recommend focusing on peer activities when working with adolescents; however, they caution to remain aware of the influence of peers on teen delinquency and substance abuse. In response, they advocate a psychoeducational approach with teens regarding these risks.

Finally, activity scheduling is included in recent online interventions designed specifically for use with teen populations who may appreciate the computer-based format, flexibility of use, and increased anonymity. Landback and colleagues (2009) teach activity scheduling as part of 10 Internet-based treatment modules (that also include elements of CBT and IPT) aimed at the prevention of depression. For each module, the authors worked to make the intervention appealing to adolescents by including stories *about* teens and *written by* teens, to aid them in learning the presented skills.

## Diversity Considerations

In addition to tailoring activity scheduling to the child's developmental level, consideration should be given to the ethnic and cultural context of the youth and family. When selecting and scheduling activities, some effort should be made to ensure that the treatment complements the family culture. For example, attending a mixed-sex school dance may not be an acceptable activity for a conservative Muslim teen. In addition, ethnic and cultural differences may affect the degree of reward that may be experienced by participation in a given situation. For some teens, helping to cook a family meal may not be enjoyable, but in some family-oriented cultures this same activity may be highly valued and rewarding. By nature, activity scheduling is highly idiographic; the therapist works with the youth to identify and schedule activities that are rewarding to that youth in particular. Therefore, activity scheduling as a treatment component is highly flexible and adaptable to individual differences in backgrounds, cultures, and values.

No studies have evaluated the efficacy of activity scheduling— considered alone—in diverse populations. However, existing empirically supported multicomponent treatment packages for depressed youth that include activity scheduling have been adapted for use with diverse groups of adolescents. The CWD-A treatment (Clarke et al., 1990) has been adapted for use with both Puerto Rican (Rosselló et al., 2008) and Haitian-American adolescents (Nicolas, Arntz, Hirsch,

& Schmiedigen, 2009). Both teams of researchers utilized the Ecological Validity and Culturally Sensitive Framework (Bernal, Bonilla, & Bellido, 1995) to guide the adaptation of the original treatment. This framework recommends an eight-pronged approach to adaptation that involves consideration of language, therapy relationship, treatment content, treatment goals, metaphors, treatment concepts, treatment methods, and context. Nicolas and colleagues (2009) also utilized input from community stakeholders and focus groups with Haitian American adolescents in designing their intervention. For example, focus group members generated new wording and examples for each treatment session in the CWD-A manual. A full report of outcomes on this project is not yet available; however, the authors state that depression symptoms were reduced at posttreatment and outcomes were maintained at follow-up (Nicolas et al., 2009).

Initial outcome data on the use of the adapted CWD-A with Puerto Rican adolescents are also promising. Rosselló and colleagues (2008) implemented an RCT to evaluate the efficacy of IPT versus CBT (adapted CWD-A) in both individual and group formats. Outcome measures included assessments of depression, self-concept, social adaptation, and broad measures of internalizing and externalizing symptoms. Both IPT and the adapted CWD-A reduced symptoms of depression over time; however, the CBT showed larger decreases in depression symptoms as well as overall internalizing and externalizing symptoms. Results indicated that there were no differences between individual and group treatment modalities. Although activity scheduling is utilized in the adapted manual in the same way as in the original, the authors recommend considering context and culture when facilitating activity scheduling. For example, the therapist should keep in mind the value of *familism*, or respect and attachment to the family, in the selection and scheduling of activities (Rosselló & Bernal, 2005). The authors conclude that cognitive-behavioral interventions may work well with Puerto Rican adolescents owing to the cultural value of *respeto*, or the deference to authority figures. They recommend that future studies evaluate cultural values as potential mediators of outcomes.

## CONCLUSIONS

Activity scheduling has a long history grounded in behavioral theory. This treatment element involves increasing the amount of pleasant activities in a depressed individual's daily routine to increase the likelihood of instilling positively reinforcing experiences, and thus benefit overall mood. Originally utilized to treat depressed adults, activity scheduling is currently often included in treatment packages for children and adolescents with depression. Several multicomponent interventions that include activity scheduling as a main component have garnered empirical support, although no study has yet evaluated the efficacy of activity scheduling alone as a treatment for depressed youth. Activity scheduling can be easily adapted to a wide range of developmental levels and modified for use with diverse groups of adolescents. Future research should focus on evaluating the relative importance of activity scheduling within a multicomponent treatment package. In addition, adaptations of activity scheduling for young children (under 9 years of age) and additional minority groups are needed.

## BOX 10.2. Illustrative Case Example

Eddie M., a 15-year-old African American male, was brought to the clinic by his mother, who was concerned about his recent behavior. According to Mrs. M., Eddie had become increasingly despondent since the fall. Eddie was in the 10th grade at his local public high school and lived with his parents and two younger sisters. His mother reported that he used to be a "busy kid." He had a group of friends in the neighborhood, and during the ninth grade he stayed active by playing basketball on the high school junior varsity basketball team and in pick-up games at the local park. Now, however, she reported that Eddie stayed largely in his room, sleeping and occasionally playing video games or watching TV. She added that Eddie rarely interacted with his parents or younger sisters and that it was difficult to get him to come out of his room for their traditional family dinner. Mrs. M. decided that Eddie needed help after one of his teachers called home to discuss his excessive amount of incomplete work.

Eddie was a tall, athletic-looking adolescent dressed in rumpled clothing. He sat slumped in the chair and occasionally closed his eyes while answering questions from the clinician. His speech was coherent as he discussed recent events in his life. He corroborated his mother's report, stating that he spent much of his time in his room and was "not really interested in friends right now." When asked about his mood, Eddie replied that he felt "nothing," and when prompted he added that it was like "the life went out of me." When asked about the school year, Eddie replied that it was "real different" because he was not playing basketball. Further inquiry revealed that Eddie had failed to make the varsity team and had quit the junior varsity team in protest of that decision. As many of his friends played basketball, Eddie found himself alone after school. For a while, he hung out with a girl he thought might be his girlfriend, but when she started dating someone else Eddie began spending more time at home. At home, Eddie stated that his family kept "bugging him" and that they "seemed more concerned about his chores than how he was feeling." Assessment revealed that Eddie met the criteria for major depressive disorder.

Eddie was resistant to a group treatment, citing concerns about sharing his feelings in front of other teens. As a result, a modified CWD-A course was conducted in an individual format. The first session included an orientation to the program, psychoeducation about depression, and training on mood monitoring. At the end of the first session, Eddie completed the PES to aid in the identification of potentially reinforcing activities. During the second session, the mood monitor was reviewed, and Eddie was introduced to the concept of tracking his baseline mood and behaviors. In this context, he was instructed on how to record his mood and engagement in pleasant events. To help Eddie understand the relation between mood and pleasant events, he was shown a sample record of mood and activity ratings transposed on a similar chart. Through Socratic questioning, the clinician guided Eddie to the conclusion that people feel worse when they do not participate in pleasant activities and feel better when they engage in more pleasant activities. Using the results from the PES and a discussion about things that Eddie used to like to do, the clinician and Eddie developed a list of about 20 enjoyable activities (e.g., play with his younger sister, make something in his dad's woodshop, take a walk) as well as activities that might make him feel competent (e.g., wash the dishes, take out the trash, complete 30 minutes of homework) to track and increase over time. At the end of the second session, the clinician trained Eddie on how to use the log to track his mood and engagement in pleasant events.

Over the next 2 weeks, Eddie continued to log his baseline levels of mood and activities. In the intervening sessions, the clinician reviewed the baseline levels and progressed with teaching other skills in the CWD-A course (e.g., communication). After a few weeks, the clinician guided Eddie in the process of charting his own mood and pleasant events daily totals on graph paper. Eddie was able to make the observation that his mood appeared to be affected by his engagement in pleasant events. He also noticed that his mood dropped a bit on the weekends when his parents often talked to him about his noncompliance with chores and decreased academic performance. Next, the clinician and Eddie worked on setting appropriate goals for pleasant events. Eddie stated that, even though he did not enjoy it, it would make him feel better to do some of his chores and homework and would likely reduce the fighting with his parents. The clinician helped Eddie to develop small, realistic goals of completing one chore per day and spending 1 hour on homework each day. In addition, the clinician suggested that Eddie consider some social activities with friends. When Eddie replied that all his friends were too busy with sports, the clinician helped Eddie to problem-solve, and together they added talking to a classmate three times per day to the list.

At the next session, the clinician noticed that Eddie was compliant with the activity scheduling at the beginning of the week but was less so at the end of the week, meeting the goals on only one of the three preceding days. When prompted, Eddie reported that he and his parents got into an argument midweek over a test that Eddie failed. Eddie stated that, following the argument, he felt "worthless" and thought "therapy is never going to work." Together, the therapist and Eddie tested his automatic thoughts. In addition, the therapist reminded Eddie of the rationale behind activity scheduling, and together they reviewed Eddie's chart of his activities and mood to reinforce the importance of completing the scheduled activities.

Over the next several sessions, Eddie continued to track his mood and engagement in pleasant events. As his compliance with chores and homework increased, Eddie's conflict with his parents decreased and his grades began to improve. As Eddie increased his social interaction, he developed a friendship with a peer in his science class, who taught Eddie how to play chess. His activity goals changed and began to include more social goals (e.g., calling one friend per day, arranging time with former friends on the weekend when they were not playing basketball) and included a few goals to reflect his new interest in becoming a competitive chess player. He also started to play pick-up basketball games in the park on weekends again. Over this period, his mood continued to improve. At the end of 15 weeks, Eddie reported feeling much better and no longer met the diagnostic criteria for major depressive disorder.

# 11

## Self–Monitoring

with Kristel Thomassin and Diana Morelen

### BACKGROUND OF THE ELEMENT

Self-monitoring (SM) is the process of self-observing and recording one's behaviors, thoughts, and/or feelings. Not only is SM useful in obtaining additional information about thoughts and behaviors, but it can also be helpful in increasing children's awareness of certain patterns of thinking, behaving, and/or feeling. Such awareness is often the first step toward positive change. For example, asking an adolescent with depression to monitor his or her mood before and after a pleasant activity may help teach the connection between doing something enjoyable and the experience of positive emotions. Though SM techniques have been used widely in both assessment and therapy contexts (Beidel, Neal, & Lederer, 1991; Kendall & Hedtke, 2006; Lewinsohn & Clarke, 1999; Shapiro & Cole, 1999), there is a surprisingly small research base supporting their use. Nonetheless, SM in some form is included in most empirically supported treatment packages for youth with internalizing problems (see Table 11.1). This chapter provides a brief history of the use of SM with youth and examines the ways that this technique has been applied in assessment contexts and treatment programs for children and adolescents experiencing internalizing problems, such as anxiety and depression. Issues of diversity

**TABLE 11.1. The Self-Monitoring Element in Representative EBT Manuals**

| | |
|---|---|
| *Coping Cat* (Kendall & Hedtke, 2006) | • The therapist explicitly teaches the use of SM and the youth complete tasks to practice the skill. The youth learn to monitor their feelings, thoughts, and efforts at facing their fears. For instance, as part of the R step of the FEAR plan, the youth rate their efforts at facing their fears. |
| *C.A.T. Project* (Kendall, Choudhury, Hudson, & Webb, 2002) | • The therapist explicitly teaches the use of SM, and the youth complete tasks to practice the skill. The youth learn to self-monitor their feelings, thoughts, and efforts at facing their fears. |
| *Family-Based Treatment for Young Children with OCD* (Freeman & Garcia, 2009) | • SM is explicitly presented and practiced. Parents keep a monitoring form to record the child's symptoms, the time spent on the task, and other relevant details. Parents are encouraged to involve the child as is developmentally appropriate. |
| *OCD in Children and Adolescents* (March & Mulle, 1998) | • The youth is taught the use of SM and completes tasks to reinforce the skill. For example, the child is encouraged to monitor times when OCD wins and times when he or she won during the preceding week. |
| *CBT of Childhood OCD: It's Only a False Alarm* (Piacentini, Langley, & Roblek, 2007) | • The therapist explicitly teaches the use of SM strategies, and the youth complete tasks to practice. For instance, the youth self-monitor ratings using a thermometer and then graph their anxiety ratings for the therapist to see. |
| *CBT for Social Phobia: Stand Up, Speak Out* (Albano & DiBartolo, 2007) | • The youth are explicitly taught about the use of SM and assigned tasks to practice the skill (e.g., the youth complete "Daily Monitoring Logs"). |
| *When Children Refuse School: A Cognitive-Behavioral Approach* (Kearney & Albano, 2007): Chapters 4 and 5 on internalizing symptoms | • The youth are taught to identify their behaviors, thoughts, and feelings associated with anxiety-provoking situations, and both the children and parents keep corresponding "logbooks." |
| *Treating Trauma and Traumatic Grief in Children and Adolescents* (Cohen, Mannarino, & Deblinger, 2006) | • The youth are encouraged to self-monitor within various components of treatment. For instance, the youth complete a "trauma narrative" that requires them to identify their thoughts and feelings associated with the event. Parents may also be encouraged to monitor their thoughts, feelings, and behaviors both in session and for homework, as necessary. |
| *Adolescent Coping with Depression* (Clarke, Lewinsohn, & Hops, 1990) | • SM is explicitly introduced and practiced during treatment. For instance, the youth keep "mood monitoring" records and are encouraged to look for patterns. |

*(continued)*

**TABLE 11.1.** (*continued*)

| | |
|---|---|
| *Interpersonal Psychotherapy for Depressed Adolescents,* 2nd edition (Mufson, Dorta, Moreau, & Weissman, 2011) | • SM is not explicitly covered during treatment, though it is implicitly included. For instance, the youth rates his or her mood at the start of each session and then reports if the mood was worse at any time during the preceding week. If so, the teen then identifies what was happening at that time. The therapist uses the opportunity to help both him- and herself and the teen identify areas to be targeted in treatment. |
| *Treating Depressed Children: Therapist Manual for "Taking Action"* (Stark & Kendall, 1996) | • SM is explicitly taught and practiced throughout the treatment. For example, youth are taught to self-monitor positive thoughts as a way to catch the positive (the C in ACTION is for "Catch the positive, and let the negative go"). |
| *Treating Depressed Youth: Therapist Manual for "Action"* (Stark et al., 2007) | • SM is explicitly taught and practiced on a weekly basis during treatment. At the beginning of treatment, the youth are asked to record positive things that happen in a Catch the Positive Diary and fill out a daily mood meter. Throughout treatment, they complete weekly homework assignments that involve recording times when their mood became more positive (i.e., "Be an Emotion Detective"), when they used problem-solving strategies (i.e., "Be a Problem Inspector"), and when they changed negative thoughts to coping thoughts (i.e., "Be a Thought Detective"). |
| *Psychotherapy for Children with Bipolar and Depressive Disorders* (Fristad, Arnold, & Leffler, 2011) | • The parents and children are explicitly taught how to monitor. For instance, the youth monitor moods using a simple scale, and the parents complete mood and mood-medication records on the child. |

*Note.* Some book titles are shortened to conserve space. See the References at the back of the book for full titles.

and developmental considerations in the use of SM are also explored. Toward the middle of the chapter readers will find a task analysis that is provided to assist with the practical application of SM. And, finally, a case example in which SM is used in the treatment of a 14-year-old Caucasian male with social anxiety disorder is also presented (at the end of the chapter).

## Brief History

An historical overview of SM provides a context for understanding its current use. One of the first studies on the use of SM with children was published in 1971 in the *Journal of Applied Behavior Analysis* (Broden, Hall, & Mitts, 1971), which reflects its strong roots in behaviorism. In their pioneering study, Broden et al. (1971) demonstrated that having two eighth-grade students self-record was helpful in increasing their study behavior and decreasing inappropriate talking in the classroom. In particular, one student was given a piece of paper and told to document each time she noticed that she was studying (appropriately) in the classroom. In contrast, the other student was instructed to document each time he talked out of turn in class. Improvements in both students' behavior were noted during times when they self-monitored their behavior but not during the baseline or when the self-monitoring forms were discontinued. These and other promising findings (Gottman & McFall, 1972; Kazdin, 1974a; Rutner & Bugle, 1969; Thomas, Abrams, & Johnson, 1971) resulted in an increased emphasis on properly understanding SM and especially its key aspects that lead to behavior change (Kanfer, 1970; Kazdin, 1974b; Mace & Kratochwill, 1985; Nelson & Hayes, 1981).

This increased focus on SM coincided with a broader interest in treating behavioral problems that require self-observation, such as smoking and overeating (Kazdin, 1974b). Such behaviors required self-observation because they often occur when individuals are alone. Self-observation provided a way to assess behaviors in real-world settings over a defined period of time and was believed to be a key step in effecting behavior change (Mahoney & Thoresen, 1974). In particular, the process of attending to and recording target behaviors was believed to increase the client's awareness of the behavior and thus facilitate positive change (Nelson, Lipinski, & Black, 1976). For instance, a child's monitoring of his or her behavior during class time would serve to increase self-awareness and result in greater periods of on-task behavior. Interestingly, however, total accuracy in recording the behaviors does not appear to be essential for SM to have positive effects (Broden et al., 1971; Nelson & Hayes, 1981). When a child's monitoring of his or her on-task behavior is inaccurate (whether over- or underendorsed as compared with objective ratings), the child will likely still make behavioral adjustments to be more on-task than before the monitoring began. In fact, research suggests that similar results may be obtained when the child is provided with directions on SM but does not actually make any physical recordings (Nelson & Hayes, 1981). Thus, the mere act of attending to target behaviors seems to be a key first step in effecting positive behavioral change. We now turn to a more in-depth discussion of the theory base behind SM, as a solid conceptual grounding is sure to facilitate the application of this core element in practice.

## Theory Base

Several different theories have been proposed to explain the useful-
ness of SM. In one of the earlier accounts, Kanfer (1970) proposed that
behavior change occurs through a series of three steps, namely, SM,
self-evaluation, and self-administered consequences. Imagine a child
who is depressed and who has just been encouraged to keep a log of
pleasant activities that she (or he) engaged in over the course of a week.
Through SM, the youth first becomes more aware of how often she is
actually involved in pleasant activities. As a result, she may feel slightly
guilty for engaging in so few activities. This evaluation may then help
motivate the child to engage in more pleasant activities, thus potentially decreasing her depressed mood. Kanfer emphasized that this
chain begins with the SM process and leads to changes in behavior
via self-evaluation and self-administered consequences. For example,
an anxious child might be coached on how to self-monitor avoidant
behavior. When the youth notices that she faced an anxiety-provoking
situation that she would typically have avoided, she could tell herself,
"Wow, I just faced my fear!"—or, alternatively, she could reward herself
by having a special snack later in the day.

The accurate SM of a target behavior can also facilitate a functional
analysis of behavior (Cone, 1997). A functional analysis helps explain
what comes before (antecedent) and after (consequence) a target behavior and serves to identify what makes the behavior more or less likely to
happen again. SM also provides the therapist with the opportunity for
repeated measurement, facilitating the assessment of the function(s) of
the behavior, which is of primary interest when developing a treatment
plan. Continuing with the previous example of an anxious youth, a
functional analysis of avoidant behavior might identify physical distress (e.g., stomachaches) as an antecedent to the avoidant behavior and
a relief in symptoms as a consequence of the behavior. In this way, the
functional analysis has assisted the clinician in identifying potential
treatment targets (e.g., physical symptoms associated with anxiety).

Nelson and Hayes (1981) elaborated upon earlier theoretical models by highlighting the importance of paying greater attention to the
steps taken prior to SM, which include providing instructions and
training in SM procedures. Mace and Kratochwill (1985) likewise noted
that clear, explicit instructions regarding SM increase the likelihood
of behavior change. Despite the notion that specific and clear instructions improve self-monitoring, research has found that SM is a fairly
robust procedure. For instance, research has found positive effects of
SM even when the actual SM recordings may be inaccurate (Broden
et al., 1971), when the client does not perform the SM recordings as

intended, and/or when the target behavior occurs very infrequently or not at all (Maletzky, 1974).

Other perspectives have also been proposed to account for the effects of SM. In particular, Bandura (1977b) proposed that the acquisition of self-efficacy (i.e., a sense of one's ability to meet goals) helps explain why behavioral change occurs when SM is implemented. Bandura postulated that perceived self-efficacy influences participation and perseverance in the face of obstacles as well as susceptibility to self-arousal (Bandura, 1969). For example, imagine two boys with a phobia of heights scheduled to go on a hiking trip to the mountains. The boy with low self-efficacy may not initiate coping strategies (i.e., avoid the trip altogether) or may give up quickly when attempting to overcome his fear because he does not believe in his ability to face the situation if he were to feel fearful. Conversely, the boy with high self-efficacy would likely still feel fear but would have more confidence in his ability to use coping skills (e.g., deep breathing, positive thinking) and would therefore be more likely to attempt and complete the hike (as compared to the boy with low self-efficacy). Not only can the process of self-monitoring provide the client with the perception of control over his or her behavior, but tracking target behaviors also provides the opportunity for building mastery. For example, having an anxious child track the completion of exposure tasks can enhance self-efficacy via accomplishments that build mastery (Suveg, Sood, Comer, & Kendall, 2009). Similarly, a child with symptoms of depression may track his or her participation in pleasurable activities, which would in turn provide evidence of performance accomplishments.

## Evidence Base

Given that SM has been used as both an assessment and treatment tool, this section reviews the literature relevant to both. Importantly, however, the distinction between assessment and treatment is not always clear. For instance, a clinician may assign an SM task to a depressed teen that requires him or her to note each time the person takes part in a social activity. Though the clinician may initially assign this task to gain assessment information, the process of monitoring activity levels may actually provide therapeutic benefits (Broden et al., 1971; Gottman & McFall, 1972).

With regard to the assessment context, Korotitsch and Nelson-Gray (1999) have argued that SM methods can be especially useful in assessing the covert (unobservable) thoughts and feelings that are often associated with internalizing symptoms. Target behaviors relevant to internalizing symptoms in youth may not be readily identified by observers, such as parents and teachers. For example, an anxious child may look inattentive in class as a result of being preoccupied with worrisome thoughts that could easily be missed by teachers. In a similar vein, a depressed child may simply look unmotivated and defiant to an outside observer while in reality the child is likely experiencing significant sadness and negative thoughts.

Though relatively scant, research does support the use of SM as an assessment tool. For example, Beidel and colleagues (1991) examined the use of SM with anxious and nonanxious youth using a paper-and-pencil diary. Third- through sixth-grade children were required to report daily for 2 weeks on how they felt during anxiety-provoking situations and what they did in response to each situation. Children were given either diaries with written response options or ones that illustrated options through symbols adapted from prior versions (Picture Communication Book by Johnson [1998] as cited in Beidel et al., 1991). Results indicated that less than half of the youth completed the diaries for a full 2 weeks, suggesting the need for external monitoring (e.g., parent or teacher involvement in the child's self-monitoring) or environmental reinforcements (e.g., earning rewards for completing the SM chart). The data that were captured appeared to be reliable, based on a 6-month test–retest examination, but the authors acknowledged several difficulties inherent in assessing reliability across time through the event-based diary method. For instance, "events" are not likely to stay stable across time, and events themselves are likely to vary in the degree to which they cause distress (e.g., a regular test vs. a final exam). Such variables make the assessment of reliability over time challenging. Regarding validity, youth with an anxiety disorder indicated greater degrees of distress than youth without anxiety disorders. This study also provided important information regarding developmental considerations for SM techniques. Specifically, younger children had greater success with the pictorial diary than the written diary, whereas there was no difference for older youth. Additional research groups have likewise successfully used SM as an assessment method for youth with specific phobias (e.g., Heard, Dadds, & Conrad, 1992; King et al., 1988).

With regard to the treatment context, modified versions of the SM diary format are a common component of various treatment programs for youth experiencing internalizing difficulties (Kendall & Hedtke, 2006; March & Mulle, 1998; Mufson et al., 2011; Ollendick, 1995). With respect to the treatment of anxiety in particular, Graziano and colleagues have incorporated SM in a self-control program for children's nighttime fear reduction (Graziano & Mooney, 1980; Graziano et al.,

1979). Children ages 7–10 years were asked to track their use of self-control exercises at nighttime. The program was successful in reducing children's problematic behaviors at bedtime. The CBT-based Coping Cat (Kendall & Hedtke, 2006) is exemplary in its use of SM through the course of treatment. Developed for children with social phobia, generalized anxiety disorder, and separation anxiety disorder, the program encourages youth to develop an awareness of somatic symptoms of anxiety, challenge "thinking traps" that may exacerbate their anxiety, and participate in exposure-based activities (i.e., tasks that enable youth to face their fears while using the skills learned in therapy). Not only are the children asked to track their completion of these tasks (with help from the therapist and parents), but the protocol also encourages self-evaluation and self-reward. Together, these components support the self-monitoring of accomplishments that build a sense of mastery (Suveg et al., 2009) while at the same time teaching the child appropriate, not overly critical, self-evaluation (e.g., "An A for effort!"). In older age groups, Ollendick (1995) reported successful use of SM in the treatment of four adolescents with panic disorder and agoraphobia. Teens were asked to keep a daily record of the time, location, symptoms, and duration of panic symptoms by using a structured record. At the start of each session, adolescents were asked to rate the degree to which they avoided anxiety-provoking situations during the preceding week, and at the end of the session they rated their likely self-efficacy in coping with panic attacks if they should occur over the coming week. The results showed that panic attacks were extinguished, avoidance was reduced, and symptoms declined to normative levels (Ollendick, 1995).

Treatment packages often consist of several different components, and researchers have thus begun to try to identify the particular components that account for positive change. In a study designed to examine the timing of treatment gains for anxious youth, Nakamura et al. (2009) found that youth benefited from SM and psychoeducation when these components were introduced early during the treatment program and prior to exposure tasks (i.e., some children showed positive change, including a reduction in anxiety symptoms, after the introduction of psychoeducation and SM but before exposure tasks were initiated). Yet, not all researchers have found such positive effects of only SM and psychoeducation for the treatment of youth anxiety disorders. Kendall and colleagues (1997) conducted an RCT of CBT for youth with anxiety disorders. Overall, results supported CBT (including psychoeducation, SM, relaxation, and exposures) as an effective treatment for youth with anxiety disorders. Exploratory analyses examined the relative efficacy (i.e., whether the component was related to treatment gains) of the first portion of treatment (i.e., the psychoeducation and skills training) versus the latter portion of treatment (i.e., exposure training) and found positive effects only for exposures. The actual mechanism of change, however, remains unclear. It is important to note that in this treatment SM is used throughout exposures and thus additional research examining it as a distinct treatment component is needed.

With regard to depression in youth, SM techniques have been used successfully as an assessment method and also in tandem with other therapeutic techniques (e.g., Lewinsohn & Clarke, 1999; Stark et al., 1987). Earlier work developed SM methods that could be used in later empirical studies. For instance, Reynolds and Stark (1985) had children complete a questionnaire of pleasant activities titled "Things that are fun to do" in which they could list activities they enjoyed and how much they enjoyed them. Based on a class- or school-wide administration of the form, a comprehensive and updated list of pleasant events was then generated, and the list was copied and bound to form a diary for the child. In an empirical study of a 5-week group CBT program for depressed teens, Reynolds and Coats (1986) had teens graphically depict the relation between the number of pleasant events the youth engaged in and their mood. Results showed a significant decline in depressive symptoms at posttreatment and follow-up.

Additional SM strategies have been used in treating depressive symptoms in older children and adolescents (e.g., CWDA; Clarke et al., 1990). In the CWDA program for adolescent depression that has been shown to reduce depressive symptoms among youth (Rohde, Lewinsohn, & Seeley, 1994), behaviors, emotions, and thoughts are emphasized as components acting and interacting to contribute to symptoms of depression. The CWDA protocol includes SM as a technique to address each of these components. For example, the teen may be taught that the thought "I won't have any fun" leads to the behavior of avoiding a school dance. The behavior (staying home rather than going to the dance) then leads to feeling lonely and sad, which leads to more negative thoughts ("I am alone and no one loves me"). Self-monitoring is used to help the teen become more aware of this process and identify potential intervention points (e.g., going to the dance or changing the negative thoughts) that would lead to decreased negative mood. In line with previous work involving younger children (e.g., Reynolds & Stark, 1985), the CWDA protocol includes self-monitoring of participation in pleasurable activities, as it has been shown that individuals with depression participate in fewer pleasurable events (Kaslow, Rehm, & Siegel, 1984). Behaviorally, engagement in pleasurable events can increase the experience of positive emotions and the willingness to engage in such activities. For instance, the adolescent chooses examples of pleasurable activities from a list developed either by the adolescent or from a list provided by the therapist, performs or takes part in the activities, and rates the level of interest in the activity as well as one's mood prior to and after completion. Over time, the tracking of these experiences can provide useful information for both the therapist and adolescent about changes in willingness to engage in pleasurable activities and changes in mood after taking part in the activities.

## THE ELEMENT IN PRACTICE

### "Core of the Core" Element

Though SM can be done in a number of ways, several procedures are often considered necessary for its effective use in therapy. Box 11.1 outlines the basic steps for administering SM, and Box 11.2 (at the end of the chapter) describes the use of SM procedures for an adolescent boy with social anxiety disorder. Like any therapy element, SM should be presented within the context of a strong therapeutic relationship. Research suggests that the strength of the therapeutic alliance is positively correlated with engagement in therapeutic tasks (Chu et al., 2004; Shirk & Saisz, 1992) and, more broadly, to treatment outcomes for youth with internalizing disorders (Chu & Kendall, 2004; McLeod & Weisz, 2005; Shirk & Karver, 2003). Obtaining full engagement in the SM task (Step 1) is facilitated by first establishing an alliance with the youth. Inviting questions and concerns from youth while describing the SM task will further build the therapeutic relationship. Importantly, the various components of SM should be presented in ways consonant with the youth's developmental level. Youth receiving treatment for internalizing disorders will vary widely in their cognitive abilities, with some able to engage in only the most concrete forms of thinking and others in the more abstract forms characterized by formal operational thought (Piaget, 1972). Attending closely to the youth's developmental level will help the therapist to use descriptions of the SM task for the subsequent devising of actual SM tasks that the child can readily comprehend (see the "Developmental Adaptations" section later for specific considerations).

Once the youth is sufficiently engaged in the process, the next steps (Steps 2–4 in Box 11.1) focus on identifying the thought, behavior, or feeling that is to be monitored and the procedure for doing so. The decision of which variable to monitor will likely be based on hypotheses about factors related to the etiology or maintenance of the youth's

## BOX 11.1. Task Analysis of Self-Monitoring

1. Obtain the youth's engagement in the activity by providing a clear rationale for the activity that is tailored to the child's developmental level. Invite questions and clarification from the youth.

2. Identify the variable to be monitored in the context of the youth's developmental level, and be as specific as possible. For example, encourage a younger child to self-monitor "nervous or worried thoughts" as opposed to "anxious cognitions." Likewise, rather than referring to "feelings," identify "anxiety" or "sadness" as specific emotions to be self-monitored.

3. Decide which method to use to monitor the variable.
   a. Consider the youth's developmental level and individual characteristics. For instance, if a youth has an expressive writing disorder, consider alternative methods of monitoring. If a youth enjoys technology, consider whether an electronic method of recording would be appropriate.
   b. Specify the frequency of recording.

4. Collaboratively create the monitoring device with the youth, where possible, to increase his or her involvement in the activity. Encourage the youth to think creatively about the self-monitoring device.

5. Identify positive reinforcements for SM. Allow the youth, in collaboration with his or her parent, to identify rewards prior to the monitoring that he or she can earn for successful completion of the SM.

6. Model for the youth how to self-monitor the identified variable. Encourage questions and clarifications from the youth.

7. Discuss and problem-solve potential difficulties that may arise during SM (e.g., the youth forgets to fill in the record at an indicated time, the log takes longer than anticipated to complete, the variable to be monitored does not actually occur during the week). Emphasize the youth's effort at SM and *attempts* to independently problem-solve difficulties rather than actual performance.

8. Have the youth self-monitor the identified behavior as directed until the next therapy session. Review the SM task with the parents when the youth is younger and/or the therapist anticipates difficulties with the task.

9. Review the SM log at the next therapy session.
   a. Emphasize the youth's *efforts*.
   b. Problem-solve issues that arose (e.g., the youth did not monitor the intended variable, did not complete the record fully or as instructed, or denied that the variable was encountered).
   c. Reinforce efforts with a preidentified reward.

10. Create a display of the SM log, where appropriate, for use with both the youth and therapist. For example, creating a pictorial representation of a decrease in an undesirable behavior may serve as a reinforcer to the youth. Visual

representations of the results of an SM log, whether it was completed for 1 week or several, can also assist in guiding future treatment directions.

11. Discuss with the child the potential use of future SM tasks.
    a. Assess the child's beliefs about the usefulness of the SM task.
    b. Collaboratively plan future SM tasks, as appropriate.

distress. For instance, if the therapist identifies a lack of engagement in pleasant activities as a contributing factor to depressive symptoms, then the therapist and youth might agree to monitor mood during preplanned activities that are expected to elicit positive affect. Regardless of the particular variable to be monitored, the therapist should be clear about the specific variable on which the youth should focus. For example, rather than having the youth monitor "feelings," the therapist should direct the youth to monitor "anxious feelings."

Once there is agreement on the particular variable to be monitored, the therapist and child can collaboratively decide how to monitor the variable and at what frequency. In this case, the youth can be encouraged to think creatively, with the therapist's assistance, about SM devices. For instance, if a youth does not like to write or is indifferent about standard paper-and-pencil measures of recording, the youth can use a voice recording device to complete the task. Such high-tech devices as data recorders or smart phones can also be used as an SM device. Younger youth may enjoy and thus respond better to pictorial SM exercises (Beidel et al., 1991). The particular device that is chosen may depend, in part, on the frequency of the SM. For example, a SM exercise that requires the youth to record a variable many times a day might benefit more from using efficient recording devices that require little writing than an SM task that requires recording just a few times in one day.

Contingent reinforcement is also a "core element" of evidence-based treatments for internalizing disorders in youth (see Chapter 9) and should be incorporated into the SM process. Recording of one's behavior and/or feelings can be highly demanding process for youth, particularly those who are experiencing distress. Initial engagement and ongoing participation in the SM tasks may be facilitated by identifying specific rewards that the youth can earn upon significant effort or successful completion of the task. The caregiver, teacher, or therapist may wish to facilitate the child's tracking of successful events (e.g., participating in a pleasant event) via a point bank or sticker chart. Also consider that the youth will likely be receiving rewards throughout the treatment program. Starting out with a very large reward will make it difficult to effectively reinforce tasks that the youth may perceive as harder later in treatment. On the other hand, the reward should be meaningful enough to be reinforcing. Generally, the child's self-monitoring of progress can serve several functions, including inducing positive affect, highlighting accomplishments and mastery, and encouraging a sense of self-efficacy for the child.

During the next steps (Steps 6 and 7), the therapist models how to self-monitor the chosen variable using the selected monitoring device and troubleshoots potential difficulties that may arise. For instance, if the therapist and youth collaboratively agree to self-monitor specified feelings during particular times of the day using pictorial representations, then the therapist should role-play that specific situation and actually complete one entry in the SM log during the session. If the youth cannot imagine potential scenarios, the therapist can provide assistance. For instance, if a youth decides to use a palm recorder to monitor his or her mood, the therapist might troubleshoot solutions if the palm recorder were to stop working during the week (e.g., begin using a paper-and-pencil diary). The clinician should help the youth to troubleshoot several issues that might arise in an effort to facilitate successful completion of the task.

The final steps (Steps 8–11) involve having the youth complete the SM task, reviewing the log with the therapist, and discussing future SM tasks. While reviewing the SM task, the therapist should be sure to praise the child's efforts in completing the task. Youth experiencing internalizing symptoms may experience difficulties in being aware of their emotions (Suveg, Hoffman, Zeman, & Thomassin, 2009), which may make the task of monitoring their mood or feelings challenging. For instance, if a child is instructed to self-monitor specific feelings but has difficulty differentiating among them, the task is likely to be difficult to complete. Likewise, monitoring "anxious thinking" may be harder for younger youth than for older children and adolescents, and so therapists should be sure to praise their best efforts. It is also important to consider difficulties that arose with the task and to problem-solve as necessary. For example, if a child had a difficult time charting specific emotions, assess whether additional coaching in emotion labeling and awareness may be necessary prior to further implementing the SM. The therapist can also process the youth's experience in completing the task—was it wholly unpleasant, or were there some parts that were fun or even informative for the child? Gauging the youth's actual experience with the task in depth will facilitate the discussion of whether and how to best implement specific SM tasks in the future.

After a few weeks of SM tasks, it might be beneficial to create a visual representation of the results. For instance, by graphing SM results, one might better discern under what conditions a youth is most likely to experience a particularly distressing emotion. Alternatively, by examining SM results on the graph, the youth and therapist might notice that a distressing behavior has actually decreased over time. Sometimes patterns or trends become more evident when displayed in a visual format. Charting the SM results may also help the youth to appreciate the significance of the task. For example, for reluctant youth, visualizing decreases in undesirable patterns of behavior or increases in desirable ones may motivate them to continue with future SM tasks that seem tedious.

## Developmental Adaptations

SM is used more frequently in the treatment of internalizing disorders for older children and adolescents as compared to younger youth, given that the ability to accurately identify and report on thoughts and feelings increases with age (King, Ollendick, & Murphy, 1997). A variety of adaptations have been used to match the developmental level of the child and increase the utility of SM techniques (Kingery et al., 2006). Younger or cognitively delayed youth might benefit from pictorial representations of the particular behavior to be monitored (Houghton, 1991). For example, imagine a child with separation anxiety who is receiving anxiety treatment because she (or he) is scared to sleep alone in her room. The therapist might print out a picture of a child in a bed or have the client bring in a picture of herself in bed. The picture can then be placed on a chart that keeps track of the target behavior (i.e., the hours/nights spent sleeping in her own bed). The use of thought bubbles (Kendall & Hedtke, 2006) or other pictorial representations can be helpful in assisting younger youth in self-monitoring their cognitions. For example, comic strips with blank thought bubbles could be used to help younger children understand the concept of recognizing thoughts. Moreover, several different thoughts could be offered up for the same situation to demonstrate how thinking affects emotions and behaviors (see Chapter 3).

Younger or cognitively delayed youth may also benefit more from parental involvement than older youth and adolescents, given their developmental differences in the need for autonomy (Kendall et al., 2002). For example, in the Kiddie Cat anxiety treatment program for young children (ages 4–7 years), parents are actively involved throughout the entire treatment and are taught skills to help the child monitor anxiety symptoms and decrease avoidant behavior (Hughes, Hedtke, Flannery-Schroeder, & Kendall, 2005). Additionally, younger and/or cognitively delayed youth may need help learning how to self-monitor (e.g., through modeling) and external reinforcement for appropriate completion of SM tasks. For example, a study examining an SM training program for adults with mental retardation found modeling and positive reinforcement to be essential components of teaching and maintaining SM behavior (Matson et al., 1980). Conversely, SM with older children and adolescents may be done without parental involvement at all (e.g., Clarke et al., 1990; Ollendick, 1995).

Simplifying the forms and scales used to self-monitor could also make them more understandable for younger children (King et al., 1997). In the Coping Cat treatment for youth with anxiety, for instance, an 8-point thermometer scale is used to help children rate their distress, giving them a concrete framework to help rate their anxiety. Adolescents and adults may be more likely to use a 10- or 100-point SUDS that does not necessarily have accompanying pictorial representations (Heard et al., 1992). Similarly, younger children could be provided with several concrete SM questions or concrete SM reminders. For example, the notion of challenging cognitive distortions with cognitive restructuring is relatively abstract. Rather than use abstract language, the idea of "thinking traps" can be used to teach younger children how to recognize maladaptive thinking patterns (Kendall & Hedtke, 2006). "Thinking traps" represent categories of cognitive distortions that "trap" children into patterns of anxious or depressed thinking. Once "thinking traps" are understood, therapists can work with young children to identify positive counterthoughts or "cheerleading statements." Physical reminders such as index cards or bracelets can be used to help young children to remember to check the accuracy of their thinking. For instance, the therapist and child can write "thinking traps" on one index card and "cheerleading statements" on another for the child to keep in his or her pocket, desk at school, or other accessible location. Similarly, the therapist and child can make a bracelet, sign, or other visual depiction as a reminder to use their coping skills or as a way to encourage cheerleading statements. For example, the bracelet could say "Skills rule!," "Think positive," "No fear!," or any other word or phrase that reminds the child to monitor his or her mood and use coping skills as needed. The sign could be a helpful motto (e.g., "No worries" or "Find the silver lining") and should be placed in a spot that the child is likely to frequently encounter (e.g., on the bathroom mirror, or on the inside of the front door so they see it as they are leaving for school). A case study by Ollendick (1981) revealed wrist counters to be an effective method of SM for two boys (ages 7 and 11 years) with nervous tics. Older youth or those with well-developed cognitive skills can complete written SM logs (Clarke et al., 1990; Ollendick, 1995). Adolescents with depression may be asked to self-monitor by using a flowchart that documents activating events, beliefs, the consequences of those beliefs, the accuracy of the beliefs, possible reinterpretations of the activating event, and subsequent consequences (Clarke et al., 1990).

The increasing use of high-tech devices in treatment and the relevant developmental factors must both be considered in determining the appropriateness of technological strategies for SM (Kendall, Khanna, Edson, Cummings, & Harris, 2011). For example, in a pilot study for adolescents with high-functioning autism, technological devices were used (e.g., iPod Touch) to help youth monitor their anxiety symptoms (Reaven, 2011). Another pilot study that used a community sample of youth ages 7–12 years found only mixed support for the use of palm pilots to monitor mood and emotion regulation (Suveg, Payne, Thomassin, & Jacob, 2010). However, Thomassin, Morelen, and Suveg (2012) found that when youth do monitor their emotions there is a perceivable therapeutic effect. In this study, school-age youth were given electronic diaries to record the emotions they were feeling and the intensity of the experience through diaries that were prompted to alert the child to make recordings at four random times of the day during after-school hours. The results indicated that girls who reported poor emotional coping or who were reluctant to express their emotions based on a parent report showed a reduction in anxiety symptoms 1 week after tracking their emotional experiences via the electronic diaries. The mechanism by which was effected was not identified, although the authors suggested that self-monitoring their mood states over the course of the week may have given the youth increased practice in identifying their emotional experiences, contributing to a sense of mastery and subsequently assisting them in adaptive emotion regulation. For youth who were previously reluctant to share their emotional experiences, the electronic diaries may have served as a non-threatening way to express their emotions. There are also newly developed Internet- and computer-based programs used in anxiety treatment with youth as young as 7 years old that teach and facilitate SM strategies (Kendall et al., 2011). For instance, Camp Cope-A-Lot is a colorful and interactive computerized version of CBT for youth (Kendall & Khanna, 2008a). The program features SM components of CBT that youth can complete at their own pace, including monitoring levels of anxiety and completing exposure tasks. Given the increasing rates of children who have or know how to use cell phones and the increasing tendency for schools to incorporate laptops/tablets into the curriculum, it seems that high-tech modes of SM will grow in popularity. The growth of various SM techniques may make them increasingly more relevant, fun, and accessible to youth than traditional paper-and-pencil methods of SM. Despite the increased technological sophistication of today's youth, no known studies have been conducted investigating developmental considerations when using high-tech devices for SM. More research is needed to ascertain the effectiveness of more technically oriented ways of implementing SM and the unique developmental considerations inherent in incorporating a new method of SM into treatment.

## Diversity Considerations

No studies have examined specific SM adaptations for ethnically diverse groups of children. Therefore, conclusions regarding diversity considerations can only be generalized from the broader treatment outcome literature. Several treatments for internalizing disorders that include an SM component have shown efficacy with diverse populations. For example, Rosselló and Bernal (1999) examined the efficacy of CBT with Puerto Rican adolescents meeting the criteria for depression. Their CBT treatment protocol included SM activities such as a daily mood scale, weekly activities schedule, and self-monitoring of thoughts and behavior. Similarly, CBT has been demonstrated to be an efficacious treatment for anxiety in Hispanic/Latino youth (Pina et al., 2003) and low-income African American adolescents (Ginsburg & Drake, 2002). The CBT in both of these studies included the self-monitoring of thoughts (to be restructured) and self-reward and were effective as individual- (Pina et al., 2003) and school-based (Ginsburg & Drake, 2002) interventions. A CBT-based depression intervention program that included SM was also found to be effective for Chinese youth (Yu & Seligman, 2002).

Although no known studies have examined specific modifications of SM with diverse youth, several general suggestions can be gathered from the broader culturally sensitive treatment literature. Cultural background and ethnic identity have been shown to influence the presentation and treatment of psychopathology as reflected by culture-bound syndromes, varying idioms of distress (i.e., how one expresses his or her distress), and differential reactions to treatment methods (Cooley & Boyce, 2004; Parron, 1997). For example, research has demonstrated that Hispanic/Latino children report more somatic symptoms than Caucasian peers but that patterns of somatic reporting vary by ethnocultural and language group (Pina & Silverman, 2004;

Umaña-Taylor & Fine, 2001). A link between somatic complaints and internalizing problems has also been documented among Asian and Asian American youth (Gee, 2004; B. Weiss, Tram, Weisz, Rescorla, & Achenbach, 2009). A tendency to report distress through somatic descriptions has implications for SM because somatic complaints are often tracked in both anxiety and depression treatments. Therapists working with youth with somatic complaints should use psychoeducation before encouraging youth to track their feelings and physiological reactions, given the possibility of mood symptoms being intertwined with physical problems. For example, therapists often observe that various physical symptoms (headaches, stomachaches) frequently accompany anxiety. Self-monitoring has the potential to increase hypervigilance regarding such symptoms if not prefaced with psychoeducation. Of course, the therapist can also use SM diaries (or other SM methods) to help the child identify patterns in symptoms and to illustrate the psychosomatic nature of their complaints. Understanding who is at risk for expressing psychological distress through somatic complaints is helpful, but it is not a substitute for empirically supported assessment, regardless of the youth's ethnic or cultural identification.

When using SM techniques with youth, cultural influences on cognitive appraisals should also be considered. For example, the value of *simpatía* in Mexican and Mexican American cultures encourages individuals to empathize, respect, and try to please others, sometimes requiring personal sacrifices (Gabrielidis, Stephan, Ybarra, Pearson, & Villareal, 1997). Collectivism, a sense of interdependence among group members and emphasis on group harmony over individualistic attention (Markus & Kitayama, 1991), is another cultural value with the potential to influence cognitive appraisals (Varela et al., 2004). Such values as *simpatía* and collectivism could result in greater attention to social evaluation because of the youth's concern with how their own behavior impacts others (Jung & Stinnett, 2005; Varela et al., 2004). When teaching youth with internalizing problems to attend to thoughts and evaluate their accuracy, cultural values should be taken into consideration. For example, a child might have the thought "If I don't do well on this exam, my parents will be ashamed of me." Depending on the cultural climate in the home, that thought may or may not be accurate. Therefore, the family climate should be assessed before using SM to challenge the reality of the youth's thoughts. If the therapist believes the thought may be accurate, then focus could then be placed on the child's thoughts regarding his or her ability to manage negative emotions that arise from the parents' expectations for him or her. Internalizing symptoms and their treatment should always be considered within the proper context, including how SM should be applied and adapted with diverse populations.

## CONCLUSIONS

Used both in assessment and therapeutic contexts, SM techniques have a long history in the psychological literature that is grounded in behavioral principles. SM tasks became increasingly popular during the early 1970s, given the *zeitgeist* of the time regarding self-control techniques that assisted individuals in acting as their own therapists. Today, SM techniques are used in the assessment context and are a common element of most EBT programs for youth experiencing anxiety and depressive disorders. Importantly, research suggests that SM techniques can be used successfully with youth of varying ages, races, and ethnicities. Some empirical evidence supports the use of SM alone, though there is surprisingly little empirical support for the inclusion of SM as part of a broader treatment package; the effort to disaggregate studies should prove helpful in this regard. Nonetheless, as the case example in Box 11.2 illustrates, SM can be used to facilitate behavior change for youth experiencing internalizing difficulties. A practical step-by-step guide was presented in Box 11.1 and the related discussion to assist therapists with the general application of SM tasks. However, particular attention must be paid to the child's developmental level and issues of diversity in order to assure the most effective implementation of this core element.

---

### BOX 11.2. Illustrative Case Example

John, a 14-year-old Caucasian male in the ninth grade, was seen for 12 sessions of individual CBT for social anxiety disorder. John's symptoms were interfering most in the school setting, where significant physiological symptoms accompanied his evaluative concerns. John would not voluntarily ask or answer questions in class, engage in class discussions, or interact with unfamiliar peers. He was frequently tardy for school or came home early from school a a result of significant physiological symptoms that mostly took the form of nausea and the feeling that he was going to vomit or that he had to use the bathroom. John, like many youth, did not come to therapy on his own volition—rather, he came to treatment as a result of his parents' and teachers' concerns.

The SM component of CBT involved John's monitoring his anxious thoughts and progress toward therapy goals, as in traditional treatment programs. In this case, John's physiological symptoms served as the primary target for self-monitoring. Upon starting therapy, John believed that his symptoms were related to an unidentified medical disorder rather than his anxiety. In fact, his parents had taken him for several medical evaluations prior to seeking psychological therapy. No known medical etiology could be identified. Nonetheless, John's resistance to acknowledge his physiological symptoms as a part of his anxiety posed a challenge. Because of this resistance, the therapist first addressed cognitive and behavioral aspects of anxiety while attempting to develop greater rapport.

To begin SM, the therapist first had John monitor his anxious thoughts. Given John's age, traditionally columned, paper-and-pencil forms were used as SM devices. Each day, John jotted down each time he had an anxious thought in one column, the situation in another, and the behavioral outcome in a final column. Though the frequency of thoughts varied greatly from day to day, John monitored his thoughts quite successfully with relatively little effort. He did note, however, that it was difficult to document each time he experienced an anxious thought because it often occurred when peers were around him. In this case, the therapist brainstormed with John ti develop potential solutions, such as putting a mark on his notebook to remind him to write the thoughts down as soon as he got home. Next, the therapist had John self-monitor his positive thoughts while in anxiety-provoking situations and the behavioral outcome. The same type of SM device was used for this purpose. Throughout the process of SM, the therapist also encouraged John to monitor his treatment progress. Though John did not evidence significant gains until the second half of treatment, he realized that increasing awareness of his thinking was helpful.

Once John was engaged in the treatment process, the therapist initiated discussions about self-monitoring his physiological symptoms. By this time in treatment, John and the therapist had developed sufficient rapport that John was willing to attempt the recommended therapy strategies. John began to self-monitor his physiological symptoms by first keeping a frequency count. All of John's physiological symptoms (nausea, feeling as though he was going to vomit, feeling as though he had to use the bathroom) were listed on a piece of paper, and John simply checked each time they occurred. After a week of keeping frequency counts, separate columns were added to the sheet for John to write a short description of what he was doing when he noticed the physiological symptoms, the time of day, severity of symptoms, and what he did once he noticed the symptoms. Upon returning the log, John and the therapist processed its contents and identified patterns. For instance, John frequently experienced physiological symptoms before school and during school hours on days that he experienced increased evaluation. He also came to recognize that when he engaged in active attempts at coping (e.g., trying to focus on something else, using positive thoughts) his symptoms usually subsided within a short period. The most difficult part for John was not acting on his symptoms, because they were quite distressing. For instance, when John initially began monitoring, he reported that as soon as he began to feel as though he needed to use the bathroom he would immediately go. Through self-monitoring John was able to identify that his symptoms were related to anxiety and that they usually subsided within a short period of time if he engaged in some sort of problem solving. Increasing self-awareness of his physiological symptoms greatly facilitated eventual treatment success.

# 12

## Goal Setting

## BACKGROUND OF THE ELEMENT

Goal setting involves defining the ideal outcomes that will occur as a result of therapy. Developing a clear, mutually agreed-upon set of overarching goals is crucial, as goals help guide the selection of intervention strategies. More formally defined, treatment goals "represent desired outcomes and they function as benchmarks of client progress" (Cormier et al., 2013, p. 269). Near the beginning of treatment, the clinician discusses broad goals with the youth and family. Continued collaborative discussion leads to a more individualized set of goals, which is often revised throughout treatment. Some manual-based treatments involve direct instruction related to goal setting. For example, several depression treatment programs cover how to set specific and realistic goals for skills such as pleasant events scheduling, and youth specify their goals in a written contract (e.g., Clarke et al., 1990). In contrast, many anxiety treatment programs do not explicitly teach goal setting. Instead, overall program goals are reviewed at the beginning of treatment, and specific goals are established more indirectly as treatment progresses (e.g., when constructing a fear hierarchy, which establishes goals for the completion of exposure tasks; Kendall & Hedtke, 2006). Despite these differences, it is possible to identify common steps for goal setting that are shared across many manual-based programs for anxious and depressed youth. These steps are outlined in the more applied second half of this chapter; but first the historical roots, theoretical background, and empirical foundation of goal setting are discussed, to place this element in a broader context.

## Brief History

Goal setting can be traced back to the early 1900s, when discussions focused on identifying the driving force behind the relationship between physiological states (e.g., hunger, sexual arousal) and subsequent behavior (e.g., searching for food, courting behavior). Psychologists initially postulated that instincts caused this behavior. In contrast, McDougall (1908) suggested that an individual experiencing a physiological need is pursuing an identifiable *goal*, and therefore the behavior is *purposeful*. As early as the 1930s and 1940s, several individuals began to challenge behaviorist views of human personality and behavior. For example, Tolman (1938, 1948) postulated that rats' behavior in mazes could not be accounted for solely by stimulus–response learning but also appeared to be influenced by such internal factors as expectations, goals, and knowledge of cause–effect in a given situation. By the 1960s, it became clear that behavioral theories were incomplete and that humans are often motivated by cognitive needs and processes (Hunt, 2007). This emphasis on cognitive mediators of behavior provides a historical foundation for goal setting.

The emergence of social learning theory during the 1950s placed further emphasis on the cognitive aspects of behavior. In general, social learning theory posits that human personality and behavior are shaped not only by which behaviors are actually rewarded but also by individuals' *beliefs or expectations* about the kinds of behaviors that will be rewarded. In his adaptation of this perspective, Julian Rotter (1954) emphasized that when particular behaviors are either rewarded or not rewarded (e.g., studying for a test results in a good grade or not) individuals develop general cognitive expectations about the types of behaviors that are likely to be rewarded in the future. In turn, these expectations influence individuals' behavior. Following Rotter, Bandura (1977a) spearheaded continued developments in social learning theory, asserting that individuals develop cognitive representations of themselves through various social experiences such as modeling and verbal discussions. He viewed individuals' self-efficacy beliefs (i.e., expectations related to mastering behavioral challenges) as a crucial component of behavior change. Bandura's (1986) contemporary version of social learning theory (i.e., social cognitive theory) remains influential even today, and his ideas surrounding self-efficacy certainly have implications for goal setting and accomplishment. For example, research indicates that individuals with higher self-efficacy tend to establish challenging goals and remain committed to them, persisting even when faced with obstacles or potential failure (Schunk & Pajares, 2005).

The field of humanistic psychology also emerged during the 1950s and 1960s, at approximately the same time as social learning theory. The humanists emphasized concepts directly related to goal setting, such as an individual's power to choose how he or she wants to behave and pursue self-fulfillment (Cormier et al., 2013). In his client-centered therapy, Carl Rogers (1951, 1961) asserted that his approach of providing an atmosphere of safety, warmth, and empathy helped clients to be self-directed, exploring feelings of their choice and accomplishing goals that they set for themselves. Rogers (1961) pointed out that the questions most often expressed by his clients were such ones as "What is my goal in life?," "What am I striving for?," and "What is my purpose?" (p. 164). Although goal setting in contemporary CBT tends to be more directive, ideas surrounding the importance of incorporating the clients' own perspective into the goals for therapy are rooted firmly in the humanistic perspective.

During the 1960s and 1970s, paralleling an explosion of research on basic cognitive processes (e.g., memory, information processing, language, reasoning) were developments in cognitive and cognitive-behavioral therapeutic methods, providing further historical context for goal setting. Influenced by early cognitive therapists, Meichenbaum emphasized the role of self-statements in directing individuals' behavior. He developed self-instructional training to teach patterns of covert verbalization that led to better control over overt verbal and motor behavior (Meichenbaum & J. Goodman, 1971). During self-instructional training, the child moves from watching an adult perform a task while verbalizing a deliberate strategy out loud to eventually being able to perform the task while repeating the instructions to him- or herself. The strategies that are verbalized during this process relate directly to the broader goals of therapy (e.g., teaching impulsive children specific steps toward the goal of being able to stop and plan before performing a behavior). Problem-solving therapy (also called social problem-solving therapy) is another cognitive-behavioral approach that focuses more explicitly on goal setting (D'Zurilla & Goldfried, 1971). After helping to identify and define problems, the therapist then assists the client in setting goals by having him or her answer the question "What must happen so that I no longer have the problem?" The goals can be either situation-focused (i.e., changing the actual situation that is causing the problem) or reaction-focused (i.e., changing the individual's affective, cognitive, and/or behavioral responses to the situation). The goals that are formulated guide the generation of possible solutions during the next stage of the problem-solving process (see Chapter 4).

Given this strong historical foundation, goal setting remains a key component of contemporary cognitive-behavioral interventions for internalizing disorders among youth. In fact, based upon a distillation and matching model employed to identify common strategies across EBTs, Chorpita and Daleiden (2009) found that goal setting was among the most frequently employed practices for the treatment of depressed mood among children and adolescents.

## Theory Base

Cognitive-behavioral theory also posits key assumptions about the content of treatment goals as well as the goal-setting process. In general, CBT takes a goal-oriented and problem-focused approach, emphasizing active participation on the part of clients (J. S. Beck, 2011). When working with children and adolescents, a collaborative approach involving shared decision making among parents, youth, and the clinician is utilized (Mash, 2006). Importantly, youth are "fully informed of the objectives of treatment and the methods that are going to be employed to achieve those objectives" (Stark, Sander, et al., 2006, p. 366). Clinicians play a key role in this collaborative endeavor by helping youth to articulate their goals for therapy and also by assisting caregivers in generating goals for their child, family, and/or parenting behavior. According to Judith Beck (2011), the process of specifying problems and setting specific goals in CBT allows the therapist and client to have a mutual understanding of what they are working on in therapy. Goals also serve as a guide for choosing intervention strategies, and they are revisited (and often revised) frequently as treatment progresses.

Within CBT, there is a broad perspective on goal setting, emphasizing that "treatment goals should focus on building skills in the child and his or her social environment that will reduce impairment and facilitate long-term adjustment, not just on the elimination of problem behaviors and/or the short-term reduction of subjective distress" (Mash, 2006, p. 12). Although reducing symptoms of psychopathology is often the primary goal of CBT with children and adolescents, several other goals are also viewed as being critical, including improving children's functioning (e.g., academic, social), enhancing family functioning, and addressing outcomes that can impact the larger society (e.g., a lower incidence of student drop-out in schools, decreased involvement in the juvenile justice system).

In addition to the theoretical foundation provided above, Cormier et al. (2013) outline six key purposes of treatment goals, highlighting the important role that goal setting plays in the therapeutic process. First, these authors assert that goals serve the purpose of providing a sense of direction for therapy by prioritizing a client's problems, clarifying clients' expectations about treatment, individualizing therapy, and (when established in a collaborative manner) helping clients to feel more invested in the treatment process. Second, goals help to promote successful performance and problem solving, because they are "usually rehearsed in our working memory and because they direct our attention to the resources and components in our environment that are most likely to help with the solution of a problem" (Cormier et al., 2013, p. 270). Third, goal setting helps to provide expectations for improvement and give clients a sense of hope, which contributes to a greater level of investment in treatment, thereby promoting client change. Fourth, goals allow a clinician to determine whether he or she has the skills required to help a client with particular goals. Fifth, they guide the clinician's selection of intervention strategies. Finally, goals serve as a standard against which to monitor progress and garner feedback to determine the effectiveness of the intervention.

## Evidence Base

Although the goal-setting treatment element has not been evaluated individually, evidence for its efficacy comes from studies examining this element as part of multicomponent CBT protocols for internalizing disorders among youth. According to guidelines published by the American Psychological Association's Division 12, CBT is "probably efficacious" for the treatment of childhood depression, "well-established" for adolescent depression, "probably efficacious" for child and adolescent anxiety disorders, and "possibly efficacious" for pediatric bipolar spectrum disorders (e.g., David-Ferdon & Kaslow, 2008; Fristad & MacPherson, 2014; Silverman, Pina, et al., 2008). In addition, interpersonal psychotherapy is a "well-established" treatment for adolescent depression (Verdeli et al., 2006), and family psychoeducation plus skills building (i.e., individual family or multifamily psychoeducational psychotherapy) is considered "probably efficacious" for pediatric bipolar disorders (Fristad & MacPherson, 2014). Table 12.1 includes a description

**TABLE 12.1. The Goal Setting Element in Representative EBT Manuals**

| | |
|---|---|
| *Coping Cat* (Kendall & Hedtke, 2006) | • Although goal setting is not explicitly taught, the clinician discusses program goals at the beginning of treatment (i.e., identifying anxious feelings/thoughts, using coping strategies). The clinician and the youth set more specific goals when constructing the fear hierarchy. Goals are also reviewed during two parent sessions. |
| *C.A.T. Project* (Kendall, Choudhury, Hudson, & Webb, 2002) | • Goal setting is not explicitly taught, but the clinician discusses program goals at the beginning of treatment, explained to the youth as "knowing when you're anxious," "knowing what to do about it," and practicing skills in real-life situations. More specific treatment goals are established through the creation of the fear hierarchy. Goals are also reviewed in two parent sessions. |
| *Family-Based Treatment for Young Children with OCD* (Freeman & Garcia, 2009) | • Goal setting is not explicitly taught, but goals of the program are discussed with the parents at the beginning of treatment (e.g., reducing OCD symptoms, increasing family problem solving). The clinician also discusses the goal of working together to fight against OCD. A symptom hierarchy, which is reviewed and revised weekly, is used to set goals for exposure tasks. |
| *OCD in Children and Adolescents* (March & Mulle, 1998) | • Goal setting is not explicitly taught, but the clinician outlines goals at the beginning of each session, and an information sheet with goals for the week is given to the youth at the end of each session. The clinician and the child discuss more specific goals when mapping OCD (i.e., identifying obsessions, compulsions, triggers, and avoidance behavior to place on a stimulus hierarchy). |
| *CBT of Childhood OCD: It's Only a False Alarm* (Piacentini, Langley, & Roblek, 2007) | • Goal setting is not explicitly taught, but the clinician and family create a symptom hierarchy at the beginning of treatment (i.e., My Symptom List), used to determine which symptoms to focus on. The hierarchy is reviewed every few sessions, and improvement ratings are completed periodically to assess the youth's progress. |
| *CBT for Social Phobia: Stand Up, Speak Out* (Albano & DiBartolo, 2007) | • At the beginning of treatment, the clinician explicitly asks the youth to list their goals related to improvements in social functioning (while referring to the Fear and Avoidance Hierarchy developed during the assessment) and discuss them with the group. Teens also complete a "What are my life goals?" sheet. Later in treatment, specific goals for the exposure portion of the treatment are defined. |
| *When Children Refuse School: A CBT Approach* (Kearney & Albano, 2007): Chapters 4 and 5 on internalizing symptoms | • Goal setting is not explicitly taught, but the clinician reviews general program goals during the pretreatment consultation (e.g., learn coping skills to reduce school avoidance). Specific goals related to the reasons why each child is avoiding school are also discussed. Goals for school attendance may also be outlined in a treatment contract. |

*(continued)*

**TABLE 12.1.** (*continued*)

| | |
|---|---|
| *Treating Trauma and Traumatic Grief in Children and Adolescents* (Cohen, Mannarino, & Deblinger, 2006) | • Goal setting is not explicitly taught; however, when providing feedback about the assessment, the clinician describes the treatment plan and how it will help the child/family overcome difficulties (e.g., learning skills for coping with trauma). General program goals are also reviewed at the beginning of treatment. |
| *Adolescent Coping with Depression* (Clarke, Lewinsohn, & Hops, 1990) | • Goal setting is explicitly taught at several points during this program. At the beginning of treatment, the teens write down weekly goals on a form in their workbook. They learn how to set specific and realistic goals for pleasant activities and develop a personal contract. Near the end of treatment, they complete a Life Plan Worksheet with specific and realistic long-term goals, discussing possible obstacles and ways to overcome them. |
| *Interpersonal Psychotherapy for Depressed Adolescents,* 2nd edition (Mufson, Pollack Dorta, Moreau, & Weissman, 2011) | • Goal setting is not explicitly taught, but after identifying one to two problem areas that will be the focus of treatment (e.g., interpersonal deficits, role transitions), the clinician helps the teen work toward the goals for that problem area. Goals and strategies for each problem area are outlined in the manual. At the beginning of treatment, a treatment contract (including goals) is reviewed with the teen and his or her parents. At termination, progress made toward the goals is reviewed. |
| *Treating Depressed Children: Therapist Manual for "Taking Action"* (Stark & Kendall, 1996) | • Goal setting is not explicitly taught, but the clinician discusses participants' expectations about the group (e.g., learn skills for coping with unpleasant feelings, solving problems) during the first session. The clinician indirectly models goal setting at the beginning of each session by writing down things he or she would like to cover, asking group members to add to the list, and setting an agenda. |
| *Treating Depressed Youth: Therapist Manual for "Action"* (Stark et al., 2007) | • Goal setting is explicitly covered throughout this program. The clinician has an individual goal setting meeting with each group participant at the beginning of treatment, followed by a review of the individual goals and corresponding action plans during group sessions to solicit peer support for the goals. At mid-treatment, the clinician holds a second individual meeting to review progress toward the goals' attainment. Several additional goal-attainment check-ins are held. |
| *Psychotherapy for Children with Bipolar and Depressive Disorders* (Fristad, Arnold, & Leffler, 2011) | • Goal setting is taught indirectly through the Family Fix-It List take-home project, which focuses on helping the family generate a list of three problems that they mutually agree to work on during treatment. The clinician first helps the child to create his or her own list and the parents are instructed to create a separate list, and then a combined Family Fix-It List is generated. Progress toward this list is reviewed periodically throughout the treatment. |

*Note.* Some book titles are shortened to conserve space. See the References at the back of the book for full titles.

of the extent to which goal setting is incorporated into several commonly used treatment manuals; a sampling of the empirical support for several programs in which goal setting is explicitly taught will be reviewed in this section.

Originally developed for depressed adults in outpatient settings, interpersonal psychotherapy for depressed adolescents focuses on interpersonal issues that are common during adolescence, such as separation from parents, loss of a loved one, romantic relationships, and conflicts with peers (Mufson et al., 2011). With respect to goal setting, the clinician and teen collaboratively develop goals for one or two of four problem areas (i.e., grief, interpersonal role disputes, interpersonal role transitions, interpersonal deficits), and those goals are specified in a written treatment contract (Mufson et al., 2004). In the first randomized controlled efficacy trial of IPT-A, 48 adolescents (ages 12–18 years) with major depressive disorder were assigned to either weekly IPT-A for 12 weeks ($N = 24$) or a clinical monitoring control group ($N = 24$; Mufson, Weissman, et al., 1999). Results of intent-to-treat analyses indicated that the IPT-A group had significantly fewer self-reported symptoms of depression as well as significantly improved social functioning and problem-solving skills at week 12, compared to the control group. They were also rated significantly more improved (i.e., less depressed) than controls by independent evaluators at posttreatment (Mufson, Weissman, et al., 1999).

More recently, the transportability and effectiveness of IPT-A (12 sessions administered across 12–16 weeks) were evaluated in comparison to treatment as usual (supportive counseling) in urban school-based mental health clinics (Mufson, Pollack Dorta, Wickramaratne, et al., 2004). Sixty-three adolescents ranging in age from 12 to 18 years (mean age = 15.1 years) from low socioeconomic backgrounds who met DSM-IV criteria for major depressive disorder, dysthymia, depressive disorder not otherwise specified, or adjustment disorder with depressed mood were randomly assigned to either IPT-A or TAU, with both treatments administered by school-based clinicians. Results were similar to those of the prior study, with IPT-A participants showing significantly greater improvement in depressive symptoms and overall functioning at posttreatment as compared to TAU. Several variations in the format of IPT-A also have been evaluated, with O'Shea, Spence, and Donovan (2015) reporting no significant differences in adolescent outcomes for group versus individually administered IPT-A at both posttreatment and a 12-month follow-up. Interestingly, Dietz, Weinberg, Brent, and Mufson (2015) found preliminary support for family-based IPT (FB-IPT) for depressed preadolescents (ages 7–12 years), with FB-IPT youth experiencing significantly greater improvement than those in a supportive counseling condition.

Another multicomponent manual-based CBT program in which goal setting is explicitly taught is the CWD-A course (Lewinsohn et al., 1985). In this group treatment program, teens learn key principles related to goal setting (e.g., "good" goals are specific and realistic), develop goals for each new skill learned during treatment (e.g., pleasant events scheduling), and receive feedback and support from the therapist and group members (Clarke et al., 1990). In the first RCT to evaluate this program (Lewinsohn, Clarke, et al., 1990), 59 youth with major depression or dysthymia were randomly assigned to either CWD-A without parents (i.e., 16 2-hour sessions over 8 weeks), CWD-A with a corresponding parent group (i.e., 2-hour parent sessions once a week for 8 weeks), or a waitlist control. At posttreatment, almost half (46%) of treated teens no longer met criteria for depression as compared to 5% of controls, with gains maintained across a 2-year follow-up. Though not significant, there was a trend toward greater improvement for the adolescent plus parent condition relative to the adolescent-only group. Expanding upon this study with a larger sample ($N$ = 123), Clarke, Rohde, Lewinsohn, Hops, and Seeley (1999) reported depression recovery rates of 64.9% and 68.8% at post-treatment for the adolescent group and adolescent plus parent group, respectively, compared to 48.1% for the control group (Clarke et al., 1999). Several additional randomized controlled trials support the efficacy of this program (e.g., Clarke et al., 2002; Lewinsohn et al., 1990; Rohde et al., 2004). Finally, another group-based intervention for depressed youth is the ACTION treatment program for depressed girls (Stark et al., 2010). In this program, the therapist collaboratively develops a list of goals and corresponding treatment strategies with each child, and progress toward those goals is assessed at the beginning of each group meeting. Evidence for the efficacy of this program is promising, though still preliminary (Stark et al., 2008, 2010).

In terms of the treatment of anxiety, the Stand Up, Speak Out program for adolescents with social phobia (Albano & DiBartolo, 2007) is a manual-based group CBT program in which goal setting is explicitly taught. At the beginning of treatment, teens are asked to list their goals for improvements in social functioning as well as broader "life goals" and then discuss them with the group. Albano, Marten, Holt, Heimberg, and Barlow (1995) reported initial support for this 16-session group treatment program with five participants (two female, three male; ages 13–17 years) who met DSM-III-R criteria for social phobia. Although there was no comparison group, there were significant improvements in both self-reported symptoms of anxiety and depression and diagnostic status (based on clinician interview) at posttreatment and a 12-month follow-up. Participants also reported significantly lower ratings of anxiety for two behavioral tasks (i.e., reading aloud, impromptu speech) at both assessments (Albano et al., 1995).

Hayward et al. (2000) expanded upon Albano et al. (1995) by randomly assigning 35 female adolescents to either the same 16-session group CBT program for adolescents ($N = 12$) or a no-treatment comparison ($N = 23$). At posttreatment, treated participants had significantly lower ratings of interference in functioning (per parent and child reports) and significantly fewer self-reported symptoms of social phobia as compared to the no-treatment group. Fifty-five percent (6 of 11) of treated participants continued to meet the criteria for social phobia at posttreatment, compared to 95% (21 of 22) of the untreated participants. At 1-year posttreatment, there were no significant differences between the groups in terms of the number of teens meeting criteria for social phobia or self-reported symptoms of social phobia; however, four comparison group participants received community-based treatment between posttreatment and follow-up. (Hayward et al., 2000).

Finally, goal setting is also an explicit component of psychoeducational psychotherapy, an evidence-based intervention for 8- to 12-year-old youth with bipolar spectrum disorders or depression that can be delivered in either a 20- to 24-week individual-family format or an 8-week multifamily group format (Fristad et al., 2011). In this program, youth brainstorm a list of problems to focus on during treatment, narrow that list down, and then generate three goals related to changing their behavior (i.e., Child Fix-It List). The youth and parents also develop a Family Fix-It List, which includes three mutually agreed-upon goals for the entire family to work on during treatment. Fristad and associates (2009) conducted one of several RCTs supporting the efficacy of MF-PEP compared to a waitlist control for depression and BSD among 8- to 12-year-old children, with gains maintained at a 1-year follow-up (see also Fristad et al., 2002, 2003). Other research supports the efficacy of IF-PEP for youth with BSD (Fristad, 2006) as well as the preliminary effectiveness of MF-PEP administered in community settings (MacPherson, Leffler, & Fristad, 2014)

Although beyond the scope of this section, there is a relatively large body of research supporting the efficacy of manual-based CBT programs that incorporate the goal-setting treatment element more indirectly, such as Coping Cat (Kendall & Hedtke, 2006) and various

OCD treatment protocols. As an important next step, researchers need to evaluate goal setting individually to determine its specific role in the treatment of anxiety and depression among children and adolescents.

## THE ELEMENT IN PRACTICE

We now turn to a discussion of practical strategies for conducting goal setting with anxious and depressed youth. The key steps of the goal-setting process are outlined in the task analysis in Box 12.1. More specific information about each step is included in the following section, along with suggested variations for particular developmental levels and cultural backgrounds. A case example describing the implementation of goal setting with a 17-year-old Hispanic female with major depressive disorder is presented in Box 12.2 at the end of the chapter.

### "Core of the Core" Element

Near the end of the initial evaluation, the clinician usually begins goal setting by discussing treatment goals in broad terms (Box 12.1, Step 1). For example, he or she may explain that the goals of treatment are to reduce anxiety or depression and improve social and/or academic functioning and then go on to connect those broad goals to specific aspects of treatment (e.g., depressed mood will be alleviated via pleasant events scheduling and cognitive restructuring). Preliminary treatment expectations, such as how long treatment will take and the frequency of sessions, are also discussed. Judith Beck (2011) emphasizes the importance of this early overview of goals in giving clients a sense of hope and better engaging them in the treatment. Prior to the first treatment session, the clinician initiates the next step of the goal-setting process (Step 2) by carefully reviewing all assessment data (e.g., clinical interview data; self-report measures from the child, parent, and teacher; and behavioral assessment, such as the role play of an anxiety-provoking situation with the clinician; Albano & DiBartolo, 2007) and developing a preliminary case conceptualization, which guides the creation of specific treatment goals, or "positively worded statements about desired outcomes" (Stark et al., 2006, p. 367). It is important to keep in mind that case conceptualization is an ongoing process, and therefore the initial conceptualization (and also the corresponding goals) will likely evolve as more is learned about the child and family during the first several treatment sessions.

Then, the clinician meets with the youth to discuss his or her concerns and to help the youth articulate his or her goals for treatment

## BOX 12.1. Task Analysis of Goal Setting

1. At the end of the initial evaluation, discuss treatment goals in broad terms with the youth and caregivers, connect the goals with treatment strategies, and set general expectations for treatment.

2. Prior to the first treatment session, review assessment data and form an initial case conceptualization that guides the development of specific treatment goals.

3. Next, meet with the youth to discuss his or her concerns and help the youth to articulate his or her goals for treatment:
   a. Ask the youth to identify problems that he or she has been experiencing; help him or her prioritize the problems and/or break them down into smaller parts.
   b. Assist the youth with translating the problems into goals for therapy by defining each goal, which involves:
      • Specifying goals in *behavioral terms.*
      • Clarifying the *conditions* under which the behaviors will occur.
      • Determining the level or *amount of change* that is needed to reach particular goals.
   c. Ensure that the goals are realistic (e.g., can be accomplished within the treatment time frame).

4. Create a mutually agreed-upon list of goals and corresponding treatment strategies:
   a. Share the clinician-generated list of goals to make sure that the youth agrees with them.
   b. Record the mutually agreed-upon goals on a single sheet of paper.
   c. Indicate the corresponding treatment strategies for each goal and/or specify goals on a treatment contract.
   d. Share the treatment goals with the group members and/or parents to receive their feedback, and discuss the ways in which these individuals can help the youth to achieve the goals.

5. Review and refine the treatment goals at the beginning of each session:
   a. Assist the youth in breaking the goals down into smaller steps (i.e., subgoals or action steps) as needed and in sequencing those steps from the easiest to the most difficult.
   b. Discuss the potential obstacles and available resources for each goal.
   c. Assess and document progress toward the attainment of each goal.
   d. Celebrate any progress that the youth has made toward accomplishing his or her goals through verbal praise, prizes, and/or sharing the accomplishments with the parents or peers.
   e. Establish new goals, if needed.
   f. Problem-solve any challenges (e.g., use cognitive restructuring, additional rewards, revised goals, and/or breaking a goal or task down into even smaller steps).

6. At the end of treatment, review all the goals accomplished, and discuss the goals to work on before a booster session, longer-term goals that extend beyond the end of treatment, and/or goals intended to prevent relapse.

(Step 3). This process often begins by asking the youth to identify the problems that brought him or her to treatment (Beck, 2011; Stark et al., 2006). During this discussion of problems, the clinician helps the youth prioritize those that are most concerning and, when needed, break larger problems down into manageable parts. For example, a depressed adolescent who expresses a problem as "I'm just feeling overwhelmed about everything" would need assistance in generating a list of more specific problems (e.g., those related to mood, activity level, schoolwork, and socializing). After identifying and clarifying the problems, the youth often needs assistance with transforming those problems into three or four goals to work on during therapy. When discussing each goal, it is important to help the youth identify *specific behavioral outcomes* for each goal, clarify the *conditions* (e.g., context, circumstances) under which the behavior will occur, and to decide on the *amount of change* that is needed to reach each goal (Cormier et al., 2013). For example, a depressed adolescent who identifies the goal of "wanting to feel happier" would need assistance with specifying in behavioral terms what "feeling happier" looks like to him or her (e.g., getting involved in previously enjoyable activities, spending time with friends) as well as deciding on factors such as when, where, with whom, and how often those activities will occur.

When defining goals in behavioral terms, the clinician can help the youth to specify desired behaviors by asking "What will you do (or how will you think/feel) differently?" Various prompts can be used to help the youth identify specific behaviors related to a particular goal, such as: "When you say you want to _____, describe what you see yourself doing"; "You say you want to be less anxious. What are the specific things you would be thinking and doing as a less anxious person?" or "Provide an example of this goal." When helping the youth specify the conditions under which a behavior will occur, it is important to identify *where, when*, and *with whom* the behaviors associated with each goal will take place. And, finally, the level or amount of change can be defined in terms of frequency (i.e., how often) or duration (i.e., the amount of time expended). For example, a child with separation anxiety may want to reduce the number of times that he or she asks a parent for reassurance or increase the amount of time that he or she spends in a room alone at home. Notably, in addition to being specific, the clinician must ensure that goals can be realistically accomplished within the treatment time frame. According to Fristad et al. (2011), it is better for the youth to accomplish a realistic goal and then set a new one than for him or her to establish goals that are too difficult and then feel frustrated when those goals are not attained.

After the clinician helps define the goals to be sought by the youth, a mutually agreed-upon list of goals and corresponding treatment strategies is created (Step 4). First, the clinician shares his or her own list of goals to make sure that the youth agrees with them. The goals generated by the child or adolescent are then merged with those of the clinician, and all of the mutually agreed-upon goals are recorded on a single sheet of paper. For example, the ACTION program uses a chart in which goals are listed in the first column and specific intervention strategies are listed at the top of other columns on the page. After recording each goal, a check mark is placed in subsequent column(s) to indicate relevant intervention strategies, also referred to as the "ACTION plans for obtaining their goals" (Stark et al., 2007, p. 31). Goals and corresponding rewards for each are often specified in a written treatment contract, which is a key component of the goal-setting process in a number of the programs (e.g., such as in CWD-A [Clarke et al., 1990], ACTION [Stark et al., 2007], Stand Up, Speak Out [Albano & DiBartolo, 2007], and IPT-A [Mufson et al., 2011]). In group treatment programs for adolescents, such as ACTION and Stand Up, Speak Out, the youth are also asked to share their treatment goals with one another (if they feel comfortable doing so) and then they discuss ways in which the group members can help one another accomplish those goals. Across treatment programs, the goals are also shared with the caregivers as well, to gain their feedback and support. Several programs incorporate periodic parent meetings to give caregivers the opportunity to provide input on the therapy's goals and to better understand their role in helping the children practice new skills that they are learning during treatment. Developmental differences in the extent of parent involvement and the level of autonomy that youth are granted in the goal-setting process will be discussed further in the next section.

Just as the case conceptualization evolves throughout the treatment, so likewise do treatment goals. After goals are established, it is important to review and refine them at the beginning of each treatment session (Step 5). During that time, therapists often assist the youth in breaking larger goals down into smaller steps. Those subgoals or action steps can then be sequenced, based on their level of difficulty. In addition to breaking the goals down into smaller steps, Cormier et al. (2013) emphasize the importance of discussing potential *obstacles* that could interfere with each goal's attainment as well as the resources that are available to help the youth accomplish his or hr goals. Potential obstacles and resources include the child's feelings or thoughts, the individuals in the child's environment, as well as whether the youth possesses the necessary knowledge or skills to complete a particular task related to a goal. When reviewing goals at the beginning of each session, it is also crucial to discuss and document progress toward the attainment of each goal, perhaps using charts with check marks or stickers to reinforce progress in a tangible way (Stark et al., 2006). Progress toward goal attainment can be assessed in various ways—for example, through discussions about homework assignments and situations encountered since the last therapy session, the review of weekly self-monitoring forms, the clinician's behavioral observations during the session (e.g., during completion of an *in vivo* exposure task for an anxious child), or through more formal assessments conducted periodically throughout the treatment (e.g., questionnaires given to the youth, parents, and/or teachers). Regardless of how it is assessed, progress toward goals should be celebrated through verbal praise, small prizes, self-administered rewards (particularly for older children and teens; see Chapter 9), and sharing progress with caregivers and peers (in group treatment programs).

As progress is made, it is important not only to review and refine goals that still need to be accomplished but also to establish new goals. For example, during the exposure portion of treatment, some anxious youth progress up their fear hierarchy more quickly than originally anticipated, and so new situations may need to be added to the hierarchy over time. When youth encounter difficulties in accomplishing their goals, it is important for the clinician to help the youth problem-solve so that they are able to move past whatever is impeding treatment progress. For example, certain items on a fear hierarchy may be more challenging than the youth and/or clinician initially thought they would be, and so the order of items may need to be shifted and/or situations may need to be broken down into even smaller steps (see Chapter 2 on exposure tasks). At times, it may be important for the clinician to implement cognitive restructuring to alter a youth's negative thoughts surrounding particular situations and prevent those thoughts from interfering with goal attainment. Alternatively, changes may be needed in the reward system (e.g., increasing the frequency or type of rewards; see Chapter 9 to provide additional encouragement for goals that are particularly difficult to accomplish.

The final step of the goal-setting process occurs near the end of treatment, when all of the goals that have been accomplished to that point are reviewed; at this important juncture, the youth is encouraged to identify goals that he or she would like to work on between the end of treatment and a booster session, or after termination (Step 6). At that time, the therapist may also suggest goals related to practicing certain skills on an ongoing basis to help prevent relapse (Beck, 2011). As will be explored in the next section, some treatment programs for anxious or depressed adolescents even encourage the teen to develop "life goals" related to his or her education or career or to social and family relationships that extend well beyond the end of treatment, discussing how to break these long-term goals into smaller steps and how the coping skills learned in treatment can help the youth to accomplish each goal.

## Developmental Adaptations

There are several aspects of the goal-setting process that need to be tailored to fit each youth's developmental level. First, it is important to consider how much assistance versus autonomy to provide the youth when developing treatment goals. Across manual-based CBT programs for anxious and depressed youth, goal setting with younger children occurs primarily during treatment sessions, tends to be more therapist-directed, and often involves caregivers. For example, in one program for children with bipolar and depressive disorders by Fristad and colleagues (2011), youth are asked to create a Child Fix-It List during the first treatment session by brainstorming a list of problems that they would like to work on in therapy, narrowing that list down, and then generating three goals related to changing their behavior. The manual specifies that clinicians should structure this discussion so that the children do not get overwhelmed; should provide ideas to get the discussion going (based upon information gathered during the assessment); and should help the children focus on specific problems and realistic goals that can be accomplished during the treatment time frame. At the end of the first session, the caregivers join in for a session review and to learn about a take-home project called the Family Fix-It List. For this project, caregivers first generate their own Parent Fix-It List of three family problems within their own control that they want to work on during treatment (e.g., less yelling, better communication between the parents). Then, the child and parents sit down together to develop a Family Fix-It List, which includes three mutually agreed-upon goals for the entire family to work on during treatment. In other programs, such as Coping Cat for the treatment of childhood anxiety (Kendall & Hedtke, 2006), the goal-setting process is not as closely prescribed; however, parents are often included in discussions of treatment goals during check-ins at the end of weekly child sessions and/or during the parent-only sessions, with the extent of the parents' involvement left to the clinician's discretion.

In contrast, older children and adolescents are typically granted more autonomy in the goal-setting process. Across several manual-based treatments for adolescents, the clinician first teaches the youth basic principles about goal setting during one of the early treatment sessions. Then, youth are asked to generate their own lists of goals for homework and discuss them with the therapist during the next treatment session. In group treatment programs for adolescent depression, individually generated goals are also discussed with other participants in the therapy group. For example, in CWD-A, part of an early treatment session is devoted to the clinician helping adolescents understand the difference between "good goals" and "poor goals." After the clinician reviews concrete examples of each type of goal, teens are taught that "good goals" (i.e., those that are specific and realistic) "lead to improvement through small, realistic steps" (Clarke et al., 1990, p. 106). Using these general principles, the teens work independently to develop their own "good goals" for increasing their involvement in pleasant activities. Then, with a group partner, each participant discusses not only the types of pleasant activities in which he or she would like to engage but also how participating in those activities could be made easier (e.g., by joining a club, taking lessons related to a new skill or hobby, inviting others to join in a particular activity). Teens go through a similar process when setting other types of goals during treatment, first generating their own goals for homework and then discussing them with the therapist and other group members to refine the list. Related to autonomy, some adolescents may disagree with the clinician (or parents) in terms of the problems or goals to prioritize during treatment. If this occurs, the therapist can suggest starting with more general goals and narrowing the focus as treatment progresses, or perhaps working on the teen's main concerns first and then addressing the clinician's concerns.

Another key developmental consideration is the extent to which treatment goals have an immediate versus long-term focus. With younger children, treatment goals tend to have a shorter-term focus (i.e., what will be accomplished during treatment, goals related to alleviating current symptoms and related difficulties), which is consistent with their relatively limited cognitive capacities in areas such as causal reasoning, memory, and attention span (Grave & Blissett, 2004). Based upon their more sophisticated cognitive abilities (Steinberg, 2013), older children and adolescents often can envision both short-term goals to be accomplished during the acute treatment phase and longer-term goals that extend beyond the treatment time frame and address concerns outside of their symptoms of anxiety or depression. For example, in the Stand Up, Speak Out program, teens are asked to complete a homework assignment titled "What Are My Life Goals" at the end of the second session and share it with the group the following week. According to Albano and DiBartolo (2007), the youth in this program typically identify goals related to their education or career (e.g., going to college, finding a good job), financial security (e.g., earning a decent salary), and positive personal relationships (e.g., finding a partner, having close friends). After specific goals have been identified, the clinician discusses ways in which adaptive social functioning (i.e., a main goal of the program) relates to accomplishing each type of long-term goal. Similarly, near the end of treatment in the CWD-A program, teens are encouraged to create a "life plan" that includes realistic long-term goals that fall into several categories, including friends, education/school, job plans, recreation, home and family, romantic relationships, and spiritual/religious matters. After identifying goals for each category, teens discuss potential obstacles for achieving these goals, plans for overcoming the obstacles, and short-term goals to help break the long-term goals into smaller steps (Clarke et al., 1990).

Also related to developmental differences in cognitive reasoning abilities, youth may differ in terms of the ways in which they conceptualize problems and goals. As younger children have more concrete reasoning abilities, they tend to think of their problems in more global ways and, as such, often need more assistance with breaking goals down into smaller steps (Friedberg & McClure, 2015). Alternatively, adolescents have more sophisticated reasoning abilities and are therefore able to discuss goals in more complex ways. For example, near the beginning of treatment in the ACTION program, adolescents are asked to make connections between treatment goals and relevant coping strategies that will be used to accomplish each goal (Stark et al., 2007). In Stand Up, Speak Out, about halfway through treatment the teens are asked to reflect on the progress that they have made toward reaching their treatment goals, discussing their accomplishments as well as any frustrations they might have if they are not as far along as they would like to be (Albano & DiBartolo, 2007).

Consistent with advances in social development and an increased focus on relationships with peers during the adolescent years, several manual-based CBT programs for internalizing disorders among adolescents use a group format that caters to the social needs of teens. In particular, during the goal setting fellow group members serve an important role as the teens complete tasks such as sharing goals with a partner, receiving feedback from peers as goals are generated, and asking group members for support in accomplishing those goals. For example, the ACTION program introduces the idea of sharing individual goals with the group early in treatment (during the first individual session), emphasizing that the group serves as a supportive team to help each member accomplish his or her goals. Although each teen completes an individual goal sheet, the form also includes a place for brainstorming specific things that group members can do to help the teen reach each goal. Prior to discussing goals with the group, the therapist and teen role-play how to ask other group members for help, and during the very next session each teen reads his or her goals aloud and asks group members for the specific assistance that they need in accomplishing each goal (e.g., Stark et al., 2007). Even when not using a group-based program, when working with older children and adolescents, clinicians may choose to involve peers to support goal accomplishment when appropriate and feasible.

## Diversity Considerations

Although manual-based CBT programs for anxiety and depression are used with youth from diverse backgrounds, there is a paucity of research examining the role of clients' ethnicity or cultural background in the implementation of ESTs (Jackson, 2002). In light of these limitations, this section includes an overview of the small body of research examining the effectiveness of goal setting for internalizing disorders with ethnically diverse samples of youth, followed by suggested guidelines for implementing goal setting in a culturally sensitive manner.

A small number of studies have examined the effectiveness of manual-based CBT programs with ethnically diverse samples as well as particular ethnic or racial groups. Some of this research has focused on manual-based treatments for anxiety (e.g., Ginsburg & Drake, 2002; Pina et al., 2003), and other studies have concentrated on programs for depressed youth (e.g., Gunlicks-Stoessel, Mufson, Jekal, & Turner, 2010; Listug-Lunde, Vogeltanz-Holm, & Collins, 2013). Across these studies, however, it is unclear what (if any) culturally sensitive modifications were made to the goal-setting aspect of treatment. One exception is Rosselló and Bernal's (1999) evaluation of the efficacy of IPT-A and CBT with a sample of Puerto Rican adolescents ($N = 71$; mean age = 14.70 years; 54% female). Rosselló and Bernal (1999) found that both IPT-A and CBT yielded significantly greater improvement in depressive symptoms as compared to a waitlist control. After 12 weeks of treatment,

82% of IPT-A adolescents and 59% of CBT adolescents in the CBT had moved from the clinical to normal range in self-reported depressive symptoms. In terms of cultural modifications to the active treatments, sensitivity to the strong Puerto Rican cultural value of *familismo* was incorporated by evaluating key issues such as family obligation and support and by including parents (either via individual meetings or in-session with the adolescents) whenever necessary. In a further description of their adaptations to IPT for Puerto Rican families, Rosselló and Bernal (1996) explain that the cultural values of "absolute parental authority and respect" are common among Puerto Rican parents and that youth often have a longer period of dependence on parents (p. 162). As such, clinicians meet with the parents and the teen together prior to the first treatment session to better understand the teen's role within the family, and they hold extra meetings with parents to discuss issues related to parental authority and family interdependence, as needed. With respect to goal setting, in addition to discussing goals with the teen, "parents' goals are also evaluated and taken into consideration" (Rosselló & Bernal, 1996, p. 163). Although it might seem that the concept of *familismo* would dictate that parents play a more active role in setting treatment goals and that goals that fit family needs (vs. those of the individual) would be favored, this is not directly specified in the cultural modifications described by Rosselló and Bernal (1996, 1999).

Also relevant to goal setting is a portion of the Chorpita and Daleiden (2009) study examining whether EBTs are characterized by unique practices when administered to youth of particular ethnic backgrounds. Although effective treatments administered to groups of Hispanic youth with depressed mood shared many common elements with those administered to other depressed youth, treatments targeting Hispanic youth were characterized by "higher frequency of psychoeducational-parent and parent coping and the notable absence of goal setting and self-reward/self-praise" (Chorpita & Daleiden, 2009, p. 573). The reason behind these findings is unclear, and the researchers note that there may simply be too few studies examining effective treatments for depression among Hispanic youth to draw definitive conclusions. Clearly, further research examining the use of goal setting across various ethnic groups of youth with internalizing disorders is needed.

In the meantime, general guidelines for conducting both the case conceptualization and goal-setting process in a culturally sensitive manner are important to keep in mind. For example, information about a child's cultural background should be used to inform the case conceptualization, including the child's and family's level of accul-turation, ethnic identity, and cultural beliefs surrounding the youth's symptoms and treatment approaches (Friedberg, McClure, & Garcia, 2009). Also, as children from diverse cultural backgrounds often face unique stressors related to poverty, prejudice, discrimination, and marginalization, it is crucial to assess these factors for each child and incorporate them into the case conceptualization whenever possible (see Friedberg & McClure, 2015, p. 17, for a list of sample questions to consider when assessing the cultural context of the child/family).

In addition to integrating culture into the case conceptualization, several suggestions have been offered for conducting goal setting in a culturally sensitive manner. First, clinicians must be culturally aware when developing treatment goals for youth. Specifically, they must be "aware of their own values and biases . . . and to avoid deliberately or inadvertently steering the client toward goals that may reflect their own cultural norms rather than the client's expressed wishes" (Cormier et al., 2013, p. 277). Second, it is important that goals be established collab-oratively between the clinician and youth/family to ensure that treat-ment goals match the youth's "cultural frame of reference" (Lo & Fung, 2003, p. 164). Lo and Fung (2003) emphasize that during this process the clinician may also need to navigate situations in which the youth's cultural group has goals that are different from those of the youth. For example, an Asian adolescent may desire a level of independence that is inconsistent with the traditional collectivist beliefs of his or her par-ents and extended family. Relatedly, it is important to keep in mind that youth from diverse ethnic/cultural backgrounds may have differ-ent ideas surrounding obedience to authority, which could cause them to be hesitant to say something when they disagree with a goal that the clinician suggests (Friedberg & McClure, 2015). Finally, clinicians need to understand what goals are acceptable to the child and family (based upon their cultural background/beliefs) and make sure that the goals are realistic for the child's unique environmental circumstances (e.g., neighborhood, family situation; Friedberg & McClure, 2015). For example, for an anxious child who lives in a dangerous neighborhood, walking to a friend's house alone may not be a feasible exposure task, owing to legitimate safety concerns.

Wood, Chiu, Hwang, Jacobs, and Ifekwunigwe (2008) offer several additional recommendations for culturally sensitive implementation of goal setting in the context of CBT with anxious Mexican American youth that could apply to youth from other ethnic/cultural back-grounds. They suggest holding an "orienting session" with the family early on in treatment to give the parents an overview of the therapy process (e.g., what is discussed during sessions) and the goals of treatment to "help demystify the process and facilitate client buy-in" (Wood et al., 2008, p. 521). Also, clinicians should ensure that treatment goals match the goals of the family and, when there is a mismatch, consider adjusting traditional therapy goals to make them more culturally sensitive. For example, when working with a child with separation anxiety, families who practice co-sleeping for cultural reasons may not feel that it is necessary for the child to sleep alone. In this situation, goals for developing independence from caregivers in other types of situations could be emphasized (e.g., attending Sunday school or an after-school activity without parents; Wood et al., 2008). Overall, additional research examining the nuances of culturally sensitive implementation of CBT and its effectiveness across various ethnic groups is needed to inform clinicians' work with youth from diverse ethnic and cultural backgrounds and their families.

## CONCLUSIONS

Based on contemporary theories of motivation and goals from the fields of cognitive and social psychology, the goal-setting treatment element also has a historical foundation in early theories of drive reduction, the humanistic perspective, and specific therapeutic methods such as problem-solving therapy. The evidence base supporting the effective use of goal setting with anxious and depressed youth includes studies evaluating multicomponent CBT programs that include goal setting as a key component. To implement goal setting effectively, clinicians should understand theories related to the cognitive processes underlying goal pursuit and the effect of monitoring and feedback on goal attainment as well as key assumptions regarding treatment goals (i.e., content, process) posited by cognitive-behavioral theory. The step-by-step procedures provided in this chapter outline how to establish goals in a collaborative manner with youth, reviewing and refining them as needed throughout treatment. It is also crucial for clinicians to consider carefully each child's developmental level and cultural background when implementing this treatment element.

## BOX 12.2. Illustrative Case Example

Victoria, a 17-year-old female from the Dominican Republic, was diagnosed with major depressive disorder and participated in a 16-session group treatment program for depressed adolescents. Victoria was a senior in high school living with her mother, father, maternal grandmother, and two younger brothers. Regarding symptoms of depression, Victoria reported experiencing sad mood, difficulty concentrating on her schoolwork, feelings of worthlessness (without suicidal ideation), sleeping more than usual and yet always feeling very tired, poor school performance during the prior few months, a loss of interest in usual activities, and avoidance of social interactions. Although she could not identify a particular event that precipitated her depression, Victoria recounted that, as she approached her senior year, she felt increasingly overwhelmed and hopeless about her post-high school plans. She had considered attending college, but, as a child of recent immigrants, there were no adults in her family who had pursued higher education; so, Victoria was unsure of where to begin with the college selection and application process. One of her teachers who had noticed her withdrawn behavior and an abrupt decline in her academic performance expressed concern to the school counselor, who referred Victoria for an evaluation and treatment at a community mental health clinic. In terms of strengths, Victoria had one very close friend whom she saw regularly at school and gatherings with family friends. In addition, she was bright and had excelled in school until recently, particularly in her science and math classes. She had participated previously in the Latin American cultural club at school and had supportive relationships in both her immediate and extended family.

After conducting a detailed assessment involving a semi-structured clinical interview and self-report questionnaires completed by Victoria and her parents, the clinician reviewed the results of the evaluation with the family and invited Victoria to participate in a group treatment program. The clinician described the program goals in general terms (e.g., to alleviate sad mood and related depressive symptoms, improve school performance, and increase involvement in social activities) as well as the general expectations for treatment (e.g., weekly group meetings along with periodic individual sessions across 16 weeks). Prior to the first treatment session, the clinician developed a detailed case conceptualization and her own list of treatment goals for Victoria, to be shared in a later discussion.

Prior to the first group meeting, the clinician met individually with Victoria to establish rapport and identify more specific treatment goals. During this session, Victoria was asked to articulate the most difficult problems that she had been experiencing. Victoria expressed concern about "always feeling sad and tired," "not being able to do anything right at school," "never having any fun," and "feeling overwhelmed about the future." As she spoke, the clinician recorded each problem on a dry-erase board. The clinician then helped Victoria to break the larger problems down into more manageable parts. For example, "not being able to do anything right at school" was broken down into difficulty concentrating in class, doing poorly on exams, and being too tired to study or complete homework during the evenings, whereas "never having any fun" related to skipping cultural club activities and withdrawing from social activities with friends. The problem of "feeling overwhelmed about the future" seemed to relate primarily to Victoria's uncertainty about how to pursue college plans. After specifying the problems, the clinician helped Victoria transform the concerns into specific treatment goals by asking her such questions as "When you say you want to socialize with friends more often, what do you see yourself doing?" and "You say you want to feel less sad and tired. What things would you be thinking and doing as a happier and more energetic person?"

Near the end of the first session, the clinician shared the goals generated from her own case conceptualization in a collaborative manner with Victoria. Victoria's list of goals was placed side by side with the clinician's list to see where the goals overlapped and to make sure that Victoria agreed with all of the clinician's recommended goals. The full list of goals was recorded on a chart, with intervention strategies specified for each goal. Some of the goals on the list included increasing Victoria's daily activity level as a first step to improving her mood, developing a homework schedule to make sure assignments were completed on a daily basis, accepting a few upcoming invitations to socialize with peers, beginning to attend cultural club meetings again, and meeting with the guidance counselor at school to learn more about the college application process.

Next, Victoria shared this list with her parents so that they could support her efforts throughout the treatment. Her parents expressed their concern that increased involvement with peers would take time away from family obligations (e.g., caring for her younger brothers, spending time with her grandmother, attending gatherings with the extended family). The clinician exhibited sensitivity to the family's cultural context by scheduling an extra meeting with Victoria and her parents to discuss these concerns. During this meeting, the parents' concerns were validated, and the two were treated with the utmost respect as the clinician reiterated how each treatment goal could help to alleviate Victoria's depression. They all discussed ways in which Victoria could increase her activity level and peer connections while yet maintaining her close ties with her family. As treatment progressed, periodic check-ins were held to revisit this issue and ensure that the treatment goals were aligned with the parents' strong cultural beliefs. Notably, Victoria's list of goals was revisited throughout treatment, particularly as treatment skills relating to each goal were introduced (e.g., pleasant events scheduling, problem solving, cognitive restructuring). The clinician helped Victoria define each goal in behavioral terms by specifying where, when, how often, and with whom the behavior was to occur.

In the first group session, Victoria shared her goals, and group members brainstormed ways in which they could support her progress toward specific goals (e.g., checking in on her homework progress via text messages, brainstorming ideas for increasing her daily activity level, sharing their experiences with the college application process). Victoria reviewed her goals at the beginning of each subsequent group session as part of the "goal attainment check-in," which involved discussing progress toward her goals over the past week, documenting progress with a check mark on her individual goal sheet, and revising and/or establishing new goals as needed. During periodic individual sessions, the clinician assisted Victoria in breaking larger goals down into smaller steps and sequencing those steps as well as problem solving any obstacles toward goal attainment (such as

*(continued)*

## BOX 12.2 (*continued*)

how to fit a meeting with her guidance counselor into her busy schedule or what to do when social invitations from friends interfered with important family obligations). Victoria's parents were involved in portions of these individual sessions as needed. Near the end of treatment, Victoria's progress was reviewed and celebrated, and she was encouraged to set several "life goals" that extended beyond the end of treatment, including getting a summer job or internship, submitting applications to 2- and 4-year colleges, and eventually pursuing a career as a science teacher. Although a posttreatment evaluation indicated that her depression was in remission, the clinician encouraged Victoria to set additional posttreatment goals for continuing to utilize skills such as pleasant events scheduling and cognitive restructuring to help prevent the return of depressive symptoms.

# 13

## Homework

## BACKGROUND OF THE ELEMENT

Homework refers to the completion of therapy assignments between actual sessions. The goal of homework is for the youth to practice skills learned in therapy, thereby facilitating the transfer of those skills to everyday life (Kazantzis & L'Abate, 2007). In fact, homework is theorized to be critical to the generalization of therapy skills to other settings (Gaynor, Lawrence, & Nelson-Gray, 2006). Homework also enables the therapist to better assess the extent to which the instructed skills have been mastered (Hudson & Kendall, 2002). This chapter focuses on the core processes related to homework, which are generally consistent across presenting problems, although it should be noted that homework assignment content varies widely. For example, homework assignments for youth with anxiety commonly include self-monitoring of anxiety symptoms, relaxation, thought diaries, problem solving, and exposure activities. For youth with mood disorders, typical homework assignments include activity scheduling, social skills training, problem solving, self-monitoring of mood, and thought diaries. The first portion of this chapter presents a summary of the history and theory underlying homework use in therapy as well as the empirical support for its effectiveness. The second half of the chapter offers practical suggestions on how best to implement homework in therapy and how to adapt the process when working with youth of different developmental levels or diverse cultural backgrounds. The chapter closes with an illustrative case study.

## Brief History

Early research on the positive effects of practice and rehearsal likely set the stage historically for the current use of homework in therapy. During the late 1800s, research on habits established that "every time we perform any action, mental or physical, we have more proneness to, and greater facility for, the performance of that action under similar circumstances than we had before" (Gordy, 1898, p. 184). Indeed, subsequent research documented that mental functions improve with practice (Thorndike, 1913). Although the first studies on practice and rehearsal focused on non-therapy-related activities (e.g., typing, learning Morse code), the positive effects of practice are often referred to as a key benefit of therapy homework. However, the systematic inclusion of homework in the therapy process did not occur until the emergence and popularity of treatments that tend to be skill-based (e.g., behavioral and cognitive therapies) during the 1950s and 1960s.

Although homework was occasionally used in early psychoanalytic therapies, the first appearance of homework as a routine therapy technique (meaning that it was included in most sessions) was likely in George Kelly's (1955) fixed role therapy, which encouraged clients to experiment with slightly different interpersonal roles between therapy sessions (Kazantzis & L'Abate, 2007). By the 1970s, homework was solidly entrenched in behavioral therapies (e.g., patients were often encouraged to practice relaxation or exposure between sessions; Sharf, 2012) and considered a core feature of cognitive therapy (A. T. Beck et al., 1979). Currently, homework is included in the majority of empirically supported treatment manuals. In addition, a national survey of therapists revealed that 68% reported routinely using homework as a therapy technique, regardless of their theoretical orientation (Kazantzis, Lampropoulos, & Deane, 2005).

In essence, homework is considered a means to help facilitate the transfer of learning between the therapy session and a client's life. In their seminal book on cognitive therapy for depression in adults, Aaron Beck and colleagues (1979) describe homework as an essential part of treatment right from the first session. Much as with current-day practices, the homework process then was structured (i.e., assigned at the end of the session and reviewed at the beginning of the next session), systematic (i.e., occurring every session), based on the skill covered during that session, and collaborative. With the proliferation of manualized treatments that contain recommended homework assignments for each session, Judith Beck (2011) makes the important point that, although each assignment is based on the session content, it is also individualized depending on the needs of the client. For example, activity scheduling may be assigned to most clients in the early sessions of CBT for depression, but the content and length of the list of pleasant activities will vary, depending on the interests and abilities of the individual client.

Although homework was first established as a useful therapy process in the treatment of adults, homework is also commonly used in EBTs for youth (e.g., Coping Cat, Kendall & Hedtke, 2006; "ACTION," Stark et al., 2007). For example, in CBT, homework is considered an "integral" way for youth to rehearse new skills learned in session and to facilitate mastery of those skills (Hudson & Kendall, 2005, p. 75). Moreover, homework is commonly used in treatments with youth with a wide range of emotional and behavioral difficulties.

## Theory Base

Although homework is frequently used as a therapy tool and there is research to support its efficacy, little is known about the mechanism(s) by which it works. Judith Beck (2011) explains that homework serves multiple functions, including the opportunity to practice skills, observe thoughts and moods, and read and process information on diagnosis and the therapy process. Hudson and Kendall (2002) emphasize the need for a child to practice challenging his or her maladaptive thoughts in order for the process to become automatic and more efficient as well as to promote mastery of skills. Kazantzis and L'Abate (2005) point out that homework can be useful for the therapist as well, as it can serve to better assess client learning, therapy progress, and outcomes. This section will focus on the transfer of learning (which may involve classical and/or operant conditioning) and the underlying social cognitive theory to help explain why homework is a core element of EBTs for youth with internalizing disorders.

One of the key rationales for homework is the need for the learning accomplished in therapy sessions to be transferred, or generalized, to the world outside of therapy. The transfer involved in the learning process can aid in firmly establishing new behaviors or help in reducing or eliminating old ones. Cormier and Cormier (1991) recommended supporting the transfer of learning by designing homework assignments that progress from practice in "low-risk" to more demanding *in vivo* situations. Both classical and operant conditioning principles likely apply in this generalization process. For example, exposure practices are designed to extinguish a classically conditioned anxiety response to a neutral stimulus. In the case of a fear of elevators, homework assignments may progress from having the youth stand and watch people getting on and off elevators, to standing in an elevator, to riding one floor, to riding to the top of a tall building. By repeatedly exposing him- or herself to the feared stimulus without experiencing the anxiety response, the youth will no longer associate the fear response with elevators.

Similarly, practicing outside of the session also affects the transfer of learning process through operant conditioning. Operant conditioning refers to the central tenet that behaviors are contingent on environmental response, and thus rewarded behaviors tend to increase while behaviors that are not rewarded tend to decrease (Skinner, 1953b). Learning is also situationally dependent in that youth may learn to behave in different ways in different situations because the consequences of the same behavior may vary by situation. Therefore, practicing a new skill in several situations (i.e., both in and out of therapy) helps to ensure the skill's generalization to a variety of settings. For example, cognitive restructuring is used to help depressed youth change their thoughts in order to affect their mood. The skill is first practiced in therapy and then practiced in several situations between therapy sessions with the assistance of a thought and mood log. If the youth notices that he or she feels better in a number of situations after challenging one's thoughts, then the behavior is rewarded and has a high chance of being repeated.

In addition to behavioral learning theories, Bandura's (1986) social cognitive theory may also help to explain the frequent use of homework in therapy. Social cognitive theory posits that all learning is mediated through cognition. In other words, the subsequent consequences of a behavior affect the youth's expectations and beliefs about that behavior, thus affecting their future conduct. From an intervention standpoint, then, changing one's cognitions about maladaptive behaviors can result in altering those behaviors. In fact, some theorists have proposed that the primary mechanism through which homework affects outcomes may be through changing the subject's thoughts (Addis & Jacobson, 2000). For instance, self-efficacy beliefs, or the perception that one can perform a task and/or obtain a goal, influence the likelihood that a youth will engage in a particular behavior. These beliefs are based largely on past experience. Thus, a teen who has made new friends before is more confident about his ability to make new friends in the future. Similarly, homework assignments that are met with success can positively affect one's self-efficacy. Returning to our elevator fear example, repeated exposures to elevators may extinguish the conditioned fear response *and* influence the self-efficacy beliefs that the youth holds about his or her ability to ride elevators. Both effects will likely decrease the probability of the youth's avoiding elevators in the future.

As the foregoing examples convey, the theoretical underpinnings of homework are multifaceted and suggestive of a dynamic process at work. That is, practice, conditioning, and cognitive processes likely work together to facilitate learning and maintaining new skills. Next, we address the empirical evidence for the effectiveness of homework in treating youth with internalizing disorders.

## Evidence Base

Reflective of its near ubiquitous inclusion in EST manuals (see Table 13.1 for a description of how homework is integrated into several noteworthy treatment manuals for internalizing disorders in youth), homework is one of the most commonly studied therapy elements. Yet, at this point, the majority of research on homework utilizes adult samples, with research on its efficacy with youth lagging behind. In addition, the particular developmental stage in question may moderate the efficacy of homework, as research with adult samples routinely finds that increased homework compliance is linked to greater treatment response, while results are mixed when looking at the relation between homework and therapy outcomes for youth. In this section, the results of a recent meta-analysis on the efficacy of homework are presented first, followed by research on the use of homework in the treatment of depression and then anxiety.

Several large meta-analytic studies have supported the positive effect of homework in the CBT process with adults (e.g., Kazantzis, Deane, & Ronan, 2000; Mausbach, Moore, Roesch, Cardenes, & Patterson, 2010). One of the most recent reviewed 46 studies (involving over 1,000 participants) and included analyses of both correlational (i.e., homework adherence related to outcome) as well as experimental studies (i.e., treatment with homework as compared to a control treatment; Kazantzis, Wittington, & Dattilio, 2010). Interestingly, the majority of studies evaluated the treatment of either depressed or anxious

TABLE 13.1. The Homework Element in Representative EBT Manuals

| | |
|---|---|
| *Coping Cat* (Kendall & Hedtke, 2006) | • Homework is explicitly mentioned, with assignments being referred to as Show-That-I-Can (STIC) tasks.<br><br>• STIC tasks are assigned at the end of each session and are reviewed at the beginning of the next session. The youth use a workbook to help track their STIC tasks. Stickers or points are awarded for STIC task completion and can be applied toward rewards. |
| *C.A.T. Project* (Kendall, Choudhury, Hudson, & Webb, 2002) | • Homework is explicitly mentioned, typically referred to as Take Home Projects.<br><br>• Take Home Projects are assigned at the end of each session and reviewed during the following session. The youth use a workbook to help guide their out-of-session practice. |
| *Family-Based Treatment for Young Children with OCD* (Freeman & Garcia, 2009) | • Homework is explicitly mentioned, being assigned at the close of each session and reviewed at the beginning of the next session.<br><br>• A treatment reward plan is established with the parents to encourage at-home practice. The families are given a workbook (oriented toward the parents' perspective) that contains helpful information as well as homework assignments. |
| *OCD in Children and Adolescents* (March & Mulle, 1998) | • Homework is explicitly mentioned in each session and is reviewed in the next session. |
| *CBT of Childhood OCD: It's Only a False Alarm* (Piacentini, Langley, & Roblek, 2007) | • Homework is explicitly mentioned in each session and is used primarily to encourage the youth to practice ERP outside of the session.<br><br>• Homework is reviewed at the beginning of each subsequent session. Rewards are given to encourage homework compliance. |
| *CBT for Social Phobia: Stand Up, Speak Out* (Albano & DiBartolo, 2007) | • Homework is explicitly mentioned in each session and is reviewed in the following session. |
| *When Children Refuse School: A CBT Approach* (Kearney & Albano, 2007): Chapters 4 and 5 on internalizing symptoms | • Homework is explicitly mentioned and is assigned at the end of each session.<br><br>• The review of homework in the following session is at times explicitly described. |
| *Treating Trauma and Traumatic Grief in Children and Adolescents* (Cohen, Mannarino, & Deblinger, 2006) | • TF-CBT uses the acronym PRACTICE to represent the components of treatment. In addition, the acronym serves to remind the youth of the importance of practicing the learned skills outside of the session.<br><br>• Homework is often implied rather than explicitly mentioned. |

**TABLE 13.1.** (*continued*)

| | |
|---|---|
| *Adolescent Coping with Depression* (Clarke, Lewinsohn, & Hops, 1990) | • Homework is explicitly mentioned, being assigned at the end of each session and reviewed in the next session.<br>• The youth document their homework completion in a personal workbook. |
| *Interpersonal Psychotherapy for Depressed Adolescents,* 2nd edition (Mufson, Pollack Dorta, Moreau, & Weissman, 2011) | • Homework or "work at home" is explicitly mentioned and is one of several techniques therapists can use when implementing IPT-A. |
| *Treating Depressed Children: Therapist Manual for "Taking Action"* (Stark & Kendall, 1996) | • Homework is explicitly mentioned and assigned at the end of most sessions; it is typically reviewed at the start of the following session.<br>• The youth complete homework assignments in a provided workbook, and a reward system is established with the parents to encourage the homework's completion. |
| *Treating Depressed Youth: Therapist Manual for "Action"* (Stark et al., 2007) | • Homework is explicitly mentioned and assigned at the end of each session. It is then reviewed at the beginning of the next session.<br>• The youth complete homework assignments with the help of a take-home workbook, and a within-session reward system is used to increase homework compliance. |
| *Psychotherapy for Children with Bipolar and Depressive Disorders* (Fristad, Goldberg Arnold, & Leffler, 2011) | • Homework is explicitly mentioned, and "take-home projects" are assigned at the end of each session, which are then reviewed at the beginning of the next session.<br>• The therapist manual includes numerous take-home project handouts. |

*Note.* Some book titles are shortened to conserve space. See the References at the back of the book for full titles.

adults. Results indicated support for the use of homework in therapy, as the pre-post treatment effect size was greater for those treatments that included homework than those that did not ($d = 1.08$ vs. $d = 0.63$).

Although there are several studies that link homework compliance in CBT to treatment outcomes for adults with depression (e.g., Burns & Spangler, 2000; Walker & Lampropoulos, 2014), the results for depressed youth are mixed. One recent study examined the relation between homework completion (partial vs. full homework completers) and treatment outcome utilizing data from the Treatment of Adolescent Depression Study (Simons et al., 2012). Results indicated that increased homework completion was associated with decreased self-reported

depression symptoms, hopelessness, and suicidality but not independent evaluator-rated depression symptoms. It should be noted that this
pattern of results was obtained only for those teens engaged in the
CBT arm of the study and not for those who received CBT and medication. In contrast, other studies have failed to find a relation between
homework and treatment outcome for depressed youth. For example,
Shirk, Crisostomo, Jungbluth, and Gudmundsen (2013) evaluated both
engagement in treatment and changes in cognitions as possible agents
of change in a study of 44 adolescents diagnosed with depression and
treated with CBT. Although Shirk and colleagues reported that change
in cognitive distortions was related to decreased symptoms of depression, associations between homework compliance or in-session engagement and depressive symptoms were not found.

Similar to the research on depression, research involving adults
with anxiety reveals an association between homework completion
and CBT outcomes at posttreatment (e.g., Kazantzis et al., 2010) and
at 12- and 18-month postbaseline assessments (Glenn et al., 2013),
while research with anxious youth yields mixed results. With anxious
youth, some studies find a significant relation between completion of
homework tasks and outcomes. Tiwari and colleagues (2013) examined
aspects of in-session exposure assignments that might predict treatment response in 61 youth with an anxiety disorder (ages 7–13 years).
Results indicated that processing of the exposure experience after it
occurred was associated with clinician rated treatment outcomes. In
addition, exploratory analyses revealed that those youth who practiced
exposures as homework were more likely to be treatment responders.
Yet other studies have found no relation between homework and treatment outcome. For example, Hughes and Kendall (2007) compared the
influence of the therapeutic relationship and homework completion
on treatment outcome with over 100 youth diagnosed with an anxiety
disorder (ages 9–13 years). Notably, when combined with therapeutic
relationship as a predictor, homework compliance did not significantly
predict clinician-rated treatment outcome at posttreatment or 1-year
follow-up assessments.

There are several possible explanations for these discrepant findings. First, perhaps developmental ability (e.g., memory, motivation,
executive functioning) is a moderator and homework a more powerful therapy tool for adults than for youth. Alternatively, the most common research approach uses a correlational design that assesses the
relationship between an overall summary score of homework adherence (e.g., overall percentage of time the client completed homework

and treatment outcome, which may not capture the complexity of the research question. Indeed, homework efficacy may be affected by the type of assignment (e.g., relaxation vs. exposure), the timing (e.g., early vs. later in treatment), and within-participant variability in its completion (Gaynor et al., 2006). In addition, overall measures of homework compliance assess the quantity (not the quality) of homework completion and treat it solely as a client variable, ignoring the possible influence of the therapist's skill in both homework assignment and review (Kazantzis & L'Abate, 2007).

Despite such mixed findings, homework is a staple ingredient in multicomponent treatments for depressed youth, and empirical evidence for the efficacy of these treatments may lend some indirect support for homework as a potential active mechanism of treatment outcome. Based on the American Psychological Association's (Division 12) criteria for empirically supported treatments, CBT is rated as "probably efficacious" for the treatment of childhood depression and as "well established" for the treatment of adolescent depression (David-Ferdon & Kaslow, 2008). In addition, psychoeducational psychotherapy is classified as "probably efficacious" for the treatment of pediatric bipolar disorders (Fristad & MacPherson, 2014). Although homework is more of an adjunctive than systematic tool in IPT, it is also considered "well established" for the treatment of adolescent depression (David-Ferdon & Kaslow, 2008). Homework is routinely used in every session of CBT for anxiety, and CBT is considered a "probably efficacious" treatment for child anxiety as well as pediatric OCD (Freeman et al., 2014; Silverman, Pina, et al., 2008).

## THE ELEMENT IN PRACTICE

This next section of the chapter focuses on the practical application of homework in therapy with youth with internalizing disorders. Included is a step-by-step description of how to implement homework, which is complemented by a task analysis in Box 13.1 as well as a case study in Box 13.2 (at the end of the chapter). In addition, developmental and diversity adaptations are discussed.

### "Core of the Core" Element

Although the content of homework assignments varies, the step-by-step implementation of homework as a therapy element is surprisingly

## BOX 13.1. Task Analysis of Homework

1. Introduce the homework assignment.
   a. Provide a rationale for the specific assignment.
   b. Discuss the collaborative nature of homework.
   c. Discuss the reward system for homework completion (if applicable).

2. Assign the homework.
   a. Provide a rationale for its assignment.
   b. Be specific as to what, when, where, how much, or how often. Consider having the youth write the assignment down.
   c. Decide on how to record the homework (e.g., in a workbook, journal, mood diary).
   d. Practice the assignment during the session.
   e. Problem-solve potential obstacles to completing the assignment.

3. Check the homework toward the beginning of the following session.
   a. Provide a reward (e.g., praise, stickers, points toward a larger reward) for completed homework.
   b. Review the homework (e.g., probe the thoughts and feelings experienced during the homework assignment, clarify any misunderstandings, reinforce the homework's lesson).

4. Take positive action if the homework is not completed.
   a. Encourage and support any attempts made to complete the assignment.
   b. Discuss the obstacles to completion, and problem-solve for the next time.
   c. Complete the homework during the session.
   d. Reinforce the rationale for the homework in a nonjudgmental manner.

consistent across authors and manuals. The process can be broken down into four basic steps: introduction/presentation of homework, assignment of homework, checking homework in the next session, and responding to the youth when homework is not fully (or not at all) completed. In some ways, the term *homework* can be misleading, as it might connote the types of school assignments that are typically delegated with little discussion or consultation with the youth. In contrast, therapy homework should be collaboratively designed and assigned. For example, if the assignment is a thought diary, the youth can be actively engaged in a conversation about the best way to keep track of their thoughts. One youth may prefer a chart posted on the refrigerator, while another may prefer to keep a private diary in the notes app on a smartphone or tablet. Collaborative development of the homework assignment ensures "buy in" from the youth and likely helps to increase homework completion (Friedberg & McClure, 2015).

In addition, the term *homework* may lead the youth to think that the work will be "graded" and that therefore there is a chance that he or she might "fail" the assignment—when, in fact, this is not the case. To aid in making the distinction between school homework and therapy homework, several authors recommend utilizing other terms, such as take-home projects, home practice, work at home, or Show-That-I-Can (i.e., STIC) tasks (Kendall & Hedtke, 2006; Mufson, 2011).

The first step of the homework process is to introduce the general concept and rationale for homework and to discuss how this common element will work in therapy (Box 13.1, Step 1). This step is typically completed during the first session and is often part of the larger process of introducing the youth to the therapy process. The simplest way to present the rationale for homework is to stress the importance of practice when learning a new skill. In this discussion, the therapist may want to make an analogy to other skills the youth has learned. For example, if the youth plays an instrument, the therapist could ask how often she practices, what happens when she (or he) practices every day, and what happens when she skips several days of practice. Through this dialogue, the therapist can point out that to learn the new skills presented in therapy—and especially to learn them well—will require regular practice. In this discussion, the distinction should be made between school and therapy homework. Collaboratively making a list of how each is similar and different could aid in this process. One important difference is the collaborative nature of therapy homework, and the therapist should clearly communicate that the youth will have considerable input in determining the homework tasks. For example, in working with anxious youth, the therapist will want to reassure the youth that homework assignments for exposures will be planned together. Finally, the therapist should discuss what homework is like in the framework of the particular therapy. For instance, if there is a reward system for homework completion (see Coping Cat, Kendall & Hedtke, 2006), then the therapist can explain the reward system and gather ideas for potential rewards from the youth. Similarly, the therapist can introduce a homework workbook if one will be used.

The second step occurs when the specific homework assignment is given, typically at the end of each session (Step 2). This process should feel both collaborative and organic, meaning that the assignment should be a logical outgrowth of the material discussed in the session. The therapist should start by sharing the rationale for the specific homework. For example, if the therapist is assigning a mood diary, a discussion of how keeping track of moods may aid in discovering triggers or patterns in thoughts or behaviors may be appropriate. Next, the therapist should discuss the specifics of the assignment including what needs to be done, how often, and how to record it. In the case of a mood diary, the therapist may ask the youth to rate his or her mood several times a day. This part of the process naturally encourages collaboration with the youth. For example, the therapist may ask the youth about the times of day when it is most convenient to record (e.g., before school, after school, immediately before bedtime), where to record (e.g., in the youth's bedroom), and the preferred means of recording (e.g., in a diary, on a computer, on a worksheet handout, with stickers, etc.). Once an assignment is agreed upon by the therapist and youth, the youth should be encouraged to write it down. Next, the therapist and youth should practice implementing the assignment. The therapist may choose to first model the task and then ask the youth to practice it. This in-session practice enables the therapist to assess the youth's understanding and determine whether there are any foreseeable barriers to completing the assignment (e.g., developmental level), adapting the assignment if needed. Finally, the therapist and youth can brainstorm possible obstacles to homework completion as well as solutions to overcome those obstacles. For instance, a teen may be concerned about keeping a mood diary at school where peers may notice and consequently decide to record his mood before and after school instead of during school.

Next, the homework assignment is reviewed toward the beginning of the following session (Step 3). Recognizing and reviewing the homework in the next session lets the youth know that it is considered important, even vital, to the therapy process. Completed homework can be rewarded to increase the likelihood of the completion of future homework assignments. Such rewards may include praise, stickers, and/or points to be collected for a larger reward (see Chapter 9). Once the homework has been recognized and positively reinforced, the therapist then reviews the specific assignment with the youth. In this process, the therapist should be attentive to the thoughts and feelings that the youth experienced while completing the assignment. This gives the therapist the opportunity to address any negative thoughts (e.g., "I won't be able to do this," "This is not going to help") that may be interfering with homework completion. The therapist can also use the homework review to assess the youth's understanding and reinforce the practiced skill. For example, if the youth is working on making connections between thoughts and feelings by keeping a thought diary, the therapist can ask about specific entries in the log and reflect

on observed themes. The therapist may also use the homework assignment to start laying the foundation for the next skill. So, while reviewing the thought diary, the therapist may discuss the link between
thoughts and feelings and then ask the youth if it might be possible to
*change* thoughts to elicit different feelings.

The final step occurs only in the case of incomplete homework
(Step 4). At times, the youth will only partially complete (e.g., carry out
three of the four scheduled exposure tasks) or not manage to complete
homework assignments. In these cases, the best response is to encourage and support any efforts made to complete the homework. Together,
the youth and the therapist can identify the obstacles that prevented the
homework's completion and collaboratively develop a plan to facilitate
its completion next time. The solution is straightforward if the youth
simply did not understand the requirements of the assignment. In this
case, the therapist and youth can review and practice the task again.
Similarly, if the youth forgot to complete the homework, the youth and
therapist can problem-solve ways to remember (e.g., engage the parents
in the process, program a reminder into a phone). However, the moti-
vations behind homework noncompliance may be multifaceted. For
example, youth may have negative thoughts related to the assignment
or homework in general, may avoid homework out of anxiety and/or
fear of making an error, or may not have a family environment that
supports the assignment. Regardless of the reason behind the incomplete homework, in most cases it is a good idea to finish the homework
before continuing with the session. By doing the homework in session, the importance of the assignment is underscored, and the youth
thereby engages in the recommended practice. If completing the homework becomes a chronic problem, the therapist might want to revisit
the reward system and further engage the parents.

Although the basic four-step process differs very little across disorders, some types of homework are also more common to certain disorders. For example, emotion monitoring, thought tracking, thought
challenging, and problem-solving homework appear in manuals for
anxiety as well as those for mood disorders. However, activity scheduling and practicing types of interpersonal interactions (as per interpersonal psychotherapy) tend to be specific to treatments for mood
disorders, whereas exposure tasks tend to be unique to anxiety treatments. In addition, youth with mood disorders may experience low
energy levels and/or feelings of overwhelmedness and may thus benefit from smaller, more frequent, homework assignments. Some anxious
youth tend to be perfectionists and complete homework to the best of

their ability out of fear of making mistakes or breaking the rules. As such, when working with anxious youth, the therapist should inquire about the motives behind complete homework and consider adding exposure tasks that deliberately involve "making mistakes" and/or turning in an incomplete assignment (e.g., skipping one day of a daily mood diary).

## Developmental Adaptations

Youth presenting with depression and/or anxiety symptoms exhibit a wide range of developmental abilities. Fortunately, the ways of implementing homework can be adapted in several ways to meet the individual needs and developmental level of the youth. Even in initial conversations about the homework process, the therapist's approach may differ, depending on the age of the youth. For example, the discussion of the rationale behind homework will be simplified for younger children and may be aided by simple slogans (e.g., "Practice makes perfect!"). Older youth and teens may benefit from a more detailed discussion of how practice helps skills to become "automatic" or the need to generalize skills outside of the session. If one is using a reward system to encourage homework compliance, younger children may be excited about a sticker chart and smaller, more immediate, rewards (e.g., fake tattoos, marbles, Matchbox cars; see Chapter 9). In contrast, older youth may appreciate the chance to earn points to redeem for larger rewards (e.g., and iTunes giftcard) or privileges (e.g., extra screen time). In addition, teens are more likely to be motivated by internal factors and may benefit from being reminded of the long-term values of learning new skills to cope with difficult emotions than younger youth.

Therapists will need to be especially sensitive to developmental level in selecting and designing specific homework assignments. Practicing homework assignments in the session allows for an assessment of the youth's ability to complete the homework and gives the therapist the opportunity to adapt the task as needed. In general, younger children are likely to benefit from simple, brief assignments, and utilizing a workbook (e.g., Coping Cat; Kendall & Hedtke, 2006) may help younger youth keep better track of their homework tasks. In addition, younger youth may benefit from greater parental involvement in the homework process. Parents can gently remind their children about the assignments, serve as out-of-session coaches when appropriate, and/or assist by modeling the new skills. In fact, one intervention designed to treat OCD in children younger than 7 years of age includes "family home assignments" to build in parental involvement (Ginsburg, Burstein, Becker, & Drake, 2011). Although there may be several benefits to involving parents in the homework process, therapists will need to weigh the costs and benefits of including parents when working with adolescents. Teens are more likely to value their own independence and for that reason may be less susceptible to or appreciative of parent reminders and coaching than younger clients. In addition to these process recommendations, there are several adaptations for specific skills that are commonly incorporated in homework assignments in the treatment of youth with internalizing symptoms (e.g., activity scheduling, self-monitoring, relaxation, problem solving, and exposure tasks), and therapists are encouraged to refer to the chapters in this book that discuss those specific skills.

Finally, noncompliance with homework assignments is frequently an issue with youth of all ages and developmental levels. However, the reasons for, and the best responses to, nonadherence may vary. Although there may be some overlap across age groups, common reasons for noncompliance for younger children include forgetting, not having sufficient time, and not wanting to or not being able to (i.e., "It was too hard!") complete the homework (Hudson & Kendall, 2005). Parents can be a helpful resource for the forgetting and not having time excuses, as they can remind the child and help create time in a busy schedule for homework completion. Lack of motivation may be addressed by reminding the child of the consequences of homework completion (e.g., reward, getting better faster) and lack of completion (e.g., no rewards, doing the homework anyway at the beginning of the session) or by altering the reward menu. Sometimes the youth attempts a homework assignment but then discovers that it is too difficult. In this case, the therapist can adapt or change those aspects of the assignment that were too challenging. For example, if the youth has trouble remembering all the steps of a problem-solving activity, the therapist and youth can create a reminder card during the session. Similarly, if the youth has trouble writing, the therapist can use a feelings log with pictures.

For teens, the therapist can increase the likelihood of homework compliance by making the homework assignments fully collaborative, relevant to the teen's problem, and clear (Friedberg & McClure, 2015). As adolescents are embracing their increased autonomy, they are much more likely to complete a homework assignment that they helped to create. In addition, they may be sensitive to assignments that do not seem relevant to their own view of the problem. Thus, further clarifying a rationale that directly links the assignment to the presenting problem may increase the likelihood of their completing the homework. In fact, in a unique prospective and observational study, Jungbluth and Shirk (2013) found that depressed teens in CBT were most likely to comply with homework assignments when the therapist presented a clear rationale, devoted more time to discussing the homework, and considered possible barriers to completion. Moreover, despite the increased cognitive level of teens as compared to their younger peers, clear step-by-step assignments continued to be most helpful. Some treatments for adolescents—similar to those for younger youth—utilize workbooks to help keep assignments maximally clear and well organized (e.g., the C.A.T. Project; Kendall et al., 2002). Gently probing the reasons for noncompliance may elicit additional possibilities, including a heightened level of distress and various skills deficits (e.g., social skills, reading ability; Friedberg & McClure, 2015). In each case, the appropriate response involves processing the situation and collaboratively generating solutions that address the specific needs of the youth.

## Diversity Considerations

Delivering treatment with sensitivity to the diversity of the client is essential for treatment efficacy (Bernal et al., 2009) and is recommended by the American Psychological Association (2003, 2006). At this time, however, there is little research to guide recommendations for adapting the homework process for different minority populations. What we do know is that interventions for internalizing disorders that incorporate homework as part of the treatment have been shown to be effective for a variety of youth. Specifically, research supports the efficacy of manualized treatments for anxiety with African American teens (Ginsburg & Drake, 2002) and Hispanic/Latino youth (Pina et al., 2003). In addition, manualized treatments for anxiety have been successfully adapted for use in other countries (e.g., Coping Koala in Australia; Barrett et al., 1991; trauma-focused CBT in Norway; Jensen et al., 2014). Treatments for depression that include homework have also been applied to diverse samples with promising results. Specifically, manualized treatments for depression have benefited Puerto Rican (Rosselló et al., 2008) and incarcerated Hispanic youth (Sanchez-Barker, 2003). Similarly, there is preliminary evidence for the use of manualized treatments for depression with Haitian American adolescents (Nicolas et al., 2009). A meta-analysis of controlled trials of treatment effectiveness revealed that there are treatments for both anxiety and depression that can be classified as "probably efficacious" or "possibly efficacious" for use with minority youth (Huey & Polo, 2008).

Several articles on adapting manualized treatments for work with diverse youth have rich descriptions of the overall adaptation process; however, very few specifically mention homework. To aid in their adaptation of the CWD-A course for Haitian American adolescents, Nicolas and colleagues (2009) created an advisory board, established relationships with the community, and held focus groups with Haitian American teens. Feedback focused on the language, metaphors, and content of the treatment. In addition, members of the focus groups also evaluated the content of session homework assignments. Nicolas et al. (2009) reported that the teens in the focus group felt that the active listening assignments included in the therapy were not likely to be conducted outside of therapy. Another specific mention of homework occurs in a study of community perspectives on the use of CBT to treat anxiety in rural Latino youth (Chavira, Bustos, Garcia, Ng, & Camacho, 2015). In this study, input was collected from both bilingual community mental health providers (focus groups) and parents of anxious youth (individual interviews). Although feedback on the CBT was mostly positive, the community mental health providers expressed concern about the amount of homework in the CBT and the diminished likelihood that the Latino youth would complete the homework.

Considering the task analysis on the homework process, general recommendations can be made to aid in its specific application to diverse minority youth. When introducing homework, a discussion of how the youth and family typically handle problems may help gauge the role of both immediate and extended family in the youth's life. If the therapist is using a reward system to encourage homework, he or she should find it useful to discuss the process with the parents or caregivers to better assess the openness/acceptability/feasibility of implementing the particular system as well as to determine appropriate rewards. For specific homework assignments, it is recommended that the therapist consult empirical resources for suggested adaptations for the specific needs of the youth. Finally, in cases of noncompliance with homework, the therapist should always maintain a nonpunitive stance and try to understand the reasons for noncompliance, being especially sensitive to unique circumstances of the youth.

## CONCLUSIONS

Homework is assigned as part of empirically supported treatments to aid in the mastery and generalization of skills taught in the therapy session. Considered a core ingredient in CBT, homework is included as a systematic and routine (used in every session) process in the majority of manual-based treatments for youth with internalizing disorders. Although the link between homework engagement and treatment outcomes is well established among adult populations, the research on homework and youth outcomes is mixed. Additional research is needed to examine potential moderators of homework effects in youth, including the specific developmental level, in-session timing, and type of assignment. Homework is relatively easy to implement, and the process may be adapted for the individual developmental needs of the youth. In addition, there are recommendations for applications of specific types of homework and the homework process for use with diverse minority youth.

## BOX 13.2. Illustrative Case Example

Theresa was a 12-year-old Caucasian girl brought to therapy owing to problems with social anxiety. Her mother reported that Theresa had "always been shy" but that her anxiety increased significantly with the transition to middle school and her parent's divorce, which occurred around the same time. Theresa confided in the therapist that she was too anxious to text or call her peers, even her best friend, for fear of "saying something wrong or embarrassing." In addition, she shared that she no longer attended sleepovers or play dates at other houses. Theresa shared that, while she used to have three or four close friends, she currently had just one close friend. Her mother stated that Theresa had recently quit playing lacrosse, a sport that she loved and had played for years, because she got too nervous during games. In addition, Theresa indicated that she was too scared to talk in her classes, would not raise her hand to ask or answer questions, and when called on would respond with "I don't know" to avoid potentially answering the question incorrectly. A broad assessment including a clinical interview and self-, parent-, and school counselor-report surveys confirmed that Theresa met the diagnostic criteria for social phobia. Theresa agreed to participate in CBT using the Coping Cat manualized treatment (Kendall & Hedtke, 2006).

In the first session, the therapist established rapport and oriented Theresa to the treatment. At the end of that session, the therapist introduced the Show-That-I-Can (STIC) tasks. First, the therapist reinforced the value of practice by asking Theresa about lacrosse. Specifically, she asked Theresa to tell her about the game, how many years she had played it, and how she had learned some of the more difficult moves. During this discussion, the therapist and Theresa came to the conclusion that practice was necessary to become a good lacrosse player. She then pointed out that practice was also needed to become really good at handling anxiety. The therapist gave Theresa a Coping Cat Workbook and explained that her STIC tasks should be completed in the workbook and that she could earn points toward rewards by completing them. Then, the therapist and Theresa spent about 5 minutes brainstorming possible rewards (e.g., playing a game with the therapist at the end of the session, a $5 gift certificate to iTunes, a trip to her favorite ice cream shop) and how many points each would be worth (see Chapter 9 for helpful information on negotiating rewards with parents).

After completing the reward menu, the therapist gave Theresa her first STIC task assignment. The therapist opened the workbook to the STIC task and explained that the first task was for Theresa to write down a time that she felt great—not at all anxious—and that this would help Theresa get used to paying attention to her different emotions. Theresa was encouraged to also write down how she felt, what helped her to feel great, and what she was thinking at the time. The therapist shared an example by stating: "Last weekend I went to the beach. I sat in the sun and felt really relaxed. I was thinking about how fun it is to spend time with my family, with no chores or work to do." The therapist then prompted Theresa to do the same. Theresa shared that she felt good when she was playing lacrosse in the backyard with her brother. The therapist helped her complete the exercise by

*(continued)*

## BOX 13.2 (continued)

asking her what helped her feel comfortable ("No one else was watching me") and what she was thinking at the time ("I was thinking that it was fun and concentrating on catching the ball"). The therapist praised Theresa's efforts and reminded her to complete the one STIC task for the next session to earn two points. The therapist asked Theresa if she could come up with a plan for remembering the STIC task. Theresa stated that she would write it on her calendar and probably complete it a day or two before the next session. The therapist asked if there were any things that Theresa thought might get in the way of doing the STIC task, but Theresa was confident that she could complete the assignment. At the end of the first session, Theresa and the therapist invited her mother into the room to share the importance of therapy, discuss the appropriateness of the rewards, and better engage her cooperation in granting some of the potential rewards.

In the second session, the therapist shared the session agenda and then asked to review Theresa's STIC task. Theresa sheepishly got out the workbook and said that she did not find time to complete the STIC task. When the therapist asked why, she learned that Theresa waited until the night before her session to complete the STIC task, forgetting that she had a research paper due the same day in school. So, instead of completing the STIC task, she completed the paper. The therapist was understanding, but she reminded Theresa of the importance of practice ("What happens if you don't practice lacrosse?") and asked her to come up with a better strategy for next week ("I guess I will put the STIC task of my calendar for a couple days before the next session and ask my mom to remind me"). Then the therapist had Theresa complete the STIC task during the session. Upon its completion, the therapist discussed the assignment and had Theresa talk more about feeling good (e.g., what her body felt like when it was relaxed), thus previewing some of the emotion labeling content that will be introduced later that same session. The therapist praised Theresa's completion of the assignment and awarded the two points to her reward menu. The therapist then continued with the session agenda. The same homework process, with different assignments, was followed in each subsequent session. As the sessions progressed over time, Theresa appeared to become more confident in her ability to complete her homework assignments and needed fewer reminders from her mother.

# 14

## Maintenance and Relapse Prevention

### BACKGROUND OF THE ELEMENT

Despite the efficacy of evidence-based practices for the acute treatment of internalizing disorders in youth (Cohen, Deblinger, et al., 2006; Freeman et al., 2008; Walkup et al., 2008), relapse rates for both anxiety and mood disorders are high (Curry et al., 2011; Ginsburg, Becker, et al., 2014; Ginsburg, Kendall, et al., 2011; Kennard, Silva, et al., 2006; Miklowitz et al., 2014). Not surprisingly then, strategies to encourage maintenance of treatment gains and relapse prevention are a common element of evidenced-based practices for internalizing disorders in youth. Most often a component of broader treatment packages, maintenance and relapse-prevention strategies have only recently garnered focused research attention (e.g., Kennard, Stewart, Hughes, Jarrett, & Emslie, 2008). This chapter begins with an overview of the historical and theoretical foundations of maintenance and relapse prevention (MRP). Empirical support for its use is reviewed and the various methods of implementation for MRP strategies are then highlighted. For instance, MRP can be addressed in the acute portion of treatment via discussion of relevant issues and review of skills (e.g., Torp et al., 2015), and it can also be administered as an entire program following the acute treatment phase (Kennard, Stewart, et al., 2008). Finally, the chapter concludes with practical considerations for implementing this core element when working with youth with anxiety and mood disorders. Key developmental and diversity issues are considered, and a case example is also provided.

## Brief History

MRP strategies have their roots, in part, in the "generalization" literature that sprouted with fervor during the 1970s. Following the accumulating empirical support for behavioral approaches, interest in generalization, or the application of skills learned in therapy to real-world situations, came into focus (Kendall, 1989; Stokes & Baer, 1977). Importantly, prior to this time, little effort was devoted to the study of the process of generalization itself. To demonstrate this notion, in their review of over 100 studies that assessed for or directly targeted generalization, Stokes and Baer (1977) identified "train and hope" as a frequently employed strategy. Train and hope implied that skills were taught in session, and although generalization was a desired outcome, it was not explicitly addressed during treatment. Although initial efforts to examine and train generalization occurred most often within the context of externalizing, academic, or social problems (Broden, Bruce, Mitchell, Carter, & Hall, 1970; Meichenbaum, Bowers, & Ross, 1968; Stokes, Baer, & Jackson, 1974), several of these early generalization strategies underlie the MRP techniques that are used today for the treatment of internalizing disorders in youth.

During the 1980s, the specific concept of *relapse prevention* became deeply embedded within the addictions literature (Marlatt & Gordon, 1985), and attempts were made to apply those principles and strategies to other problem behaviors among adults, including depression (Overholser, 1998). Definitional and conceptual dilemmas abounded during this time regarding the nature and operationalization of relapse (see the "Evidence Base" section of this chapter and Brownell, Marlatt, Lichenstein, & Wilson, 1986). Regardless of the particular definition, however, relapse was typically considered an undesirable outcome of therapy. In contrast, Kendall (1989) proposed the "no-cure criticism" (p. 360), suggesting that psychological therapy assists individuals to manage, *but not cure*, problem behavior. He called for therapists to have reasonable expectations regarding therapeutic outcomes; relapses should be expected *and* specifically planned for in therapy sessions. This was an important notion, because explicitly planning for behavioral setbacks with patients helped to ward off notions that treatment was ineffective and to discourage personal feelings of failure when symptoms reemerged following therapy.

Emerging data from early clinical trials evaluating treatment programs for internalizing disorders in youth provided further support for the need to consider MRP strategies as core elements of these programs. Early studies supported the use of CBTs for both anxiety and depression in youth, but a meaningful percentage of participants either did not respond to the treatment or experienced a relapse at some point following a positive response to therapy (Clarke et al., 1999; Kendall, 1994). Acknowledging these data, many programs for internalizing disorders in youth incorporated some discussion of ways to maintain therapeutic gains following the acute phase of treatment (e.g., March & Mulle, 1998), and some even implemented booster sessions (e.g., Clarke et al., 1999) as a means of preventing relapse.

Notably, early efforts to include MRP strategies most often incorporated them within the context of the acute, or active, phase of treatment, reflecting a review or expansion of already learned content and techniques. Typically, when MRP is addressed during the acute phase of treatment, it is done toward the end of the treatment and includes a review of the skills that were learned in treatment (e.g., challenging negative thoughts) and a discussion of potential barriers (e.g., the transition to middle school) that might interfere with the maintenance of gains. MRP can also take the form of booster sessions, or meetings with the therapist that occur following the standard course of treatment and focus primarily on reinforcement and further generalization of skills (March & Mulle, 1998).

Only relatively recently have efforts focused specifically on the development and empirical evaluation of MRP strategies themselves within the context of internalizing disorders for youth. For example, West, Henry, and Pavuluri (2007) published a feasibility study examining a maintenance model of psychosocial therapy for bipolar disorder in youth. Similarly, Kennard and colleagues (Kennard, Stewart, et al., 2008) developed a CBT program to prevent depression relapse in youth. Programs that are specifically focused on the maintenance of treatment gains and relapse prevention tend to be fairly comprehensive, often expanding the content beyond that which was learned during the acute treatment phase. Collectively, empirical investigations of MRP programs for youth with internalizing disorders are contributing to a more nuanced understanding of these processes and the ways in which they can be best implemented; such studies are reviewed in the "Evidence Base" section of this chapter.

## Theory Base

Empirical data are emerging to support the use of MRP strategies for the treatment of internalizing disorders in youth (Cox et al., 2012; Gearing, Schwalbe, Lee, & Hoagwood, 2013). Yet, exactly how such strategies exert their positive effects is not clear, particularly because of the great variability in how MRP is conceptualized and operationalized across treatment programs. Nonetheless, their broad use is grounded in theory, suggesting that the skills learned during the acute phase of treatment are not always sufficient for maintaining long-term behavioral change.

At the most basic level, the MRP treatment element provides opportunities for therapists to reinforce application of the skills learned during treatment. For instance, booster sessions are often used to review skills that are learned during treatment and to assess how the youth is applying them in new situations. When the youth fails to apply the skills to situations beyond those directly addressed in therapy, MRP can provide an opportunity for the therapist to "train" generalization. Efforts reflecting generalization can be rewarded and reinforced, thereby increasing the probability of their occurrence (Stokes & Baer, 1977). Bandura's social learning theory suggests that the belief in oneself to successfully carry out a behavior greatly increases the chances that the behavior will be performed. The reinforcement of applying one's skills across a broad range of situations, in particular, is likely to build a sense of self-efficacy that can, in turn, further contribute to positive long-term outcomes (Bandura, 1977b).

The notion of focusing on the youth's application of skills as an MRP strategy is also consistent with the transfer of control model (Silverman, Ginsburg, & Kurtines, 1995), which posits that a transfer of control from the therapist, to parent, and then to child is necessary for long-term behavioral change. Control begins with the therapist, who is knowledgeable about the skills needed to effect change. The therapist then transfers control of these skills and methods to parents, who subsequently transfer them to the child. Ultimately, children must feel knowledgeable about and confident (i.e., to have control) in applying skills themselves in order to maintain treatment gains and prevent relapse.

In addition to training generalization, MRP also provides opportunities for targeting contextual factors involved in the etiology, maintenance, or recurrence of symptoms (Negreiros & Miller, 2014; Weinstein, Henry, Katz, Peters, & West, 2015; West et al., 2007). Steinberg and Avenevoli (2000) suggest that context is a powerful influence on the course of psychopathology because the particular pattern of disorder is a result of the extent to which the context allows the constellation of behavioral, emotional, and cognitive influence relating to the psychopathology to be repeated. For example, the role of family stress and negative emotional communication in bipolar disorder is well established (Miklowitz, 2007). In their maintenance model for the treatment of bipolar disorder in youth, West and colleagues (2007) directly address such family issues, encouraging parents to engage in self-care and teaching them how to collaboratively problem-solve and offer emotional support to their child. In so doing, stressful family interactions are likely to be reduced along with the negative cognitions and feelings the child may experience and that contribute to his or her depression. Theoretically, targeting variables known to negatively influence the course of psychopathology can reduce opportunities for the behavioral, emotional, and cognitive components of the disorder to be repeated, thereby improving longer-term outcomes.

Not only are broad contextual factors addressed during MRP programs, but other risk factors associated with relapse (e.g., negative attributional style) are likewise targeted in a flexible way that is tailored to individual needs. Most recently, MRP work has included a wellness component in addition to its traditional elements. For instance, Kennard, Stewart, et al. (2008) adapted Ryff and Singer's model (1996) that focuses on various areas of wellness, including the generation of optimism, gratitude, altruism, and a sense of purpose. Though not well articulated in the literature, a focus on strengths and positivity in MRP work is consistent with the broaden-and-build theory of positive emotions (Fredrickson, 1998). According to this theory, positive emotions broaden individuals' thought–action repertoires and, in so doing, build enduring personal resources. For example, a depressed child who is able to generate the positive emotion of interest is more likely to engage in academic endeavors, social outings, and/or individual activities that are stimulating. Over time, this child who experiences interest, and perhaps additional positive emotions, is more likely to show gains across intellectual, social, and emotional domains, which in turn help to build enduring personal resources that can contribute to warding off a relapse. The role of positive affect in children's emotional adjustment is gaining increased attention (see Davis & Suveg, 2014, for a review), and initial efforts to incorporate wellness components into MRP programs are promising (Kennard, Stewart, et al., 2008).

Given the relatively recent focus on MRP as an active rather than passive process, much work is needed to better understand how this element works and to identify moderators of its effectiveness. Despite its relatively recent inclusion as a process worthy of study in its own right, there is an emerging body of empirical work supporting the use of MRP strategies for youth with internalizing disorders that will now be reviewed.

## Evidence Base

Research supports the use of CBT approaches for anxiety, trauma, and obsessive–compulsive disorders (Freeman, Garcia, et al., 2014; Silverman, Pina, et al., 2008) and the use of both CBT and IPT treatments for child and adolescent depression (Birmaher et al., 2007; David-Ferdon & Kaslow, 2008; West et al., 2014), all of which address MRP in some way (see Table 14.1). Nonetheless, both depressive and bipolar disorders in youth are chronic and have high rates of recurrence and relapse following treatment (Kennard, Emslie, et al., 2006; Miklowitz et al., 2014). Relapse rates for anxious youth are likewise high (Ginsburg et al., 2014; Ginsburg, Kendall, et al., 2011), suggesting the need for a greater focus on MRP. In fact, a recent meta-analysis indicated that CBT packages that offer booster sessions are more effective in treating anxiety and depression in youth from pretreatment to a follow-up period than those that do not offer the sessions ($r = .64$ and .48, respectively; Gearing et al., 2013). This section will review the evidence base for MRP strategies, and because "package" treatments as a whole have been well reviewed and evaluated elsewhere, the focus will primarily be on studies that have examined MRP strategies distinct from other treatment components.

Prior to reviewing the evidence base for MRP strategies for youth with internalizing disorders, a few caveats are in order. First, the criteria and terminology that are used to assess and define treatment outcomes are widely variable across studies (Prien, Carpenter, & Kupfer, 1991). Typically, response is used to refer to an improvement in symptoms, whereas remission implies symptom-free status (Frank et al., 1991). Recovery, also referred to as sustained remission (Kennard, Stewart, et al., 2008), reflects a sustained period of remission of at least 4 months (Rush et al., 2006). Recurrence refers to the new onset of the disorder after a recovery period, whereas relapse reflects an increase of symptoms before full recovery is achieved (Frank et al., 1991). The second caveat is that MRP has been carried out in a variety of ways. Some research integrates MRP into a part of the acute treatment phase (i.e., that which is intended to reduce symptoms), whereas others have designed programs specifically to maintain treatment gains and

TABLE 14.1. The Maintenance and Relapse Prevention Element in Representative EBT Manuals

| | |
|---|---|
| *Coping Cat* (Kendall & Hedtke, 2006) | • The therapist explicitly discusses the maintenance of treatment gains and relapse prevention with the caregiver and child. The therapist explains that they will call to check in on how the child is doing a few weeks after treatment has ended. |
| *C.A.T. Project* (Kendall, Choudhury, Hudson, & Webb, 2002) | • The therapist explicitly discusses the maintenance of treatment gains and relapse prevention. The therapist tells the adolescent that he or she will call and check in on him or her in about 4 weeks. The therapist gives the adolescent his or her contact information and encourages the teen to call to schedule a booster session if he or she feels that it is needed, even before the therapist calls to check in. The inclusion of parents in the discussion on MRP is optional. |
| *OCD in Children and Adolescents* (March & Mulle, 1998) | • The use of MRP strategies is explicit. Parents are encouraged to call the therapist to schedule a booster session, if needed. |
| *CBT of Childhood OCD: It's Only a False Alarm* (Piacentini, Langley, & Roblek, 2007) | • MRP is explicitly addressed. The chronic nature of OCD is addressed, and ways to manage future symptoms are discussed. Caregivers are encouraged to seek future treatment for symptoms that are complicated. |
| *Family-Based Treatment for Young Children with OCD* (Freeman & Garcia, 2009) | • MRP is explicitly discussed. The therapist discusses the chronicity of OCD and the option of future booster sessions as needed. |
| *CBT for Social Phobia: Stand Up, Speak Out* (Albano & DiBartolo, 2007) | • MRP is explicitly addressed, and booster sessions are offered as needed (e.g., during times of transition such as the start of school). |
| *Treating Trauma and Traumatic Grief in Children and Adolescents* (Cohen, Mannarino, & Deblinger, 2006) | • The therapist addresses the maintenance of treatment gains by offering future treatment sessions, particularly for those youth who anticipate future stressors related to the trauma. |
| *Adolescent Coping with Depression* (Clarke, Lewinsohn, & Hops, 1990) | • MRP strategies are explicitly addressed. The youth are encouraged to recognize when they can use the tools learned in treatment to manage symptoms and when they should seek treatment again. |
| *Interpersonal Psychotherapy for Depressed Adolescents*, 2nd edition (Mufson, Pollack Dorta, Moreau, & Weissman, 2011) | • The maintenance of treatment gains is emphasized throughout treatment and during a termination phase. For instance, the therapist is encouraged to emphasize throughout treatment that the adolescents are learning skills that will be maintained after treatment. Several options for follow-up treatment are discussed, including monthly maintenance sessions that are time-limited. |

*(continued)*

**TABLE 14.1.** (*continued*)

| | |
|---|---|
| *Treating Depressed Youth: Therapist Manual for "Action"* (Stark et al., 2007) | • MRP is addressed by reviewing the skills learned throughout the treatment and the progress made by each group participant. A process for scheduling booster sessions is also discussed. |
| *Psychotherapy for Children with Bipolar and Depressive Disorders* (Fristad, Arnold, & Leffler, 2011) | • MRP is an explicit component of this treatment program. Both the children and parents are given "Take-home Messages" sheets that include reminders of the skills learned during the sessions and ways to maximize the child and family's functioning. |

*Note.* Some book titles are shortened to conserve space. See the References at the back of the book for full titles.

prevent relapse. Studies that have specifically evaluated continuation (i.e., maintenance of treatment gains) and maintenance (i.e., prevention of new episodes) phases of treatment will be reviewed in this section (Frank et al., 1991; Kennard, Stewart, et al., 2008). Finally, MRP is a core element of evidence-based psychosocial treatments for internalizing disorders in youth, but it is also empirically supported in the context of pharmacological interventions for these disorders. That is, sometimes nonpharmacological MRP strategies are implemented after a positive response to medications in an attempt to maintain treatment gains and prevent relapse. In fact, the majority of research investigating the effects of nonpharmacological MRP strategies has been in the context of pharmacological treatment alone or in combination with psychosocial treatment; thus, those studies are included in this review.

Acknowledging the high rates of relapse following treatment for depressed youth, Kennard, Stewart, et al. (2008) developed relapse prevention CBT (RP-CBT). RP-CBT is designed to be administered after an acute phase of medication treatment pursuant to the rationale that, though both medications and CBT have similar outcomes over longer-term follow-up periods, the time to response is faster with medications (Kennard, Stewart, et al., 2008; Treatment for Adolescents with Depression Study [TADS], 2004). RP-CBT, which consists of 8–11 sessions, is intended for use with youth who have shown a positive response to the acute phase of pharmacological treatment. Treatment was designed to be less intense than an acute phase of CBT and to be delivered flexibly, allowing the therapist to modify the content based on the youth's individual needs. Core CBT skills are taught and practiced during the first few sessions, concentrating in particular on the child's key symptoms. In addition to core CBT skills (e.g., cognitive restructuring), the various modules cover emotion regulation, social skills, and asser-tiveness training, and the therapists assist the youth in applying their skills to such common challenges as boredom, self-esteem, irritability, and adherence. The family component serves to gain the caregivers' insights on the youth's progress, address family emotional commu-nication styles (e.g., expressed emotion), and encourage family well-ness. Finally, during the wellness component, the youth are introduced to the concept that wellness occurs on a continuum and is likely to fluctuate over time. Six general areas of wellness are also covered: self-acceptance, social relations, success (autonomy and mastery), self-goals, spiritual (optimism, gratitude, and altruism), and soothing rem-edies (relaxation activities). Families are offered three optional booster sessions at the end, depending on their need. The particular timing of treatment components is based on the number of residual symptoms the youth exhibits at the end of the acute phase of treatment. For youth with a greater number of symptoms, more sessions are allotted for the practice and application of CBT skills.

Kennard, Stewart, et al. (2008) piloted the RP-CBT program with six adolescents between the ages of 11 and 18 years, all of whom were considered responders to antidepressant medications. Participants demonstrated a decrease in self-reported depressive symptoms and reported high satisfaction with the treatment. Based on the initial pilot, Kennard and colleagues further refined the treatment approach and the methods used to assess outcomes. Since the initial development of the program, Kennard and colleagues have used randomized designs to provide further evidence that relapse rates are significantly lower when clinically depressed youth receive RP-CBT in combination with medication management than medication management only (Kennard, Becker, et al., 2014; Kennard, Emslie, et al., 2008).

West and colleagues (2007) likewise developed a maintenance model for the treatment of bipolar disorder in youth, given its refrac-tory course. The maintenance program is designed to be implemented after successful participation in the child- and family-focused CBT pro-gram (CFF-CBT). CFF-CBT consists of 12 60- to 90-minute sessions that include psychoeducation, content to improve child self-esteem and par-ent self-efficacy, cognitive restructuring and mindfulness, and social problem solving, as well as other content to address the psychosocial and interpersonal stress that often accompanies bipolar disorder. Dur-ing the acute treatment phase of this study, participants received CFF-CBT in combination with medication management. The maintenance phase of CCF-CBT treatment consisted of 50-minute booster sessions that were held from once per week to once every 3 months over a 3-year period with youth, the vast majority of whom were still taking medications. The content of the booster sessions focused on the core treatment strategies that were learned during the acute phase of treatment, with the particular emphasis and timing of the treatment elements based on each child's individual needs. Barriers to recovery were identified for participants (e.g., uncontrolled aggression, family conflict) and were addressed within the core treatment strategies of CFF-CBT. For example, aggression was framed within the affect regulation skills that were learned in CFF-CBT. Results following the 3-year maintenance phase showed that the youth maintained their posttreatment gains, with 83% of the youth experiencing minimal or no symptoms.

The MRP literature for anxiety-based disorders is less well developed than that for depression in youth. Only one study was identified that specifically examined relapse prevention in the treatment of anxiety (Scott & Feeny, 2006). In this case study, a 9-year-old girl with separation anxiety disorder and anxiety disorder not otherwise specified was seen for 20 sessions of CBT. The first 15 sessions included standard CBT content, such as psychoeducation, relaxation, exposure, and cognitive restructuring, whereas the final five sessions addressed relapse prevention. During the final sessions, the therapist and child created a relapse prevention book that reviewed each component of therapy. For instance, in one section of the book the child wrote about all of the coping skills that were learned throughout therapy. Toward the end of the book was a section titled "Planning for My Future," which identified future anxiety-related stressors and tools to manage each stressor. The child experienced only minimal symptoms at posttreatment and reportedly had no symptoms at the 12-month follow-up period. Importantly, the relapse prevention book is very similar to that which is used in the Coping Cat program (Kendall & Hedtke, 2006), both of which help to reinforce and review skills that were learned in the therapy. The difference with the relapse prevention book, however, was that it was created over several sessions at the end of therapy and thus was perhaps a relatively well focused component of the treatment.

## THE ELEMENT IN PRACTICE

With a theoretical and empirical base for MRP established, the second half of this chapter turns to the practical aspects of this core element.

The section begins with a narrative description of the key components related to implementing MRP (Box 14.1). Then, developmental and diversity issues are discussed. The chapter ends with a case summary (Box 14.2) that highlights the use of MRP strategies with an 11-year-old boy with an anxiety disorder.

## BOX 14.1. Task Analysis of Maintenance and Relapse Prevention

1. Set the foundation for the use of maintenance and relapse-prevention strategies by setting realistic expectations at the beginning of treatment.
   a. Normalize the experience of symptoms. Share with the child that everyone experiences symptoms from time to time to some degree.
   b. Emphasize that the goal of therapy is a significant reduction in, but not complete amelioration of, symptoms.

2. Near the end of treatment, initiate MRP by reviewing the youth's progress in treatment.
   a. Have the youth think back to when treatment started, specifically recall the severity of the symptoms, and reflect on his or her current levels of functioning.
   b. Collaboratively create a list of all of the youth's accomplishments since therapy began.
   c. Create a graph of the child's symptoms from the start of therapy to the time of termination.
   d. If booster sessions are not already formally integrated within the treatment program, determine whether MRP is best addressed toward the end of the acute phase of treatment or as booster sessions once the treatment is over.

3. Review the skills learned in therapy to assure a solid understanding of them.
   a. Create a book or worksheets that the youth can reference as needed during future situations.
   b. Provide the caregivers with worksheets or similar materials that likewise review the skills that were learned in therapy so that they can help the youth to maintain treatment gains.
   c. Have the youth practice the skills that were learned in therapy during potential stressful situations that might occur in the future.

4. Address factors that might interfere with the maintenance of treatment gains.
   a. Identify potential interfering variables (e.g., psychopathology affecting the parents).
   b. Formulate a plan to minimize the potential negative impacts that those variables could have on the maintenance of treatment gains.
   c. Identify additional ameliorative services as necessary (e.g., treatment for the parents' psychopathology).

## "Core of the Core" Element

MRP is addressed in a variety of ways across treatment programs, with some briefly addressing this core element and others being entirely focused on maintenance and relapse-prevention content. Given this, there is no single "right" way to implement MRP that is supported by empirical data; nevertheless, key components of this core element appear to be included in some capacity in *most* EBTs for internalizing disorders in youth (see Table 14.1).

Though not explicitly labeled as such, therapists often build a foundation for MRP during the first few sessions of treatment (see Box 14.2, Step 1). Specifically, during the psychoeducation phase of treatment, therapists normalize the experience of anxiety and depression and provide education about the chronicity of the symptoms. When implementing Coping Cat (Kendall & Hedtke, 2006), for example, therapists describe their own anxious experiences, thereby normalizing the feelings. The notion that everyone experiences at least occasional feelings of sadness or anxiety helps to set realistic goals for therapy, with improvement, not complete amelioration of symptoms, being the most likely outcome (Kendall, 1989). Normalizing the experience of anxiety and setting realistic goals are important in facilitating a favorable treatment outcome as well as warding off feelings of self-blame when symptoms reappear after therapy has ended. With reasonable expectations, both the children and caregivers are better able to identify when a reemergence of symptoms requires further treatment or when they can apply the skills learned on their own.

Once MRP is explicitly introduced, it is often helpful to begin by praising youth lavishly for their efforts in therapy and to acknowledge all that they have accomplished (Step 2). Therapists can highlight a youth's progress in a variety of ways. For instance, a fear hierarchy was likely created during the treatment for anxious youth. Therapists and youth can review the fear hierarchy, noting how the youth could not imagine overcoming fears on the top of the hierarchy at the start of treatment. In the Coping Cat treatment for anxious youth (Kendall & Hedtke, 2006), a videotaped commercial is created and directed by the child to provide an opportunity for him or her to showcase the successes. Youth are given a copy of the commercial to take home with them. For both anxious and depressed youth, the therapists can plot their symptom levels over time so that they can clearly see their improvement. The therapist and each client can also make a list together of how the youth has improved. A depressed youth, for example, might note feeling more comfortable with activities such as planning social events with friends. Regardless of the ways that the therapist and the youth collaboratively reflect on progress, it is very important to do so. Highlighting the youth's accomplishments can help to build his or her self-efficacy, which in turn can help him or her to apply the skills learned whenever symptoms reemerge (Bandura, 1977b).

Also during Step 2, the therapist can collaboratively determine with the youth and his family whether they will participate in booster sessions. Sometimes booster sessions might already be formally integrated into the program, whereas at other times they will be optional. If optional, the therapist can initiate a discussion about whether booster sessions might be helpful for the youth and his or her family and, if so, determine how frequently they will occur and for how long.

Reviewing the skills that were learned during therapy is the next key component in MRP (Step 3), regardless of whether it occurs during the acute portion of treatment or during a booster session. This process helps to consolidate all that was learned during therapy and helps to solidify the insights for the youth. The review of skills can happen in a variety of ways. For instance, during ITP-A (Mufson et al., 2011), the therapist spends the final session reviewing the strategies that the depressed adolescent has learned for successfully negotiating his or her interpersonal relationships following the therapy. The goal in doing so is to improve the skills' application in future situations. In OCD treatment for youth (March & Mulle, 1998), therapists have children imagine a "slip" that is likely to occur at some future juncture and discuss how they could apply the tools they learned during therapy. The therapist assists the child in making the exposure feel as real as possible and then coaches the child in applying the learned strategies. In treatment for anxious youth (Kendall & Hedtke, 2006), skills can be reviewed by using a workbook that was created during the course of therapy. The youth take the workbook home with them so that they can reference the skills as needed. Similarly, in treating youth with depressive and bipolar disorders, the parents and children are given individual "Take-Home Messages" sheets that provide reminders of key treatment concepts. Regardless of the particular way that skills are reviewed, the goal is to help the youth internalize them so that they can be implemented readily when needed during future situations.

The final step of MRP is to address lingering stressors that can negatively impact the maintenance of treatment gains (Step 4). For instance, the role of expressed emotion is well established in bipolar disorders (Miklowitz, 2007), and therapists may need to address it, if relevant, during treatment. West et al. (2007), for instance, explicitly teach the parents how to offer emotional support to their child. Likewise, Fristad, et al. (2011) spend considerable time facilitating adaptive communication among family members of children with depressive and bipolar disorders. In addition to absorbing explicit teaching about communication, families complete a number of out-of-session tasks that provide opportunities to practice skills. For example, families complete the "Out with the Old Communication, In with the New" worksheet that requires them to document old (hurtful) communication, how they were able to catch themselves using the old communications, and then identify what is the new (helpful) communication. Parental accommodation also can interfere with the maintenance of treatment gains. Parents' anxiety, for example, about observing their child in distress can interfere with his or her successful completion of exposure tasks outside of treatment. Consequently, therapists can address parents' own anxiety and behaviors either in session or perhaps by referring them for their own individual treatment. There can be a wide of variety of variables that can interfere with the maintenance of treatment gains, and therapists need to be alert to these throughout the course of treatment so that they can be adequately addressed prior to termination.

## Developmental Adaptations

MRP strategies are easily adapted for use with youth of all developmental levels. Younger children are likely to need more assistance in maintaining treatment gains and monitoring symptoms than older youth, who may appreciate more autonomy in relapse prevention. Regardless of the particular level of involvement by youth and caregivers, however, the broad strategies involved in MRP can easily be modified as needed.

Freeman and colleagues developed a family-based CBT program for 5- to 8-year-old children with OCD (Freeman & Garcia, 2009; Freeman, Sapyta, et al., 2014). Given the young age of the children involved in this program, parents are active participants in all phases of treatment. With regard to the relapse-prevention component of treatment, there is a specific focus on reviewing the tools that parents have learned through the treatment. For instance, the therapist reviews skills such as differential attention, modeling appropriate behaviors, and scaffolding children's adaptive emotional responses. Therapists also review tools that the parents are expected to encourage their children to use. Parents are coached in how to help their child boss back OCD as well as develop a hierarchy of exposure tasks and then implement them.

Parents are also taught how to monitor the child's symptoms and what to do if they reappear. Importantly, the discussion of MRP is directive: "Do not overprotect your child from stress" or "Watch more carefully for a return of symptoms during stressful periods." Initial empirical support for this developmentally modified program is positive (Freeman, Sapyta, et al., 2014), though long-term follow-up is needed.

When one is treating other anxiety disorders in youth, various versions of EBT manuals can be modified, based on the child's developmental level. For instance, Coping Cat (Kendall & Hedtke, 2006) is designed for school-age children, and the workbook that accompanies treatment consists of cartoons, thought bubbles, and other pictorial images to facilitate the youth's understanding of CBT concepts. The discussion of MRP occurs at the end of treatment with both the parents and children. The skills learned in therapy are reviewed with the parents, and the therapist helps to set reasonable expectations for the future. In particular, parents are reminded that the child may have difficulties with anxiety again in the future, and during such times he or she should be encouraged to practice the skills learned. The C.A.T. Project is a parallel version of Coping Cat that is used with adolescents. Adolescents are given much more autonomy throughout the program, and with regard to MRP, in particular, the therapist may be flexible with whether they discuss these issues with parents and adolescents together or just with the teen (Kendall et al., 2002).

Regardless of whether parents are present for the discussion of MRP, the therapist can readily modify relevant strategies based on the child's developmental level. For instance, when reviewing treatment progress, both younger and older youth might appreciate a visual representation of how their symptoms have changed over time. For younger youth, the therapist can create a very simple graph with verbal descriptors (e.g., "*lots* of anxiety," "just a little anxiety") instead of numbers. Adolescents might prefer a more technical graph that depicts changes in actual anxiety symptom scores (e.g., based on self-report measures) over time.

Kennard, Stewart, et al. (2008) explicitly noted the need to attend to developmental differences when piloting RP-CBT for youth with depressive disorders. Mood monitoring is a key feature of this program; yet, it may be difficult for younger youth, given that this activity requires cognitive skills that may not yet be adequately developed. Consequently, Kennard et al. implemented a behavioral approach to monitoring mood in which children were encouraged to measure their mood before and after a fun activity. In contrast, older youth might be asked to recall an event and their corresponding feelings and thoughts. Metacognition is required for this activity, and thus it would be difficult for younger youth (Flavell, Green, & Flavell, 2009). The focus on behavioral activities for younger youth is not only consistent with their cognitive abilities but also more likely to maintain the youth's attention and keep them engaged in the therapy process. Many strategies used in MRP can be presented behaviorally. For instance, when helping youth to identify treatment progress, the therapist might have older youth think back to how they felt at the start of treatment and how they feel now when faced with an anxiety-provoking situation. For younger youth, the therapist might have the youth act out what they did before treatment when in an anxiety-provoking situation and what they do now.

## Diversity Considerations

No studies could be identified that specifically examined the effectiveness of MRP strategies when implemented with diverse groups of individuals. The meta-analysis by Gearing and colleagues (2013) indicated that CBT for internalizing disorders in youth is more effective when booster sessions are included than when not; however, the findings were not broken down by racial group or socioeconomic status. Similarly, Silverman, Pina, et al. (2008) reported that CBT is efficacious for treating anxiety in youth; yet, they emphasized that whether the findings generalize to minority populations was unknown, given the relative dearth of data that were available. With regard to relapse prevention programs for youth with mood disorders, research has likewise included mostly Caucasian middle-class samples (West et al., 2007).

Despite the lack of research examining the effectiveness of MRP strategies specifically, such strategies are a common element of EST packages, many of which have been examined with diverse samples of youth with internalizing disorders (Ferrell, Beidel, & Turner, 2004; Ginsburg & Drake, 2002; Gordon-Hollingsworth et al., 2015; Pina et al., 2003; Rosselló, Bernal, & Rivera-Medina, 2012; Southam-Gerow, Kendall, & Weersing, 2001). Further, as reviewed by Huey and Polo (2008), CBT-based programs, which include at least some consideration of MRP, should be considered a first-line treatment approach when working with youth of diverse backgrounds.

Nonetheless, issues of diversity are essential considerations for the therapist when implementing ESTs and research suggests that socioeconomic diversity, in particular, may be an important variable to consider in the context of MRP. Ginsburg et al. (2014), for example, examined predictors of remission (i.e., being free of all anxiety disorders that were present at pretreatment) at a mean of 6 years after randomization in a treatment study for youth ages 7–17 years with an anxiety disorder. No differences were found by treatment condition (CBT, medication, or combination treatment); however, higher socioeconomic status predicted lower anxiety severity and better functioning at follow-up, whereas better family functioning predicted remission status. Similarly, Gordon-Hollingsworth et al. (2015) recently reported that African American youth with anxiety disorders were less likely to remit than their Caucasian counterparts, perhaps in part because African American families were more likely to be from single-parent homes and to report lower socioeconomic status than Caucasian participants. Relapse rates at 24 weeks were similar across racial groups, though the very small sample size for the relapse analyses may have precluded detection of group differences.

Low socioeconomic status tends to co-occur with other family risk factors such as maternal psychopathology that can have a negative cumulative effect on youth (Evans, 2003). In the context of treatment outcomes specifically, these risk factors may interfere with treatment gains and their maintenance via a variety of pathways. In the context of financial stress or psychopathology, caregivers may be less able to provide the logistical (e.g., accessing good care, traveling to appointments) and emotional support to youth that is necessary for relapse prevention. Findings by Weinstein et al. (2015) are consistent with the notion that attending to family-level variables during treatment may be associated with better outcomes, both in terms of initial treatment response as well as maintenance of gains and relapse prevention. In their study of bipolar youth, CFF-CBT, which includes up to six monthly follow-up sessions over a 9-month treatment-maintenance phase, performed better than treatment as usual when the child had a parent with higher baseline depressive symptoms and who was economically disadvantaged. CFF-CBT includes a distinct focus on parental self-care and family problem solving and communication that may be particularly important when working with samples experiencing multiple psychosocial stressors.

Collectively, findings from research examining EBTs (of which MRP is a part) suggest that these approaches can be used with diverse groups of youth experiencing internalizing disorders. However, the specific strategies that might be most helpful with diverse groups of youth have yet to be examined. Nonetheless, the examination of family risk factors, such as parental psychopathology and low socioeconomic status, is consistent with the broader MRP literature that calls for attention to broader contextual variables that can affect long-term treatment gains.

## CONCLUSIONS

MRP strategies are a core element of EBT practices for internalizing disorders in youth of all ages. Though long included in treatments for internalizing disorders in youth, only recently have researchers examined the efficacy of specific relapse-prevention programs. Given the high relapse rates for both depression and anxiety in youth, the examination of programs designed specifically to facilitate the maintenance of treatment gains and prevent relapse is clearly a significant undertaking. Preliminary data suggest that programs that specifically address maintenance issues, possibly by offering booster sessions and focusing on the broader psychosocial context of the child and his or her family, are positively associated with favorable long-term treatment outcomes. Tailoring MRP strategies to the child and family's individual needs is important for all youth, but particularly those who present with multiple stressors that can negatively impact treatment gains.

# BOX 14.2. Illustrative Case Example

Andrew, an 11-year-old caucasian boy with separation anxiety disorder, was treated with CBT for 12 sessions. When Andrew first presented at the clinic, he was experiencing severe impairment from his symptoms. Most significantly, he rarely attended a complete school day; either arriving at school late or leaving early. He cited a variety of reasons for missing school, though mostly he complained of stomachaches and headaches. Andrew developed a relationship with the school nurse as a result of his frequent visits to her office, and it was she who eventually contacted Andrew's parents with concern about his frequent somatic symptoms. After a thorough evaluation with Andrew's pediatrician that revealed no apparent cause for his symptoms, his parents, the school nurse, and the pediatrician decided that he needed to have a psychological evaluation. Though reluctant, Andrew acknowledged the interference he was experiencing as a result of his anxiety and agreed to begin treatment.

The MRP component of CBT began during the first treatment session, when the therapist normalized the experience of anxiety for Andrew. First, she elaborated that everyone experiences anxiety sometimes and that the emotion can be adaptive. Next, she and Andrew discussed the various ways in which anxiety and fear can be helpful. For instance, the therapist noted how anxiety before presentations had led her to prepare for them. Andrew was also able to identify several ways that anxiety could be helpful, such as in prepping for a soccer game or studying for a test. The therapist then noted that, because anxiety can be adaptive, the goal of treatment was to reduce his anxiety so that at a more helpful level it would no longer interfere with his life. She emphasized that some level of anxiety is adaptive, and thus the goal of treatment is not to *completely* eliminate the emotion.

Next, the therapist discussed that everyone experiences anxiety and fear at different levels, for a variety of reasons. During the intake interview, both Andrew and his parents noted that he was always a bit nervous for as long as they could remember. The therapist brought this information to the fore during the first therapy session as ways of focusing on temperamental differences. She explained that some people experience anxiety more quickly and intensely than others, and that this is not good or bad—it is just a temperamental difference. Andrew noted that he was always more anxious about things than his friends appeared to be. Collaboratively, the therapist and Andrew reiterated that the goal of therapy would be to reduce his anxiety so that it no longer interfere with his life unduly but that he would probably always have a higher level of anxiety than many of his friends.

When Andrew's treatment neared termination, the focus shifted more explicitly to MRP. The therapist started by reflecting genuinely on the remarkable gains that Andrew had made. In particular, she noted that Andrew had not missed even one day of school since beginning treatment, was regularly engaging in social activities outside of his home, and no longer called to talk to his parents when he was at a friend's house. Andrew took great pride in his accomplishments and seemed to enjoy the process of describing them in detail. Though he readily acknowledged his parents' support in the therapy process, he took ownership of his treatment gains. Andrew noted that, at the beginning of treatment, he did not really believe

*(continued)*

## BOX 14.2 (continued)

he would ever be able to be away from his parents comfortably, but he chuckled as he discussed how much fun it was to be away from them occasionally now. The therapist also plotted Andrew's self- and parent-reported anxiety levels at pre-, mid-, and end of treatment, compared to age-appropriate norms, to show him that he now experienced anxiety at levels similar to his same-aged peers.

Following the therapist's reflection on treatment gains, the two collaboratively reviewed the skills that Andrew had learned during his treatment. A workbook that he had used throughout the treatment greatly facilitated this review. Andrew looked back through his book, noting which skills seemed most useful and which were least useful. The therapist explained that skills can be more or less useful at different times and encouraged Andrew to consider giving those that seemed to be less useful so far another try at a later time. He and the therapist also brainstormed several situations that might cause him significant anxiety in the future. For instance, Andrew would be starting middle school the following year; the therapist and Andrew discussed how we would likely feel in great detail. Then the therapist coached Andrew through describing what he could think and do in the situation to manage his anxious feelings. Imagining an anxiety-provoking situation and successfully using his skills helped to solidify a sense of confidence for Andrew.

Throughout the treatment it became clear that Andrew's parents had accommodated his anxiety in various ways. For instance, when Andrew woke in the mornings with a stomachache, his parents would often let him go into school late or stay home altogether. Andrew's parents, and his mother in particular, noted how difficult it was for her to discern whether his somatic symptoms were anxiety-related or really caused by a physical illness. The therapist discussed this issue with Andrew's parents at length, encouraging them to think through the consequences of the choice to let him stay home from school or not. For instance, the therapist asked the parents, "What is the worst case scenario if you send Andrew to school with a stomachache?" and "How many times has Andrew had a stomachache that the doctor clearly linked to a physical cause?" Andrew's parents also noted that he had a much tougher time going back to school after he was out for a few days and that it was probably best for him to go every day. The therapist reinforced the parents' insights and encouraged them to be a source of support for each other whenever they were having difficulty setting limits with Andrew.

At the end of the treatment, the therapist explained to Andrew and his parents that she would call to check in on how he was doing in about a month but that they should call sooner if needed. A couple of weeks after termination, the therapist received a call from Andrew's mother, who related that he had had to change schools. She feared that the transition might cause him to experience severe anxiety. The therapist first validated the mother's belief that the school transition was likely to evoke anxiety for Andrew, but then she coached Andrew's mother on ways to support him and encourage him to use his skills as needed. The therapist also offered to conduct a booster session if needed. Andrew's mother called back several months later to check in, noting that Andrew had made a successful transition to the new school and was managing his anxiety levels well.

# References

Abramowitz, J. S., Whiteside, S. P., & Deacon, B. J. (2005). The effectiveness of treatment for pediatric obsessive–compulsive disorder: A meta-analysis. *Behavior Therapy, 36,* 55–63.

Addis, M. E., & Jacobson, N. S. (2000). A closer look at the treatment rationale and homework compliance in cognitive-behavioral therapy for depression. *Cognitive Therapy and Research, 24,* 313–326.

Albano, A. M., & Dibartolo, P. M. (2007). *Cognitive-behavioral therapy for social phobia in adolescents: Stand up, speak out, therapist guide.* New York: Oxford University Press.

Albano, A. M., Marten, P. A., Holt, C. S., Heimberg, R. G., & Barlow, D. H. (1995). Cognitive-behavioral group treatment for social phobia in adolescents: A preliminary study. *Journal of Nervous and Mental Disease, 183,* 649–656.

Allen, J. P., Hauser, S. T., Bell, K. L., & O'Connor, T. G. (1994). Longitudinal assessment of autonomy and relatedness in adolescent–family interactions as predictors of adolescent ego development and self-esteem. *Child Development, 65,* 179–194.

American Psychological Association. (2003). Guidelines on multicultural education, training, research, practice, and organizational change for psychologists. *American Psychologist, 58,* 377–402.

American Psychological Association. (2006). Evidence-based practice in psychology. *American Psychologist, 61,* 271–285.

Anderson, C. M., Hogarty, D. G., & Reiss, D. J. (1980). Family treatment of adult schizophrenic patients: A psycho-educational approach. *Schizophrenia Bulletin, 6,* 490–505.

Angold, A., Costello, E. J., & Erklani, A. (1999). Comorbidity. *Journal of Child Psychology and Psychiatry, 40,* 57–87.

Azrin, N. H., Vinas, V., & Ehle, C. T. (2007). Physical activity as reinforcement for classroom calmness of ADHD children: A preliminary study. *Child and Family Behavior Therapy, 29,* 1–7.

Baer, D. M., Peterson, R. F., & Sherman, J. A. (1967). The development of imitation by reinforcing behavioral similarity to a model. *Journal of the Experimental Analysis of Behavior, 10,* 405–416.

Bandura, A. (1961). Psychotherapy as a learning process. *Psychological Bulletin, 58,* 143–159.

Bandura, A. (1962). Social learning through imitation. In M. R. Jones (Ed.), *Nebraska Symposium on Motivation* (pp. 211–269). Lincoln, NE: University of Nebraska Press.

Bandura, A. (1969). *Principles of behavior modification.* New York: Holt, Rinehart & Winston.

Bandura, A. (1977a). *Self-efficacy: The exercise of control.* San Francisco: Freeman.

Bandura, A. (1977b). Self-efficacy: Toward a unifying theory of behavioral change. *Psychological Review, 84,* 191–215.

Bandura. A. (1977c). *Social learning theory.* Englewood Cliffs, NJ: Prentice-Hall.

Bandura, A. (1978). The self system in reciprocal determinism. *American Psychologist, 33,* 344–358.

Bandura, A. (1986). *Social foundations of thought and action: A social cognitive theory.* Englewood Cliffs, NJ: Prentice-Hall.

Bandura, A. (2004). Swimming against the mainstream: The early years from chilly tributary to transformative mainstream. *Behaviour Research and Therapy, 42,* 613–630.

Bandura, A., Adams, N. E., & Beyer, J. (1977). Cognitive processes mediating behavioral change. *Journal of Personality and Social Psychology, 35,* 125–139.

Bandura, A., Blanchard, E. B., & Ritter, B. (1969). Relative efficacy of desensitization and modeling approaches for inducing behavioral, affective, and attitudinal changes. *Journal of Personality and Social Psychology, 13,* 173–199.

Bandura, A., Grusec, J. E., & Menlove, F. L. (1967). Vicarious extinction of avoidance behavior. *Journal of Personality and Social Psychology, 5,* 16–23.

Bandura, A., & Menlove, F. L. (1968). Factors determining vicarious extinction of avoidance behavior through symbolic modeling. *Journal of Personality and Social Psychology, 3,* 99–108.

Bandura, A., Reese, L., & Adams, N. E. (1982). Microanalysis of action and fear arousal as a function of differential levels of perceived self-efficacy. *Journal of Personality and Social Psychology, 43,* 5–21.

Bandura, A., Ross, D., & Ross, S. A. (1961). Transmission of aggression through imitation of aggressive models. *Journal of Abnormal and Social Psychology, 63,* 575–582.

Bandura, A., & Walters, R. H. (1959). *Adolescent aggression: A study of the influence of child-training practices and family interrelationships.* New York: Ronald Press.

Bandura, A., & Walters, R. H. (1963). *Social learning and personality development.* New York: Holt, Rinehart & Winston.

Banks, R., Hogue, A., Timberlake, T., & Liddle, H. (1996). An Afrocentric approach to group social skills training with inner-city African American adolescents. *Journal of Negro Education, 65,* 414–423.

Barrett, L. F. (1998). Discrete emotions or dimensions?: The role of valance focus and arousal focus. *Cognition and Emotion, 12,* 579–599.

Barrett, P. M. (1998). Evaluation of cognitive-behavioral group treatments for childhood anxiety disorders. *Journal of Clinical Child Psychology, 27,* 459–468.

Barrett, P. M. (2000). Treatment of childhood anxiety: Developmental aspects. *Clinical Psychology Review, 20,* 479–494.

Barrett, P. M., Dadds, M. R., & Rapee, R. M. (1991). *Coping Koala workbook*. Unpublished manuscript, School of Applied Psychology, Griffith University, Nathan, Australia.

Barrett, P. M., Dadds, M. R., & Rapee, R. M. (1996). Family treatment of childhood anxiety: A controlled trial. *Journal of Consulting and Clinical Psychology, 64,* 333–342.

Barrett, P. M., Duffy, A. L., Dadds, M. R., & Rapee, R. M. (2001). Cognitive–behavioral treatment of anxiety disorders in children: Long-term (6-year) follow-up. *Journal of Consulting and Clinical Psychology, 69,* 135–141.

Barrett, P. M., Healy-Farrell, L., & March, J. S. (2004). Cognitive-behavioral family treatment of childhood obsessive–compulsive disorder: A controlled trial. *Journal of the American Academy of Child and Adolescent Psychiatry, 43,* 46–62.

Barrett, P. M., Moore, A. F., & Sonderegger, R. (2000). The FRIENDS program for young former-Yugoslavian refugees in Australia: A pilot study. *Behaviour Change, 17,* 124–133.

Barrett, P. M., & Shortt, A. L. (2003). Parental involvement in the treatment of anxious children. In A. E. Kazdin & J. R. Weisz (Eds.), *Evidence-based psychotherapies for children and adolescents* (pp. 101–119). New York: Guilford Press.

Barrett, P. M., Sonderegger, R., & Sonderegger, N. L. (2001). Evaluation of an anxiety-prevention and positive coping program (FRIENDS) for children and adolescents of non-English speaking background. *Behaviour Change, 18,* 78–91.

Beal, D., Kopec, A. M., & DiGiuseppe, R. (1996). Disputing patients' irrational beliefs. *Journal of Rational-Emotive and Cognitive-Behavioral Therapy, 14,* 215–229.

Beck, A. T. (1964). Thinking and depression: II. Theory and therapy. *Archives of General Psychiatry, 10,* 561–571.

Beck, A. T. (1967). *Depression: Clinical, experimental and theoretical aspects.* New York: Hoeber.

Beck, A. T. (1976). *Cognitive therapy and the emotional disorders.* New York: International Universities Press.

Beck, A. T. (1987). Cognitive models of depression. *Journal of Cognitive Psychotherapy, 1,* 5–37.

Beck, A. T., Emery, G., & Greenberg, R. L. (1985). *Anxiety disorders and phobias: A cognitive perspective.* New York: Basic Books.

Beck, A. T., Rush, A. J., Shaw, B. F., & Emery, G. (1979). *Cognitive therapy of depression.* New York: Guilford Press.

Beck, A. T., & Shaw, B. F. (1977). Cognitive approaches to depression. In A. Ellis & R. Grieger (Eds.), *Handbook of rational-emotive therapy* (pp. 119–134). New York: Springer.

Beck, J. S. (2011). *Cognitive behavior therapy: Basics and beyond* (2nd ed.). New York: Guilford Press.

Beelman, A., Pfingsten, U., & Losel, F. (1994). Effects of training social competence in children: A meta-analysis of recent evaluation studies. *Journal of Clinical Child Psychology, 23,* 260–271.

Beidas, R. S., Benjamin, C. L., Puleo, C. M., Edmunds, J. M., & Kendall, P. C. (2010). Flexible applications of the Coping Cat Program for anxious youth. *Cognitive and Behavioral Practice, 17,* 142–153.

Beidel, D. C., Neal, A. M., & Lederer, A. S. (1991). The feasibility and validity of a daily diary for the assessment of anxiety in children. *Behavior Therapy, 22,* 505–517.

Beidel, D. C., Turner, S. M., & Morris, T. L. (2000). Behavioral treatment of child-hood social phobia. *Journal of Consulting and Clinical Psychology, 68,* 1072–1080.

Beidel, D. C., Turner, S. M., & Morris, T. L. (2004). *Social effectiveness therapy for children and adolescents (SET-C).* North Tonawanda, NY: Multi-Health Systems.

Beidel, D. C., Turner, S. M., & Young, B. J. (2006). Social effectiveness therapy for children: Five years later. *Behavior Therapy, 37,* 416–425.

Beidel, D. C., Turner, S. M., Young, B. J., Ammerman, R. T., Sallee, F. R., & Crosby, L. (2007). Psychopathology of adolescent social phobia. *Journal of Psychopathology and Behavioral Assessment, 29,* 47–54.

Bell-Dolan, D., & Wessler, A. E. (1994). Attributional style of anxious children: Extensions from cognitive theory and research on adult anxiety. *Journal of Anxiety Disorders, 8,* 79–86.

Benjamin, C. L., Harrison, J. P., Settipani, C. A., Brodman, D. M., & Kendall, P. C. (2013). Anxiety and related outcomes in young adults 7 to 19 years after receiving treatment for child anxiety. *Journal of Consulting and Clinical Psychology, 81,* 865–876.

Benson, H. (1975). *The relaxation response.* New York: Avon Books.

Berger, K. S. (2012). *The developing person through childhood* (6th ed.). New York: Worth.

Berger, K. S. (2014). *The developing person through the lifespan* (9th ed.). New York: Worth.

Bernal, G., Bonilla, J., & Bellido, C. (1995). Ecological validity and cultural sensitiv-ity for outcome research: Issues for the cultural adaptation and development of psychosocial treatments with Hispanics. *Journal of Abnormal Child Psychology, 23,* 67–82.

Bernal, G., Jiménez-Chafey, M. I., & Domenech Rodríguez, M. M. (2009). Cultural adaptation of treatments: A resource for considering culture in evidence-based practice. *Professional Psychology: Research and Practice, 40,* 361–368.

Bernstein, D. A., & Borkovec, T. D. (1973). *Progressive relaxation training: A manual for the helping profession.* Champaign, IL: Research Press.

Best, J. R., & Miller, P. H. (2010). A developmental perspective on executive func-tion. *Child Development, 81,* 1641–1660.

Bierman, K. L., & Furman, W. (1984). The effects of social skills training and peer involvement on the social adjustment of preadolescents. *Child Development, 55,* 151–162.

BigFoot, D. S., & Schmidt, S. R. (2012). American Indian and Alaska Native Chil-dren: Honoring children—mending the circle. In J. A. Cohen, A. P. Manna-rino, & E. Deblinger (Eds.), *Trauma-focused CBT for children and adolescents: Treatment applications* (pp. 280–300). New York: Guilford Press.

Bilek, E. L., & Ehrenreich-May, J. T. (2012). An open trial investigation of a transdi-agnostic group treatment for children with anxiety and depression. *Behavior Therapy, 43,* 887–897.

Birmaher, B., Brent, D., Bernet, W., Bukstein, O., Walter, H., Benson, R. S., . . . Medi-cus, J. (2007). Practice parameter for the assessment and treatment of children and adolescents with depressive disorders. *Journal of the American Academy of Child and Adolescent Psychiatry, 46,* 1503–1526.

Bornstein, M. R., Bellack, A. S., & Hersen, M. (1977). Social-skills training for unas-sertive children: A multiple-baseline analysis. *Journal of Applied Behavior Anal-ysis, 10,* 183–195.

Bornstein, M., Bellack, A. S., & Hersen, M. (1980). Social skills training for highly aggressive children: Treatment in an inpatient psychiatric setting. *Behavior Modification, 4,* 173–186.

Bouton, M. E. (2007). *Learning and behaviors: A contemporary synthesis.* Sunderland, MA: Sinauer Associates.

Bradlyn, A. S., Himadi, W. G., Crimmins, D. B.. Christoff, K. A., Graves, K. G., & Kelly, J. A. (1983). Conversational skills training for retarded adolescents. *Behavior Therapy, 14,* 314–325.

Breinholst, S., Esbjørn, B. H., Reinholdt-Dunne, M. L., & Stallard, P. (2012). CBT for the treatment of child anxiety disorders: A review of why parental involvement has not enhanced outcomes. *Journal of Anxiety Disorders, 26,* 416–424.

Broden, M., Bruce, C., Mitchell, M. A., Carter, V., & Hall, R. V. (1970). Effects of teacher attention on attending behavior of two boys at adjacent desks. *Journal of Applied Behavior Analysis, 3,* 205–211.

Broden, M., Hall, R. V., & Mitts, B. (1971). The effect of self-recording on the classroom behavior of two eighth-grade students. *Journal of Applied Behavior Analysis, 4,* 191–199.

Brownell, K. D., Marlatt, G. A., Lichtenstein, E., & Wilson, G. T. (1986). Understanding and preventing relapse. *American Psychologist, 41,* 765–782.

Burns, D. D., & Spangler, D. L. (2000). Does psychotherapy homework lead to improvements in depression in cognitive-behavioral therapy or does improvement lead to increased homework compliance? *Journal of Consulting and Clinical Psychology, 68,* 46–56.

Cannon, W. B. (1939). *The wisdom of the body.* New York: Norton.

Carey, M. P., Kelley, M., L., Buss, R. R., & Scott, W. O. N. (1986). Relationship of activity to depression in adolescents: Development of the adolescent activities checklist. *Journal of Consulting and Clinical Psychology, 52,* 774–783.

Cartledge, G., & Loe, S. A. (2001). Cultural diversity and social skill instruction. *Exceptional Children, 9,* 33–46.

Cartwright-Hatton, S., Tschernitz, N., & Gomersall, H. (2005). Social anxiety in children: Social skills deficit, or cognitive distortion? *Behaviour Research and Therapy, 43,* 131–141.

Casey, R. J., & Berman, J. S. (1985). The outcome of psychotherapy with children. *Psychological Bulletin, 98,* 388–400.

Cautela, J., & Groden, J. (1978). *Relaxation: A comprehensive manual for adults, children, and children with special needs.* Champaign, IL: Research Press.

Chambless, D. L., & Hollon, S. D. (1998). Defining empirically supported therapies. *Journal of Consulting and Clinical Psychology, 66,* 7–18.

Chambless, D. L., & Ollendick,T. H. (2001). Empirically supported psychological interventions: Controversies and evidence. *Annual Review of Psychology, 52,* 685–716.

Chavira, D. A., Bustos, C. E., Garcia, M. S., Ng, B., & Camacho, A. (2015, June 29). Delivering CBT to rural Latino children with anxiety disorders: A qualitative study. *Community Mental Health Journal.* Epub ahead of print. PMID: 26119534.

Chertock, S. L., & Bornstein, P. H. (1979). Covert modeling treatment of children's dental fears. *Child Behavior Therapy, 1,* 249–255.

Chittenden, G. F. (1942). An experimental study in measuring and modifying assertive behavior in young children. *Monographs of the Society for Research in Child Development, 7*(1, Serial No. 31).

Chorpita, B. F. (2006). *Modular cognitive-behavioral therapy for childhood anxiety disorders*. New York: Guilford Press.

Chorpita, B. F., Albano, A. M., & Barlow, D. H. (1996). Cognitive processing in children: Relation to anxiety and family influences. *Journal of Clinical Child Psychology, 25*, 170–176.

Chorpita, B. F., Becker, K. D., & Daleiden, E. L. (2007). Understanding the common elements of evidence-based practice: Misconceptions and clinical examples. *Journal of the American Academy of Child and Adolescent Psychiatry, 46*, 647–652.

Chorpita, B. F., & Daleiden, E. L. (2009). Mapping evidence-based treatments for children and adolescents: Application of the distillation and matching model to 615 treatments from 322 randomized trials. *Journal of Consulting and Clinical Psychology, 77*, 566–579.

Chorpita, B. F., Daleiden, E. L., & Weisz, J. R. (2005). Identifying and selecting the common elements of evidence-based interventions: A distillation and matching model. *Mental Health Services Research, 7*, 5–20.

Chorpita, B. F., & Southam-Gerow, M. A. (2006). Fears and anxieties. In E. J. Mash & R. A. Barkley (Eds.), *Treatment of childhood disorders* (3rd ed., pp. 271–335). New York: Guilford Press.

Chorpita, B. F., Taylor, A. A., Francis, S. E., Moffitt, C., & Austin, A. A. (2004). Efficacy of modular cognitive behavior therapy for childhood anxiety disorders. *Behavior Therapy, 35*, 263–287.

Christoff, K. A., Scott, W. O. N., Kelley, M. L., Schlundt, D., Baer, G., & Kelly, J. A. (1985). Social skills and social problem-solving training for shy young adolescents. *Behavior Therapy, 16*, 468–477.

Christopher, J. S., Hansen, D. J., & MacMillan, V. M. (1991). Effectiveness of a peer-helper intervention to increase children's social interactions: Generalization, maintenance, and social validity. *Behavior Modification, 15*, 22–50.

Christopher, J. S., Nangle, D. W., & Hansen, D. J. (1993). Social-skills interventions with adolescents. *Behavior Modification, 17*, 313–338.

Chu, B. C., Choudhury, M. S., Shortt, A. L., Pincus, D. B., Creed, T. A., & Kendall, P. C. (2004). Alliance, technology, and outcome in the treatment of anxious youth. *Cognitive and Behavioral Practice, 11*, 44–55.

Chu, B. C., & Kendall, P. C. (2004). Positive association of child involvement and treatment outcome within a manual-based cognitive-behavioral treatment for children with anxiety. *Journal of Consulting and Clinical Psychology, 72*, 821–829.

Chu, B. C., Skriner, L., & Zandberg, L. J. (2013). Trajectory and predictors of alliance in cognitive behavioral therapy for youth anxiety. *Journal of Clinical Child & Adolescent Psychology, 43*, 1–14.

Clarke, G. N., & DeBar, L. L. (2010). Group cognitive-behavioral treatment for adolescent depression. In J. R. Weisz & A. E. Kazdin (Eds.), *Evidence-based psychotherapies for children and adolescents* (2nd ed., pp. 110–125). New York: Guilford Press.

Clarke, G. N., DeBar, L. Lynch, F., Powell, J., Gale, J., O'Connor, E., . . . & Hertert, S. (2005). A randomized effectiveness trial of brief cognitive-behavioral therapy for depressed adolescents receiving antidepressant medication. *Journal of the American Academy of Child and Adolescent Psychiatry, 44*, 888–898.

Clarke, G. N., Hawkins, W., Murphy, M., Sheeber, L., Lewinsohn, P. M., & Seeley, J. (1995). Targeted prevention of unipolar depressive disorder in an at-risk sample of high school adolescents: A randomized trial of a group cognitive intervention. *American Academy of Child and Adolescent Psychiatry, 34,* 312–321.

Clarke, G. N., Hops, H., & Lewinsohn, P. M. (1992). Cognitive-behavioral group treatment of adolescent depression: Prediction of outcome. *Behavior Therapy, 23,* 341–354.

Clarke, G. N., Lewinsohn, P. M., & Hops, H. (1990). *Adolescent coping with depression course.* Eugene, OR: Castalia Press.

Clarke, G., Reid, E., Eubanks, D., O'Connor, E., DeBar, L. L., Kelleher, C., Nunley, S. (2002). Overcoming depression on the Internet (ODIN): A randomized controlled trial of an Internet depression skills intervention program. *Journal of Medical Internet Research, 4*(3), e14.

Clarke, G. N., Rohde, P., Lewinsohn, P. M., Hops, H., & Seeley, J. R. (1999). Cognitive-behavioral treatment of adolescent depression: Efficacy of acute group treatment and booster sessions. *Journal of the American Academy of Child and Adolescent Psychiatry, 38,* 272–279.

Cloitre, M., Cohen, L. R., & Koenen, K. C. (2006). *Treating survivors of childhood abuse: Psychotherapy for the interrupted life.* New York: Guilford Press.

Cohen, J. A., Deblinger, E., Mannarino, A. P., & Steer, R. A. (2004). A multisite, randomized controlled trial for children with sexual abuse-related PTSD symptoms. *Journal of the American Academy of Child and Adolescent Psychiatry, 43,* 393–402.

Cohen, J. A., Deblinger, E., Mannarino, A. P., & Steer, R. A. (2006). A follow-up study of a multisite, randomized controlled trial for children with sexual abuse-related PTSD symptoms. *Journal of the American Academy of Child and Adolescent Psychiatry, 45,* 1474–1484.

Cohen, J. A., & Mannarino, A. P. (2008). Trauma-focused cognitive behavioral therapy for children and parents. *Child and Adolescent Mental Health, 13,* 158–162.

Cohen, J. A., Mannarino, A. P., & Deblinger, E. (2006). *Treating trauma and grief in children and adolescents.* New York: Guilford Press.

Cohen, J. A., Mannarino, A. P., & Deblinger, E. (2010). Trauma-focused cognitive-behavioral therapy for traumatized children. In J. R. Weisz & A. E. Kazdin (Eds.), *Evidence-based psychotherapies for children and adolescents* (2nd ed., pp. 295–311). New York: Guilford Press.

Cohen, J. A., Mannarino, A. P., & Deblinger, E. (Eds.). (2012). *Trauma-focused CBT for children and adolescents: Treatment applications.* New York: Guilford Press.

Compton, S. N., Peris, T. J., Almirall, D., Birmaher, B., Sherrill, J., Kendall, P. C., Albano, A. M. (2014). Predictors and moderators of treatment response in childhood anxiety disorders: Results from the CAMS Trial. *Journal of Consulting and Clinical Psychology, 82,* 212–224.

Cone, J. D. (1997). Issues in functional analysis in behavioral assessment. *Behavioral Research and Therapy, 35,* 259–275.

Connolly, J., Geller, S., Marton, P., & Kutcher, S. (1992). Peer responses to social interaction with depressed adolescents. *Journal of Clinical Child Psychology, 21,* 365–370.

Constantino, G., Malgady, R. G., & Rogler, L. H. (1986). Cuento therapy: A culturally sensitive modality for Puerto Rican children. *Journal of Consulting and Clinical Psychology, 54,* 639–645.

Cooley, M. R., & Boyce, C. A. (2004). An introduction to assessing anxiety in child and adolescent multiethnic populations: Challenges and opportunities for enhancing knowledge and practice. *Journal of Clinical Child and Adolescent Psychology, 33,* 210–215.

Cooley-Quille, M., Boyd, R. C., & Grados, J. J. (2004). Feasibility of an anxiety prevention intervention for community violence exposed children. *Journal of Primary Prevention, 25,* 105–123.

Cormier, W. H., & Cormier, L. S. (1991). *Interviewing strategies for helpers: Fundamental skills and cognitive behavioral interventions* (3rd ed.). Pacific Grove, CA: Brooks/Cole.

Cormier, S., Nurius, P. S., & Osborn, C. J. (2009). *Interviewing and change strategies for helpers: Fundamental skills and cognitive-behavioral interventions* (6th ed.). Pacific Grove, CA: Brooks/Cole.

Cormier, S., Nurius, P. S., & Osborn, C. J. (2013). *Interviewing and change strategies for helpers: Fundamental skills and cognitive-behavioral interventions* (7th ed.). Pacific Grove, CA: Brooks/Cole.

Costello, E. J., Mustillo, S., Erkanil, A., Keeler, G., & Angold, A. (2003). Prevalence and development of psychiatric disorders in childhood and adolescence. *Archives of General Psychiatry, 60,* 837–844.

Costigan, G. (1965). *Sigmund Freud: A short biography.* New York: Macmillan.

Coué, E. (1922). *Self mastery through conscious autosuggestion.* New York: American Library Service.

Cox, G. R., Fisher, C. A., De Silva, S., Phelan, M., Akinwale, O. P., Simmons, M. B., & Hetrick, S. E. (2012). Interventions for preventing relapse and recurrence of a depressive disorder in children and adolescents. *Cochrane Database of Systematic Reviews, 11.* CD007504.

Craske, M. G., & Barlow, D. H. (2014). Panic disorder and agoraphobia. In D. H. Barlow (Ed.), *Clinical handbook of psychological disorders: A step-by-step treatment manual* (5th ed., pp. 1–61). New York: Guilford Press.

Crawley, S. A., Beidas, R. S., Benjamin, C. L., Martin, E., & Kendall, P. C. (2008). Treating socially phobic youth with CBT: Differential outcomes and treatment considerations. *Behavioural and Cognitive Psychotherapy, 36*(4), 379–389.

Creed, T. A., & Kendall, P. C. (2005). Therapist alliance-building behavior within a cognitive-behavioral treatment for anxiety in youth. *Journal of Consulting and Clinical Psychology, 73,* 498–505.

Cuijpers, P., Muñoz, R. F., Clarke, G. N., & Lewinsohn, P. M. (2009). Psychoeducational treatment and prevention of depression: The "coping with depression" course thirty years later. *Clinical Psychology Review, 29,* 449–458.

Curry, J., Rohde, P., Simons, A., Silva, S., Vitiello, B., Kratochvil, C., . . . the TADS Team. (2006). Predictors and moderators of acute outcome in the Treatment for Adolescents with Depression Study (TADS). *Journal of the American Academy of Child and Adolescent Psychiatry, 45,* 1427–1439.

Curry, J., Silva, S., Rohde, P., Ginsburg, G., Kratochvil, C., Simons, A., . . . March, J. (2011). Recovery and recurrence following treatment for adolescent major depression. *Archives of General Psychiatry, 68,* 263–270.

Curry, J. F., Wells, K. C., Brent, D. A., Clarke, G. N., Rohde, P., Albano, A. M., . . . March, J. S. (2000). *Treatment for Adolescents with Depression Study (TADS) cognitive behavior therapy manual: Introduction, rationale, and adolescent sessions.* Unpublished manuscript, Duke University Medical Center, Durham, NC.

David-Ferdon, C., & Kaslow, N. J. (2008). Evidence-based psychosocial treatments for child and adolescent depression. *Journal of Clinical Child and Adolescent Psychology, 37,* 62–104.

Davis, A. F., Rosenthal, T. L., & Kelley, J. E. (1981). Actual fear cues, prompt therapy, and rationale enhance participant modeling with adolescents. *Behavior Therapy, 12*, 536–542.

Davis, M., & Suveg, C. (2014). Focusing on the positive: A review of the role of child positive affect in developmental psychopathology. *Clinical Child and Family Psychology Review, 17*, 97–124.

de Arellano, M. A., Danielson, C. K., & Felton, J. W. (2012). Children of Latino descent: Culturally modified TF-CBT. In J. A. Cohen, A. P. Mannarino, & E. Deblinger (Eds.), *Trauma-focused CBT for children and adolescents: Treatment applications* (pp. 253–279). New York: Guilford Press.

De Cuyper, S., Timbremont, B., Braet, C., De Backer, V., & Wullaert, T. (2004). Treating depressive symptoms in schoolchildren. *European Child and Adolescent Psychiatry, 13*, 105–114.

de Haan, E., Hoogduin, K. A., Buitelaar, J. K., & Keijsers, G. P. (1998). Behavior therapy versus clomipramine for the treatment of obsessive–compulsive disorder in children and adolescents. *Journal of the American Academy of Child and Adolescent Psychiatry, 37*, 1022–1029.

de Souza, M. A. M., Salum, G. A., Jarros, R. B., Isolan, L., Davis, R., Knijnik, D., Manfro, G. G., & Heldt, E. (2013). Cognitive-behavioral group therapy for youths with anxiety disorders in the community: Effectiveness in low and middle income countries. *Behavioural and Cognitive Psychotherapy, 41*, 255–264.

Deblinger, E., & Heflin, A. H. (1996). *Treating sexually abused children and their nonoffending parents: A cognitive behavioral approach.* Thousand Oaks, CA: Sage.

Deffenbacher, J. L. (2000). Social skills training. In A. E. Kazdin (Ed.), *Encyclopedia of psychology* (Vol. 7, pp. 370–373). Washington, DC: American Psychological Association/Oxford University Press.

Delprato, D. J., & McGlynn, F. D. (1984). Behavioral theories of anxiety disorders. In S. M. Turner (Ed.), *Behavioral theories and treatment of anxiety* (pp. 1–49). New York: Plenum Press.

Dietz, L. J., Weinberg, R. J., Brent, D. A., & Mufson, L. (2015). Family-based interpersonal psychotherapy for depressed preadolescents: Examining efficacy and potential treatment mechanisms. *Journal of the American Academy of Child and Adolescent Psychiatry, 54*, 191–199.

Dollard, J., & Miller, N. E. (1950). *Personality and psychotherapy.* New York: McGraw-Hill.

Drysdale, A. T., Hartley, C. A., Pattwell, S. S., Ruberry, E. J., Somerville, L. H., Compton, S. N., . . . Walkup, J. T. (2014). Fear and anxiety from principle to practice: Implications for when to treat youth with anxiety disorders. *Biological Psychiatry, 75*, e19–e20.

Dugas, M., Latarte, H., Rheaume, J., Freeston, M. H., & Ladouceur, R. (1995). Worry and problem solving: Evidence of a specific relationship. *Cognitive Therapy and Research, 19*, 109–120.

Durlak, J. A., Fuhrman, T., & Lampman, C. (1991). Effectiveness of cognitive-behavior therapy for maladapting children: A meta-analysis. *Psychological Bulletin, 110*, 204–214.

D'Zurilla, T. J., & Goldfried, M. R. (1971). Problem solving and behavior modification. *Journal of Abnormal Psychology, 78*, 107–126.

D'Zurilla, T. J., & Nezu, A. M. (1982). Social problem solving in adults. In P. C. Kendall (Ed.), *Advances in cognitive-behavioral research and therapy* (Vol.1, pp. 201–274). New York: Academic Press.

D'Zurilla, T. J., & Nezu, A. M. (2007). *Problem solving therapy: A positive approach to clinical intervention.* New York: Springer.

D'Zurilla, T. J., & Nezu, A. M. (2010). Problem-solving therapy. In K. S. Dobson (Ed.), *Handbook of cognitive-behavioral therapies* (3rd ed., pp. 197–225). New York: Guilford Press.

Ehrenreich, J. T., Buzzella, B. A., Tosper, S. E., Bennett, S. M., Wright, L. A., & Barlow, D. H. (2008). *Unified protocol for the transdiagnostic treatment of emotional disorders in adolescence.* Unpublished treatment manual, University of Miami and Boston University.

Ehrenreich-May, J. T., & Bilek, E. (2009). *Emotion Detectives treatment protocol.* Unpublished treatment manual, University of Miami.

Ehrenreich-May, J. T., Bilek, E. L., Queen, A. H., & Rodriguez, J. H. (2012). A unified protocol for the group treatment of childhood anxiety and depression. *Spanish Journal of Clinical Psychology, 17,* 219–236.

Eisen, A. R., & Silverman, W. K. (1993). Should I relax or change my thoughts?; A preliminary examination of cognitive therapy, relaxation training, and their combination with overanxious children. *Journal of Cognitive Psychotherapy, 7,* 265–279.

Ellis, A. (1971). *Growth through reason.* Palo Alto, CA: Science & Behavior Books.

Ellis, A. (1977). The basic clinical theory of rational-emotive therapy. In A. Ellis & R. Grieger (Eds.), *Handbook of rational-emotive therapy* (pp. 3–34). New York: Springer Publishing.

Ellis, A., & Bernard, M. E. (1985). *Clinical applications of rational-emotive therapy.* New York: Plenum Press.

Ellis, A., & Dryden, W. (1987). *The practice of rational-emotive therapy (RET).* New York: Springer.

Evans, G. W. (2003). A multimethodological analysis of cumulative risk and allostatic load among rural children. *Developmental Psychology, 39,* 924–933.

Eysenck, H. J. (1952). The effects of psychotherapy. *Quarterly Bulletin of the British Psychological Society, 3,* 41.

Faust, J., Olson, R., & Rodriguez, H. (1991). Same-day surgery preparation: Reduction of pediatric patient arousal and distress through participant modeling. *Journal of Consulting and Clinical Psychology, 59,* 475–478.

Ferster, C. B. (1973). A functional analysis of depression. *American Psychologist, 28,* 857–870.

Ferrell, C. B., Beidel, D. C., & Turner, S. M. (2004). Assessment and treatment of socially phobic children: A cross cultural comparison. *Journal of Clinical Child and Adolescent Psychology, 33,* 260–268.

Flannery-Schroeder, E. C., & Kendall, P. C. (2000). Group and individual cognitive-behavioral treatments for youth with anxiety disorders: A randomized clinical trial. *Cognitive Therapy and Research, 24,* 251–278.

Flatt, N., & King, N. (2010). Brief psycho-social interventions in the treatment of specific childhood phobias: A controlled trial and a 1-year follow-up. *Behaviour Change, 27,* 130–153.

Flavell, J. H., Green, F. L., & Flavell, E. R. (2009). Development of children's awareness of their own thoughts. *Journal of Cognition and Development, 1,* 97–112.

Foa, E. B., & Kozak, M. J. (1986). Emotional processing of fear: Exposure to corrective information. *Psychological Bulletin, 99,* 20–35.

Foa, E. B., McLean, C. P., Capaldi, S., & Rosenfield, D. (2013). Prolonged exposure vs. supportive counseling for sexual abuse-related PTSD in adolescent girls: A randomized clinical trial. *Journal of the American Medical Association, 310,* 2650–2657.

Foster, S. L., Kendall, P. C., & Guevremont, D. C. (1988). Cognitive and social learning theories. In J. E. Matson (Ed.), *Handbook of treatment approaches in childhood psychopathology* (pp. 79–117). New York: Plenum Press.

Frame, C., Matson, J. L., Sonis, W. A., Falkov, M. J., & Kazdin, A. E. (1982). Behavioral treatment of depression in a prepubertal child. *Journal of Behavior Therapy and Experimental Psychiatry, 13,* 239–243.

Frank, E., Prien, R. F., Jarrett, R. B., Keller, M. B., Kupfer, D. J., Lavori, P. W., . . . Weissman, M. M. (1991). Conceptualization and rationale for consensus definitions of terms in major depressive disorder: Remission, recovery, relapse, and recurrence. *Archives of General Psychiatry, 48,* 851–855.

Fredrickson, B. L. (1998). What good are positive emotions? *Review of General Psychology, 2,* 300–319.

Freeman, J. B., & Garcia, A. M. (2009). *Family-based treatment for young children with OCD: Therapist guide.* New York: Oxford University Press.

Freeman, J. B., Garcia, A. M., Coyne, L., Ale, C., Przeworski, A., Himle, M., . . . Leonard, H. L. (2008). Early childhood OCD: Preliminary findings from a family-based cognitive-behavioral approach. *Journal of the American Academy of Child and Adolescent Psychiatry, 47,* 593–602.

Freeman, J., Garcia, A., Frank, H., Benito, K., Conelea, C., Walther, M., & Edmunds, J. (2014). Evidence-base update for psychosocial treatments for pediatric obsessive–compulsive disorder. *Journal of Clinical Child and Adolescent Psychology, 43,* 7–26.

Freeman, J., Sapyta, J., Garcia, A., Compton, S., Khanna, M., Flessner, C., . . . Franklin, M. (2014). Family-based treatment of early childhood obsessive–compulsive disorder: The Pediatric Obsessive–Compulsive Disorder Treatment Study for Young Children (POTS Jr)—a randomized clinical trial. *Journal of the American Medical Association Psychiatry, 71,* 689–698.

Fried, R. (1993). The role of respiration in stress and stress control: Toward a theory of stress as a hypoxic phenomenon. In P. M. Lehrer & R. L. Woolfolk (Eds.), *Principles and practice of stress management* (2nd ed., pp. 301–331). New York: Guilford Press.

Friedberg, R. D., & McClure, J. M. (2015). *Clinical practice of cognitive therapy with children and adolescents: The nuts and bolts* (2nd ed.). New York: Guilford Press.

Friedberg, R. D., McClure, J. M., & Garcia, J. H. (2009). *Cognitive therapy techniques for children and adolescents: Tools for enhancing practice.* New York: Guilford Press.

Fristad, M. A. (2006). Psychoeducational treatment for school-aged children with bipolar disorder. *Development and Psychopathology, 18,* 1289–1306.

Fristad, M. A., Goldberg Arnold, J. S., & Gavazzi, S. M. (2002). Multi-family psychoeducation groups (MFPG) for families of children with bipolar disorder. *Bipolar Disorders, 4,* 254–262.

Fristad, M. A., Goldberg Arnold, J. S., & Gavazzi, S. M. (2003). Multi-family psychoeducation groups in the treatment of children with mood disorders. *Journal of Marital and Family Therapy, 29,* 491–504.

Fristad, M. A., Goldberg Arnold, J. S., & Leffler, J. M. (2011). *Psychotherapy for children with bipolar and depressive disorders.* New York: Guilford Press.

Fristad, M. A., & McPherson, H. A. (2014). Evidence-based psychosocial treatments for child and adolescent bipolar spectrum disorders. *Journal of Clinical Child & Adolescent Psychology, 43,* 339–355.

Fristad, M. A., Verducci, J. S., Walters, K., & Young, M. E. (2009). Impact of multifamily psychoeducational psychotherapy in treating children aged 8 to 12 years with mood disorders. *Archives of General Psychiatry, 66,* 1013–1020.

Frye, A. A., & Goodman, S. H. (2000). Which social problem-solving components buffer depression in adolescent girls? *Cognitive Therapy and Research, 24,* 637–650.

Fuchs, C. Z., & Rehm, L. P. (1977). A self-control behavior therapy program for depression. *Journal of Consulting and Clinical Psychology, 45,* 206–215.

Gabrielidis, C., Stephan, W. G., Ybarra, O., Pearson, V., & Villareal, L. (1997). Preferred styles of conflict resolution: Mexico and the United States. *Journal of Cross-Cultural Psychology, 28,* 661–677.

Galassi, M. D., & Galassi, J. P. (1977). *Assert yourself!: How to be your own person.* New York: Human Sciences Press.

Garcia-Lopez, L. J., Olivares, J., Beidel, D., Albano, A. M., Turner, S. M., & Rosa, A. I. (2006). Efficacy of three treatment protocols for adolescents with social anxiety disorder: A 5-year follow-up assessment. *Journal of Anxiety Disorders, 20,* 175–191.

Garland, A. F., Accurso, E. C., Haine-Schlagel, R., Brookman-Frazee, L., Roesch, S., & Zhang, J. J. (2014). Searching for elements of evidence-based practices in children's usual care and examining their impact. *Journal of Clinical Child & Adolescent Psychology, 43,* 201–215.

Garland, A. F., Hawley, K. M., Brookman-Frazee, L., & Hurlbut, M. S. (2008). Identifying common elements of evidence-based psychosocial treatments for children's disruptive behavior problems. *Journal of the American Academy of Child and Adolescent Psychiatry, 47,* 505–514.

Gaynor, S. T., & Harris, A. (2008). Single-participant assessment of treatment mediators: Strategy description and examples from a behavioral activation intervention for depressed adolescents. *Behavior Modification, 32,* 372–402.

Gaynor, S. T., Lawrence, P. S., & Nelson-Gray, R. O. (2006). Measuring homework compliance in cognitive-behavioral therapy for adolescent depression: Review, preliminary findings, and implications for theory and practice. *Behavior Modification, 30,* 647–672.

Gearing, R. E., Schwalbe, C. J., Lee, R., & Hoagwood, K. E. (2013). The effectiveness of booster sessions in CBT treatment for child and adolescent mood and anxiety disorders. *Depression and Anxiety, 30,* 800–808.

Gee, C. B. (2004). Assessment of anxiety and depression in Asian American youth. *Journal of Clinical Child and Adolescent Psychology, 33,* 269–271.

Ginsburg, G. S., Becker, E. M., Keeton, C. P., Sakolsky, D., Piacentini, J., Albano, A. M., . . . Kendall, P. C. (2014). Naturalistic follow-up of youth treated for pediatric anxiety disorders. *JAMA Psychiatry, 71,* 310–318.

Ginsburg, G. S., Becker, K. D., Drazdowski, T. K., & Tein, J. (2012). Treating anxiety disorders in inner city schools: Results from a pilot randomized controlled trial comparing CBT and usual care. *Child and Youth Care Forum, 41,* 1–19.

Ginsburg, G. S., Burstein, M., Becker, K. D., & Drake, K. L. (2011). Treatment of obsessive–compulsive disorder in young children: An intervention model and case series. *Child and Family Behavior Therapy, 33,* 97–122.

Ginsburg, G. S., & Drake, K. L. (2002). School-based treatment for anxious

African-American adolescents: A controlled pilot study. *Journal of the American Academy of Child and Adolescent Psychiatry, 41,* 768–775.

Ginsburg, G. S., Kendall, P. C., Sakolsky, D., Compton, S. N., Piacentini, J., Albano, A. M., . . . March, J. (2011). Remission after acute treatment in children and adolescents with anxiety disorders: Findings from the CAMS. *Journal of Consulting and Clinical Psychology, 79,* 806–813.

Ginsburg, G. S., Silverman, W. K., & Kurtines, W. K. (1995). Family involvement in treating children with phobic and anxiety disorders: A look ahead. *Clinical Psychology Review, 15,* 457–473.

Gittelman, M. (1965). Behavior rehearsal as a technique in child treatment. *Journal of Child Psychology and Psychiatry, 6,* 251–255.

Glaser, R. (1971). *The nature of reinforcement.* New York: Academic Press.

Glenn, D., Golinelli, D., Rose, R. D., Roy-Byrne, P., Stein, M. B., Sullivan, G., . . . Craske, M. G. (2013). Who gets the most out of cognitive behavioral therapy for anxiety disorders?: The role of treatment dose and patient engagement. *Journal of Consulting and Clinical Psychology, 81,* 639–649.

Goldfried, M. R., & Davison, G. C. (1976). *Clinical behavior therapy.* New York: Holt, Rinehart & Winston.

Gordon-Hollingsworth, A. T., Becker, E. M., Ginsburg, G. S., Keeton, C., Compton, S. N., Birmaher, B. B., . . . March, J. S. (2015). Anxiety disorders in Caucasian and African American children: A comparison of clinical characteristics, treatment process variables, and treatment outcomes. *Child Psychiatry and Human Development, 46,* 643–655.

Gordy, J. P. (1898). *New psychology.* New York: Hinds, Noble & Eldridge.

Gosch, E. A., Flannery-Schroeder, E., Mauro, C. F., & Compton, S. N. (2006). Principles of cognitive-behavioral therapy for anxiety disorders in children. *Journal of Cognitive Psychotherapy, 20,* 247–262.

Gottman, J. M., & McFall, R. M. (1972). Self-monitoring effects in a program for potential high school dropouts: A time-series analysis. *Journal of Consulting and Clinical Psychology, 39,* 273–281.

Gould, M. S., Greenberg, T., Velting, D. M., & Shaffer, D. (2003). Youth suicide risk and preventive interventions: A review of the past 10 years. *Journal of the American Academy of Child and Adolescent Psychiatry, 42,* 386–405.

Grave, J., & Blissett, J. (2004). Is cognitive behavior therapy developmentally appropriate for young children?: A critical review of the evidence. *Clinical Psychology Review, 24,* 399–420.

Graziano, A. M., & Mooney, K. C. (1980). Family self-control instruction for children's nighttime fear reduction. *Journal of Consulting and Clinical Psychology, 48,* 206–213.

Graziano, A. M., Mooney, K. C., Huber, C., & Ignasiak, D. (1979). Self-control instruction for children's fear-reduction. *Journal of Behavior Therapy and Experimental Psychiatry, 10,* 221–227.

Greenberger, D., & Padesky, C. A. (2015). *Mind over mood: Change how you feel by changing the way you think* (2nd ed.). New York: Guilford Press.

Gresham, F. M. (1981). Social skills training with handicapped children: A review. *Review of Educational Research, 51,* 139–176.

Gresham, F. M. (2002). Best practices in social skills training. In A. Thomas & J. Grimes (Eds.), *Best practices in school psychology* (Vol. 2, pp. 1029–1040). Bethesda, MD: National Association of School Psychologists.

Gresham, F. M., & Nagle, R. J. (1980). Social skills training with children: Responsiveness to modeling and coaching as a function of peer orientation. *Journal of Consulting and Clinical Psychology, 48,* 718–729.

Gross, J., & Thompson, R. A. (2007). Conceptual foundations for the field. In J. J. Gross (Ed.), *Handbook of emotion regulation* (pp. 3–24). New York: Guilford Press.

Grosscup, S. J., & Lewinsohn, P. M. (1980). Unpleasant and pleasant events, and mood. *Journal of Clinical Psychology, 36,* 252–259.

Grover, R. L., Hughes, A. A., Bergman, R. L., & Kingery, J. N. (2006). Treatment modifications based on childhood anxiety disorders: Demonstrating the flexibility in manualized treatment. *Journal of Cognitive Psychotherapy: An International Quarterly, 20,* 275–286.

Gryczkowski, M. R., Tiede, M. S., Dammann, J. E., Jacobsen, A. B., Hale, L. R., & Whiteside, S. H. (2013). The timing of exposure in clinic-based treatment for childhood anxiety disorders. *Behavior Modification, 37,* 113–127.

Gunlicks-Stoessel, M., Mufson, L., Jekal, A., & Turner, J. B. (2010). The impact of perceived interpersonal functioning on treatment for adolescent depression: IPT-A versus treatment as usual in school-based health clinics. *Journal of Consulting and Clinical Psychology, 78,* 260–267.

Hammond, R., & Yung, B. (1991). Preventing violence in at-risk African-American youth. *Journal of Health Care for the Poor and Underserved, 2,* 359–373.

Hannesdottir, D. K., & Ollendick, T. H. (2007). The role of emotion regulation in the treatment of child anxiety disorders. *Clinical Child and Family Psychology Review, 10,* 275–293.

Hanrahan, M., Gitlin, B, Martin, J., Leavy, A., & Francis, A. (1984). Behavior therapy of anxiety disorders: Motivating the resistant patient. *American Journal of Psychotherapy, 38,* 533–540.

Hansen, D. J., Christopher, J. S., & Nangle, D. W. (1992). Adolescent heterosocial interactions and dating. In V. B. Van Hasselt & M. Hersen (Eds.), *Handbook of social development: A lifespan perspective* (pp. 371–394). New York: Plenum Press.

Hansen, D. J., MacMillan, V. M., & Shawchuck, C. R. (1990). Social isolation. In E. L. Feindler & G. R. Kalfus (Eds.), *Adolescent behavior therapy handbook* (pp. 165–190). New York: Springer.

Hansen, D. J., Nangle, D. W., & Meyer, K. A. (1998). Enhancing the effectiveness of social skills interventions with adolescents. *Education and Treatment of Children, 21,* 489–513.

Hansen, D. J., St. Lawrence, J. S., & Christoff, K. A. (1989). Group conversational-skills training with inpatient children and adolescents. *Behavior Modification, 13,* 4–31.

Hansen, D. J., Zamboanga, B. L., & Sedlar, G. (2000). Cognitive behavior therapy with ethnic-minority adolescents: Broadening our perspectives. *Cognitive and Behavioral Practice, 7,* 54–60.

Harmon, H., Langley, A., & Ginsburg, G. S. (2006). The role of gender and culture in treating youth with anxiety disorders. *Journal of Cognitive Psychotherapy, 20,* 301–310.

Hawker, D. S. J., & Boulton, M. J. (2000). Twenty years' research on peer victimization and psychosocial maladjustment: A meta-analytic review of cross-sectional studies. *Journal of Clinical Psychology and Psychiatry, 41,* 441–455.

Hayward, C., Varady, S., Albano, A. M., Thienemann, M., Henderson, L., & Schatzberg, A. F. (2000). Cognitive-behavioral group therapy for social phobia in female adolescents: Results of a pilot study. *Journal of the American Academy of Child and Adolescent Psychiatry, 39,* 721–726.

Heard, P. M., Dadds, M. R., & Conrad, P. (1992). Assessment and treatment of simple phobias in children: Effects on family and marital relationships. *Behaviour Change, 9,* 73–82.

Hedtke, K. A., Kendall, P. C., & Tiwari, S. (2009). Safety-seeking and coping behavior during exposure tasks with anxious youth. *Journal of Clinical Child and Adolescent Psychology, 38,* 1–15.

Herschell, A. D., McNeil, C. B., & McNeil, D. W. (2004). Clinical child psychology's progress in disseminating empirically supported treatments. *Clinical Psychology: Science and Practice, 11,* 267–287.

Hersen, M., & Bellack, A. S. (1976). A multiple baseline analysis of social skills training in chronic schizophrenics. *Journal of Applied Behavioral Analysis, 9,* 239–245.

Hirshfeld-Becker, D. R., Masek, B., Henin, A., Blakely, L. R., Pollock-Wurman, R. A., McQuade, J., . . . Biederman, J. (2010). Cognitive behavioral therapy for 4- to 7-year-old children with anxiety disorders: A randomized clinical trial. *Journal of Consulting and Clinical Psychology, 78,* 498–510.

Hoffman, E. C., & Mattis, S. G. (2000). A developmental adaptation of panic control treatment for panic disorder in adolescence. *Cognitive and Behavioral Practice, 7,* 253–261.

Houghton, S. J. (1991). Promoting generalisation of appropriate behaviour across special and mainstream settings: A case study. *AEP (Association of Educational Psychologists) Journal, 7,* 49–54.

Houston, J. P. (1991). *Fundamentals of learning and memory* (4th ed.). Philadelphia: Harcourt Brace.

Hudson, J. L., Hughes, A. A., & Kendall, P. C. (2004). Treatment of generalized anxiety disorders in children and adolescents. In P. M. Barrett & T. H. Ollendick (Eds.), *Handbook of interventions that work with children and adolescents: Prevention and treatment* (pp. 115–144). West Sussex, UK: Wiley.

Hudson, J. L., & Kendall, P. C. (2002). Showing you can do it: Homework in therapy for children and adolescents with anxiety disorders. *Journal of Clinical Psychology, 58,* 525–534.

Hudson, J. L., & Kendall, P. C. (2005). Children. In N. Kazantzis, F. P. Deane, K. R. Ronan, & L. L'Abate (Eds.), *Using homework assignments in cognitive behavior therapy* (pp. 75–94). New York: Routledge Taylor & Francis.

Huey, S. J., & Polo, A. J. (2008). Evidence-based psychosocial treatments for ethnic minority youth. *Journal of Clinical Child & Adolescent Psychology, 37,* 262–301.

Hughes, A. A., Hedtke, K. A., Flannery-Schroeder, E., & Kendall, P. C. (2005). *Kiddie Cat therapist manual.* Unpublished manual.

Hughes, A. A., & Kendall, P. C. (2007). Prediction of cognitive behavior treatment outcome for children with anxiety disorders: Therapeutic relationship and homework compliance. *Behavioural and Cognitive Psychotherapy, 35,* 487–494.

Hull, C. L. (1943). *Principles of behavior.* New York: Appleton.

Hunt, M. (2007). *The story of psychology* (2nd ed.). New York: Anchor Books.

Hymel, S., Wagner, E., & Butler, L. J. (1990). Reputational bias: View from the peer group. In S. R. Asher & J. D. Coie (Eds.), *Peer rejection in childhood* (pp. 156–186). New York: Cambridge University Press.

Jackson, Y. (2002). Exploring empirically supported treatment options for children: Making the case for the next generation of cultural research. *Clinical Psychology: Science and Practice, 9,* 220–222.

Jacobson, E. (1925). Progressive relaxation. *American Journal of Psychology, 36,* 73–87.

Jacobson, E. (1938). *Progressive relaxation.* Chicago: University of Chicago Press.

Jacobson, N. S., Dobson, K. S., Truax, P. A., Addis, M. E., Koerner, K., Gollan, J. K., . . . Prince, S. E. (1996). A component analysis of cognitive-behavioral treatment for depression. *Journal of Consulting and Clinical Psychology, 64,* 295–304.

Jacobson, N. S., Martell, C. R., & Dimidjian, S. (2001). Behavioral activation treatment for depression: Returning to contextual roots. *Clinical Psychology: Science and Practice, 8,* 255–270.

Jensen, T. K., Holt, T., Ormhaug, S. M., Egeland, K., Granly, L. Hoaas, L. C., . . . Wentzel-Larsen, T. (2014). A randomized effectiveness study comparing trauma-focused cognitive behavioral therapy with therapy as usual for youth. *Journal of Clinical Child & Adolescent Psychology, 43,* 356–369.

Jones, M. C. (1924). A laboratory study of fear: The case of Peter. *Journal of Genetic Psychology: Research and Theory on Human Development, 152,* 462–469.

Jung, W., & Stinnett, T. A. (2005). Comparing judgements of social, behavioural, emotional and school adjustment functioning for Korean, Korean American and Caucasian American children. *School Psychology International, 26,* 317–329.

Jungbluth, N. J., & Shirk, S. R. (2013). Promoting homework adherence in cognitive-behavioral therapy for adolescent depression. *Journal of Clinical Child & Adolescent Psychology, 42,* 545–553.

Kahn, J. S., Kehle, T. J., Jenson, W. R., & Clark, E. (1990). Comparison of cognitive-behavioral relaxation, and self-modeling interventions for depression among middle-school students. *School Psychology Review, 19,* 196–212.

Kane, M. T., & Kendall, P. C. (1989). Anxiety disorders in children: A multiple-baseline evaluation of a cognitive-behavioral treatment. *Behavior Therapy, 20,* 499–508.

Kanfer, F. H. (1970). Self-monitoring: Methodological limitations and clinical applications. *Journal of Consulting and Clinical Psychology, 35,* 148–152.

Kanter, J. W., Manos, R. C., Bowe, W. M., Baruch, D. E., Busch, A. M., & Rusch, L. C. (2010). What is behavioral activation?: A review of the literature. *Clinical Psychology Review, 30,* 608–620.

Kaslow, N. J., Rehm, L. P., & Siegel, A. W. (1984). Social-cognitive and cognitive correlates of depression in children. *Journal of Abnormal Child Psychology, 12,* 605–620.

Kaufman, N. K., Rohde, P., Seeley, J. R., Clarke, G. N., & Stice, E. (2005). Potential mediators of cognitive-behavioral therapy for adolescents with comorbid major depression and conduct disorder. *Journal of Consulting and Clinical Psychology, 73,* 38–46.

Kazantzis, N., Deane, F. P., & Ronan, K. R. (2000). Homework assignments in cognitive and behavioral therapy: A meta-analysis. *Clinical Psychology: Science and Practice, 7,* 189–202.

Kazantzis, N., & L'Abate, L. (2005). Theoretical foundations. In N. Kazantzis, F. P. Deane, K. R. Ronan, & L. L'Abate (Eds.), *Using homework assignments in cognitive behavior therapy* (pp. 9–34). New York: Routledge Taylor & Francis.

Kazantzis, N., & L'Abate, L. (2007). Introduction and historical overview. In N.

Kazantzis & L. L'Abate (Eds.), *Handbook of homework assignments in psychotherapy: Research, practice, and prevention* (pp. 1–15). New York: Springer.

Kazantzis, N., Lampropoulos, G. L., & Deane, F. P. (2005). A national survey of practicing psychologists' use and attitudes towards homework in psychotherapy. *Journal of Consulting and Clinical Psychology, 73*, 742–748.

Kazantzis, N., Wittington, C., & Dattilio, F. (2010). Meta-analysis of homework effects in cognitive and behavioral therapy: A replication and extension. *Clinical Psychology: Science and Practice, 17*, 144–156.

Kazdin, A. E. (1973). Covert modeling and the reduction of avoidance behavior. *Journal of Abnormal Psychology, 81*, 87–95.

Kazdin, A. E. (1974a). Reactive self-monitoring: The effects of response desirability, goal setting, and feedback. *Journal of Consulting and Clinical Psychology, 5*, 704–716.

Kazdin, A. E. (1974b). Self-monitoring and behavior change. In M. J. Mahoney & C. E. Thoresen (Eds.), *Self-control: Power to the person* (pp. 218–246). Monterey, CA: Brooks/Cole.

Kazdin, A. E. (1974c). The effect of model identity and fear-relevant similarity on covert modeling. *Behavior Therapy, 5*, 624–635.

Kazdin, A. E. (2000). *Psychotherapy for children and adolescents: Directions for research and practice.* New York: Oxford University Press.

Kearney, C. A., & Albano, A. M. (2007). *When children refuse school: A cognitive-behavioral therapy approach, therapist guide* (2nd ed.). New York: Oxford University Press.

Keller, M. F., & Carlson, P. M. (1974). The use of symbolic modeling to promote social skills in preschool children with low levels of social responsiveness. *Child Development, 45*, 912–918.

Kelly, G. A. (1955). *The psychology of personal constructs.* New York: Norton.

Kelly, J. A. (1982). *Social-skills training: A practical guide for interventions.* New York: Springer.

Kendall, P. C. (1989). The generalization and maintenance of behavior change: Comments, considerations, and the "No-cure" criticism. *Behavior Therapy, 20*, 357–364.

Kendall, P. C. (1990). *Coping cat workbook.* Ardmore: PA: Workbook.

Kendall, P. C. (1994). Treating anxiety disorders in children: Results of a randomized clinical trial. *Journal of Consulting and Clinical Psychology, 62*, 100–110.

Kendall, P. C. (Ed.). (2012). *Child and adolescent therapy: Cognitive-behavioral procedures* (4th ed.). New York: Guilford Press.

Kendall, P. C., & Beidas, R. S. (2007). Smoothing the trail for dissemination of evidence-based practices for youth: Flexibility within fidelity. *Professional Psychology: Research and Practice, 38*,13–20.

Kendall, P. C., Choudhury, M., Hudson, J., & Webb, A. (2002). *"The C.A.T. Project" manual for the cognitive behavioral treatment of anxious adolescents.* Ardmore, PA: Workbook.

Kendall, P. C., Comer, J. S., Marker, C. D., Creed, T. A., Puliafico, A. C., Hughes, A. A., Hudson, J. (2009). In-session exposure tasks and therapeutic alliance across the treatment of childhood anxiety disorders. *Journal of Consulting and Clinical Psychology, 77*, 517–525.

Kendall, P. C., Cummings, C. M., Villabo, M. A., Narayanan, M. K., Treadwell, K., Birmaher, B., . . . Albano, A. M. (2016). Mediators of change in the Child/

Adolescent Anxiety Multimodal Treatment Study. *Journal of Consulting and Clinical Psychology, 84*, 1–14.

Kendall, P. C., Flannery-Schroeder, E., Panichelli-Mindel, S. M., Southam-Gerow, M., Henin, A., & Warman, M. (1997). Therapy for youths with anxiety disorders: A second randomized clinical trial. *Journal of Consulting and Clinical Psychology, 65*, 366–380.

Kendall, P. C., Furr, J. M., & Podell, J. L. (2010). Child-focused treatment of anxiety. In J. R. Weisz & A. E. Kazdin (Eds.), *Evidence-based psychotherapies for children and adolescents* (2nd ed., pp. 45–60). New York: Guilford Press.

Kendall, P. C., & Hedtke, K. (2006). *Cognitive-behavioral therapy for anxious children: Therapist manual* (3rd ed.). Ardmore, PA: Workbook.

Kendall, P. C., Howard, B. L., & Epps, J. (1988). The anxious child: Cognitive-behavioral treatment strategies. *Behavior Modification, 12*, 281–310.

Kendall, P. C., Hudson, J. L., Choudhury, M., Webb, A., & Pimentel, S. (2005). Cognitive-behavioral treatment for childhood anxiety disorders. In E. D. Hibbs & P. S. Jensen (Eds.), *Psychosocial treatments for child and adolescent disorders: Empirically based strategies for clinical practice* (2nd ed., pp. 47–73). Washington, DC: American Psychological Association.

Kendall, P. C., Hudson, J. L., Gosch, E., Flannery-Schroeder, E., & Suveg, C. (2008). Cognitive behavioral therapy for anxiety disordered youth: A randomized clinical trial evaluating child and family modalities. *Journal of Consulting and Clinical Psychology, 76*, 282–297.

Kendall, P. C., Kane, M., Howard, B., & Siqueland, L. (1990). *Cognitive-behavioral therapy for anxious children: Treatment manual.* (Available from the first author, Temple University, Department of Psychology, Philadelphia, p. 19122.)

Kendall, P. C., & Khanna, M. S. (2008a). *Camp Cope-a-Lot: The Coping Cat CD-ROM* [Software]. Ardmore, PA: Workbook.

Kendall, P. C., & Khanna, M. S. (2008b). *Coach's manual for Camp Cope-a-Lot: The Coping Cat CD-ROM* [Software]. Ardmore, PA: Workbook.

Kendall, P. C., Khanna, M. S., Edson, A., Cummings, C., & Harris, M. (2011). Computers and psychosocial treatment for child anxiety: Recent advances and ongoing efforts. *Depression and Anxiety, 28*, 58–66.

Kendall, P. C., Robin, J. A., Hedtke, K. A., Suveg, C., Flannery-Schroeder, E., & Gosch, E. (2005). Considering CBT with anxious youth?: Think exposures. *Cognitive and Behavioral Practice, 12*, 136–150.

Kendall, P. C., Safford, S., Flannery-Schroeder, E., & Webb, A. (2004). Child anxiety treatment: Outcomes in adolescence and impact on substance use and depression at 7.4-year follow-up. *Journal of Consulting and Clinical Psychology, 72*, 276–287.

Kendall, P. C., & Southam-Gerow, M. A. (1996). Long-term follow-up of a cognitive-behavioral therapy for anxiety-disordered youth. *Journal of Consulting and Clinical Psychology, 64*, 724–730.

Kendall, P. C., & Suveg, C. (2006). Treating anxiety disorders in youth. In P. C. Kendall (Ed.), *Child and adolescent therapy: Cognitive-behavioral procedures* (3rd ed., pp. 243–294). New York: Guilford Press.

Kennard, B. D., Emslie, G. J., Mayes, T. L., & Hughes, J. L. (2006). Relapse and recurrence in pediatric depression. *Child and Adolescent Psychiatric Clinics of North America, 15*, 1057–1079.

Kennard, B. D., Emslie, G. J., Mayes, T. L., Nightingale-Teresi, J., Nakonezny, P. A.,

Hughes, J. L., . . . Jarrett, R. B. (2008). Cognitive-behavioral therapy to prevent relapse in pediatric responders to pharmacotherapy for major depressive disorder. *Journal of the American Academy of Child and Adolescent Psychiatry, 47*, 1395–1404.

Kennard, B. D., Silva, S. G., Vitiello, B., Curry, J., Kratochvil, C., Simons, A., . . . March, J. (2006). Remission and residual symptoms after short-term treatment in the Treatment of Adolescents with Depression Study (TADS). *Journal of the American Academy of Child and Adolescent Psychiatry, 45*, 1404–1411.

Kennard, B. D., Stewart, S. M., Hughes, J. L., Jarrett, R. B., & Emslie, G. J. (2008). Developing cognitive behavioral therapy to prevent depressive relapse in youth. *Cognitive and Behavioral Practice, 15*, 387–399.

Khanna, M. S., & Kendall, P. C. (2009). Exploring the role of parent training in the treatment of childhood anxiety. *Journal of Consulting and Clinical Psychology, 77*, 981–986.

Khanna, M. S., & Kendall, P. C. (2010). Computer-assisted cognitive behavioral therapy for child anxiety: Results of a randomized clinical trial. *Journal of Consulting and Clinical Psychology, 78*, 737–745.

King, N. J., Hamilton, D. I., & Ollendick, T. H. (1988). *Children's phobias: A behavioural perspective*. Chichester, UK: Wiley.

King, N. J., & Ollendick, T. H. (1997). Treatment of childhood phobias. *Journal of Child Psychology and Psychiatry, 38*, 389–400.

King, N. J., Ollendick, T. H., & Murphy, G. C. (1997). Assessment of childhood phobias. *Clinical Psychology Review, 17*, 667–687.

Kingery, J., Roblek, T. L., Suveg, C., Grover, R. L., Sherrill, J. T., & Bergman, R. (2006). They're not just "little adults": Developmental considerations for implementing cognitive-behavioral therapy with anxious youth. *Journal of Cognitive Psychotherapy, 20*, 263–273.

Kingery, J. N., Kepley, H. O., Ginsburg, G. S., Walkup, J. T., Silva, S. G., Hoyle, R. H., . . . March, J. S. (2009). Factor structure and psychometric properties of the children's negative cognitive error questionnaire with a clinically depressed adolescent sample. *Journal of Clinical Child and Adolescent Psychology, 38*, 768–780.

Klingman, A., Melamed, B. G., Cuthbert, M. I., & Hermecz, D. A. (1984). Effects of participant modeling on information acquisition and skill utilization. *Journal of Consulting and Clinical Psychology, 52*, 414–422.

Koeppen, A. S. (1974). Relaxation training for children. *Elementary School Guidance and Counseling, 9*, 14–21.

Kornhaber, R. C., & Shroeder, H. E. (1975). Importance of model similarity on extinction of avoidance behavior in children. *Journal of Consulting and Clinical Psychology, 43*, 601–607.

Korotitsch, W. J., & Nelson-Gray, R. O. (1999). An overview of self-monitoring research in assessment and treatment. *Psychological Assessment, 11*, 415–425.

Kupersmidt, J. B., Coie, J. D., & Dodge, K. A. (1990). In S. R. Asher & J. D. Coie (Eds.), *Peer rejection in childhood* (pp. 274–305). Cambridge, UK: Cambridge University Press.

Ladd, G. W. (1981). Effectiveness of a social learning method for enhancing children's social interaction and peer acceptance. *Child Development, 52*, 171–178.

Ladd, G. W., & Mize, J. (1983). A cognitive-social learning model of social-skill training. *Psychological Review, 90*, 127–157.

Landback, J., Prochaska, M., Ellis, J., Dmochowska, K., Kuwabara, S. A., Gladstone,

T., . . . Van Voorhees, B. W. (2009). From prototype to product: Development of a primary care/Internet based depression prevention intervention for adolescents (CATCH-IT). *Community Mental Health Journal, 45,* 349–354.

La Roche, M. J., Batista, C., & D'Angelo, E. (2011). A culturally competent relaxation intervention for Latino/as: Assessing a culturally specific match model. *American Journal of Orthopsychiatry, 81,* 535–542.

Last, C., Hansen, C., & Franco, N. (1998). Cognitive-behavioral treatment of school phobia. *Journal of the American Academy of Child and Adolescent Psychiatry, 37,* 404–411.

Lau, W., Chan, C. K., Li, J. C., & Au, T. K. (2010). Effectiveness of group cognitive-behavioral treatment for childhood anxiety in community clinics. *Behaviour Research and Therapy, 48,* 1067–1077.

Lazarus, A. A. (1971). *Behavior therapy and beyond.* New York: McGraw-Hill.

Lazarus, A. A. (1973). Multimodal behavior therapy: Treating the BASIC ID. *Journal of Nervous and Mental Disease, 156,* 404–411.

Lazarus, A. A., & Rachman, S. (1957). The use of systematic desensitization in psychotherapy. *South African Medical Journal, 31,* 334–337.

Leitenberg, H., & Callahan, E. J. (1973). Reinforced practice and reduction of different kinds of fears in adults and children. *Behaviour Research and Therapy, 11,* 19–30.

Lejuez, C. W., Hopko, D. R., & Hopko, S. D. (2001). A brief behavioral activation treatment for depression: Treatment manual. *Behavior Modification, 25,* 255–286.

Levendosky, A. A., Okun, A., & Parker, J. G. (1995). Depression and maltreatment as predictors of social competence and social problem-solving skills in school-age children. *Child Abuse and Neglect, 19,* 1183–1195.

Leventhal, H. (1984). A perceptual-motor theory of emotion. In L. Berkowitz (Ed.), *Advances in experimental social psychology* (Vol. 17, pp. 117–182). New York: Academic Press.

Lewinsohn, P. M. (1975). Engagement in pleasant activities and depression level. *Journal of Abnormal Psychology, 84,* 729–731.

Lewinsohn, P. M. (1975). The behavioral study and treatment of depression. In M. Hersen, R. M. Eisler, & P. M. Miller (Eds.), *Progress in behavior modification* (Vol. 1, pp. 19–64). New York: Academic Press.

Lewinsohn, P. M., & Amenson, C. S. (1978). Some relations between pleasant and unpleasant mood-related events and depression. *Journal of Abnormal Psychology, 87,* 644–654.

Lewinsohn, P. M., & Clarke, G. N. (1999). Psychosocial treatment for adolescent depression. *Clinical Psychology Review, 19,* 329–342.

Lewinsohn, P. M., Clarke, G. N., Hops, H., & Andrews, J. A. (1990). Cognitive-behavioral treatment for depressed adolescents. *Behavior Therapy, 21,* 385–401.

Lewinsohn, P. M., & Graf, M. (1973). Pleasant activities and depression. *Journal of Consulting and Clinical Psychology, 41,* 261–268.

Lewinsohn, P. M., Hoberman, H. M., Teri, L., & Hautzinger, M. (1985). An integrative theory of unipolar depression. In S. Reiss & R. R. Bootzin (Eds.), *Theoretical issues in behavioral therapy* (pp. 313–359). New York: Academic Press.

Lewinsohn, P. M., & Libet, J. (1972). Pleasant events, activity schedules, and depressions. *Journal of Abnormal Psychology, 79,* 291–295.

Lewinsohn, P. M., Sullivan, J. M., & Grosscup, S. J. (1980). Changing reinforcing events: An approach to the treatment of depression. *Psychotherapy: Theory, Research, and Practice, 17,* 322–334.

Lewis, S. (1974). A comparison of behavior therapy techniques in the reduction of fearful avoidance behavior. *Behavior Therapy, 5,* 648–655.

Liddle, B., & Spence, S. H. (1990). Cognitive-behaviour therapy with depressed primary school children: A cautionary note. *Behavioural Psychotherapy, 18,* 85–102.

Listug-Lunde, L., Vogeltanz-Holm, N., & Collins, J. (2013). A cognitive-behavioral treatment for depression in rural American Indian middle school students. *American Indian and Alaska Native Mental Health Research, 20,* 16–34.

Lo, H., & Fung, K. P. (2003). Culturally competent psychotherapy. *Canadian Journal of Psychiatry/Revue Canadienne de Psychiatrie, 48,* 161–170.

Lonigan, C. J., Elbert, J. C., & Bennett Johnson, S. (1998). Empirically supported psychosocial interventions for children: An overview. *Journal of Clinical Child Psychology, 27,* 138–145.

Lovaas, O. I., Berberich, J. P., Perloff, B. F., & Schaeffer, B. (1966). Acquisition of imitative speech by schizophrenic children. *Science, 151,* 705–707.

Lukens, E. P., & McFarlane, W. R. (2004). Psychoeducation as evidence-based practice: Considerations for practice, research, and policy. *Brief Treatment and Crisis Intervention, 4,* 205–225.

Lyneham, H. J., & Rapee, R. M. (2006). Evaluation of therapist-supported parent-implemented CBT for anxiety disorders in rural children. *Behaviour Research and Therapy, 44,* 1287–1300.

Mace, F. C., & Kratochwill, T. R. (1985). Theories of reactivity in self-monitoring. *Behavior Modification, 9,* 323–343.

MacPherson, H. A., Leffler, J. M., & Fristad, M. A. (2014). Implementation of multi-family psychoeducational psychotherapy for childhood mood disorders in an outpatient community setting. *Journal of Marital and Family Therapy, 40,* 193–211.

MacPhillamy, D. J., & Lewinsohn, P. M. (1982). The Pleasant Events Schedule: Studies on reliability, validity, and scale intercorrelation. *Journal of Consulting and Clinical Psychology, 50,* 363–380.

Mahoney, M. J., & Thoresen, C. E. (1974). *Self-control: Power to the person.* Monterey, CA: Brooks/Cole.

Maletzky, B. M. (1974). Behavior recording as treatment. *Behavior Therapy, 5,* 107–111.

Malgady, R. G., Rogler, L. H., & Constantino, G. (1990). Culturally sensitive psychotherapy for Puerto Rican children and adolescents: A program of treatment outcome research. *Journal of Consulting and Clinical Psychology, 58,* 704–712.

Manassis, K. (2012). *Problem solving in child and adolescent psychotherapy: A skills-based, collaborative approach.* New York: Guilford Press.

Mann, J., & Rosenthal, T. L. (1969). Vicarious and direct counter-conditioning of test anxiety through individual and group desensitization. *Behaviour Research and Therapy, 31,* 9–15.

March, J. S., & Benton, C. M. (2007). *Talking back to OCD: The program that helps kids and teens say "no way"—and parents say "way to go."* New York: Guilford Press.

March, J. S., & Mulle, K. (1998). *OCD in children and adolescents: A cognitive-behavioral treatment manual.* New York: Guilford Press.

Marks, I. M. (1987). *Fears, phobias, and rituals: Panic, anxiety, and their disorders.* New York: Oxford University Press.

Markus, H. R., & Kitayama, S. (1991). Culture and the self: Implications for cognition, emotion, and motivation. *Psychological Review, 98,* 224–253.

Marlatt, G. A., & Gordon, J. R. (Eds.). (1985). *Relapse prevention: Maintenance strategies in addictive behavior change.* New York: Guilford Press.

Martell, C. R., Addis, M. E., & Jacobson, N. S. (2001). *Depression in context: Strategies for guided action.* New York: Norton.

Mash, E. J. (2006). Treatment of child and family disturbance: A cognitive-behavioral systems perspective. In E. J. Mash & R. A. Barkley (Eds.), *Treatment of childhood disorders* (3rd ed., pp. 3–62). New York: Guilford Press.

Mash, E. J., & Barkley, R. A. (Eds.). (2006). *Treatment of childhood disorders* (3rd ed.). New York: Guilford Press.

Masia-Warner, C., Klein, R. G., Dent, H. C., Fisher, P. H., Alvir, J., Albano, A. M., & Guardino, M. (2005). School-based intervention for adolescents with social anxiety disorder: Results of a controlled study. *Journal of Abnormal Child Psychology, 33,* 707–722.

Masters, J. C., Burish, T. G., Hollon, S. D., & Rimm, D. C. (1987). *Behavior therapy: Techniques and empirical findings* (3rd ed.). Orlando, FL: Harcourt Brace Jovanovich.

Mathur, S. R., Kavale, K. A., Quinn, M. M., Forness, S. R., & Rutherford, R. B. (1998). Social skills interventions with students with emotional and behavioral problems: A quantitative synthesis of single-subject research. *Behavioral Disorders, 23,* 193–201.

Matson, J. L., Ollendick, T. H., & Adkins, J. (1980). A comprehensive dining program for mentally retarded adults. *Behaviour Research and Therapy, 18,* 107–112.

Mausbach, B. T., Moore, R., Roesch, S., Cardenes, V., & Patterson, T. L. (2010). The relationship between homework compliance and therapy outcomes: An updated meta-analysis. *Cognitive Therapy and Research, 34,* 429–438.

McDougall, W. (1908). *An introduction to social psychology.* London: Methuen.

McFarlane, W. R., Dixon, L., Lukens, E., & Lucksted, A. (2003). Family psychoeducation and schizophrenia: A review of the literature. *Journal of Marital and Family Therapy, 29*(2), 223–245.

McLeod, B. D., & Weisz, J. R. (2005). The Therapy Process Observational Coding System—Alliance Scale: Measure characteristics and prediction of outcome in usual clinical practice. *Journal of Consulting and Clinical Psychology, 73,* 323–333.

McSweeney, F. K., & Swindell, S. (2002). Common processes may contribute to extinction and habituation. *Journal of General Psychology, 129,* 364–400.

Meichenbaum, D. H., Bowers, K. S., & Ross, R. R. (1968). Modification of classroom behavior of institutionalized female adolescent offenders. *Behaviour Research and Therapy, 6,* 343–353.

Meichenbaum, D. H., & Goodman, J. (1971). Training impulsive children to talk to themselves: A means of developing self-control. *Journal of Abnormal Psychology, 77,* 115–126.

Melamed, B. G., Hawes, R. R., Heiby, E., & Glick, J. (1975). Use of filmed modeling to reduce uncooperative behavior of children during dental treatment. *Journal of Dental Research, 54,* 797–801.

Melamed, B. G., & Siegel, L. J. (1975). Reduction of anxiety in children facing hospitalization and surgery by use of filmed modeling. *Journal of Consulting and Clinical Psychology, 43,* 511–521.

Mendenhall, A. N., Fristad, M. A., & Early, T. J. (2009). Factors influencing service utilization and mood symptom severity in children with mood disorders:

Effects of multifamily psychoeducation groups (MFPGs). *Journal of Consulting and Clinical Psychology, 77,* 463–473.

Micco, J. A., Choate-Summers, M. L., Ehrenreich, J. T., Pincus, D. B., & Mattis, S. G. (2007). Efficacious treatment components of panic control treatment for adolescents: A preliminary examination. *Child and Family Behavior Therapy, 29,* 1–23.

Michelson, L., Mannarino, A. P., Marchione, K. E., Stern, M., Figueroa, J., & Beck, S. (1983). A comparative outcome study of behavioral social-skills training, interpersonal-problem-solving and non-directive control treatments with child psychiatric outpatients. *Behaviour Research and Therapy, 21,* 545–556.

Mifsud, C., & Rapee, R. M. (2005). Early intervention for childhood anxiety in a school setting: Outcomes for an economically disadvantaged population. *Journal of the American Academy of Child and Adolescent Psychiatry, 44,* 996–1004.

Miklowitz, D. J. (2007). The role of the family in the course and treatment of bipolar disorder. *Current Directions in Psychological Science, 16,* 192–196.

Miklowitz, D. J., Schneck, C. D., George, E. L., Taylor, D. O., Sugar, C. A., Birmaher, B., . . . Axelson, D. A. (2014). Pharmacotherapy and family-focused treatment for adolescents with bipolar I and II disorders: A 2-year randomized trial. *American Journal of Psychiatry, 171,* 658–667.

Miller, N. E., & Dollard, J. (1941). *Social learning and imitation.* New Haven, CT: Yale University Press.

Mize, J., & Ladd, G. W. (1990). A cognitive-social learning approach to social skill training with low-status preschool children. *Developmental Psychology, 26,* 388–397.

Monroe, S. M., Rohde, P., Seeley, J. R., & Lewinsohn, P. M. (1999). Life events and depression in adolescence: Relationship loss as a prospective risk factor for first onset major depressive disorder. *Journal of Abnormal Psychology, 108,* 606–614.

Morris, T. L. (2004). Treatment of social phobia in children and adolescents. In P. M. Barrett & T. H. Ollendick (Eds.), *Handbook of interventions that work with children and adolescents: Prevention and treatment* (pp. 171–186). West Sussex, UK: Wiley.

Mowrer, O. H. (1947). On the dual nature of learning—a reinterpretation of condition and problem solving. *Harvard Education Review, 17,* 102–148.

Mufson, L. K., Moreau, D., Weissman, M. M., & Garfinkel, R. (1999). Efficacy of interpersonal psychotherapy for depressed adolescents. *Archives of General Psychiatry, 56,* 573–579.

Mufson, L. K., Pollack Dorta, K., Moreau, D., & Weissman, M. M. (2011). *Interpersonal psychotherapy for depressed adolescents* (2nd ed.). New York: Guilford Press.

Mufson, L. K., Pollack Dorta, K., Olfson, M., Weissman, M. M., & Hoagwood, K. (2004). Effectiveness research: Transporting interpersonal psychotherapy for depressed adolescents (IPT-A) from the lab to school-based health clinics. *Clinical Child and Family Psychology Review, 7,* 251–261.

Mufson, L. K., Pollack Dorta, K. P., Wickramaratne, P., Nomura, Y., Olfson, M., & Weissman, M. M. (2004). A randomized effectiveness trial of interpersonal psychotherapy for depressed adolescents. *Archives of General Psychiatry, 61,* 577–584.

Mufson, L. K., Weissman, M. M., Moreau, D., & Garfinkel, R. (1999). Efficacy of interpersonal psychotherapy for depressed adolescents. *Archives of General Psychiatry, 56,* 573–579.

Mullins, L. L., Siegel, L. J., & Hodges, K. (1985). Cognitive problem-solving and life events correlates of depressive symptoms in children. *Journal of Abnormal Child Psychology, 20*, 523–542.

Muñoz, R. F., & Mendelson, T. (2005). Toward evidence-based interventions for diverse populations: The San Francisco General Hospital prevention and treatment manuals. *Journal of Consulting and Clinical Psychology, 73*, 790–799.

Muris, P., Merckelbach, H., Holdrinet, I., & Sijsenaar, M. (1998). Treating phobic children: Effects of EMDR versus exposure. *Journal of Consulting and Clinical Psychology, 66*, 193–198.

Nakamura, B. J., Pestle, S. L., & Chorpita, B. F. (2009). Differential sequencing of cognitive-behavioral techniques for reducing child and adolescent anxiety. *Journal of Cognitive Psychotherapy, 23*, 114–135.

Nangle, D. W., & Hansen, D. J. (1998). Adolescent heterosocial competence revisited: Implications of an expanded conceptualization for the prevention of high-risk sexual interactions. *Education and Treatment of Children, 21*, 431–446.

Nangle, D. W., Hansen, D. J., Erdley, C. A., & Norton, P. J. (Eds.). (2010). *Practitioner's guide to empirically based measures of social skills*. New York: Springer.

Nangle, D. W., Erdley, C. A., Adrian, M., & Fales, J. (2010). A conceptual basis in social learning theory. In D. W. Nangle, D. J. Hansen, C. A. Erdley, & P. J. Norton (Eds.), *Practitioner's guide to empirically based measures of social skills* (pp. 37–48). New York: Springer.

Negreiros, J., & Miller, L. D. (2014). The role of parenting in childhood anxiety: Etiological factors and treatment implications. *Clinical Psychology: Science and Practice, 21*, 3–17.

Neisser, U., Boodoo, G., Bouchard, T. J., Boykin, A., Brody, N., Ceci, S. J., ... Urbina, S. (1996). Intelligence: Knowns and unknowns. *American Psychologist, 51*, 77–101.

Nelson, R. O., & Hayes, S. C. (1981). Theoretical explanations for reactivity in self-monitoring. *Behavior Modification, 5*, 3–14.

Nelson, R. O., Lipinski, D. P., & Black, J. L. (1976). The relative reactivity of external observations and self-monitoring. *Behavior Therapy, 7*, 314–321.

Nezu, A. M. (1986). Negative life stress and anxiety: Problem solving as a moderator variable. *Psychological Reports, 58*, 279–283.

Nezu, A. M. (1987). A problem-solving formulation of depression: A literature review and proposal of a pluralistic model. *Clinical Psychology Review, 7*, 121–144.

Nicolas, G., Arntz, D. L., Hirsch, B., & Schmiedigen, A. (2009). Cultural adaptation of a group treatment for Haitian American adolescents. *Professional Psychology: Research and Practice, 40*, 378–384.

Obler, M., & Terwilliger, R. F. (1970). Pilot study on the effectiveness of systematic desensitization with neurologically impaired children with phobic disorders. *Journal of Consulting and Clinical Psychology, 34*, 314–318.

O'Connor, R. D. (1972). Relative efficacy of modeling, shaping, and the combined procedures for modification of social withdrawal. *Journal of Abnormal Psychology, 79*, 327–334.

Oden, S., & Asher, S. R. (1977). Coaching children in social skills for friendship making. *Child Development, 48*, 495–506.

Olivares, J., Garcia-Lopez, L. J., Beidel, D. C., Turner, S. M., Albano, A. M., & Hidalgo, M. D. (2002). Results at long-term among three psychological treatments for adolescents with generalized social phobia (I): Statistical significance. *Psicología Conductual, 10*, 147–164.

Ollendick, T. H. (1981). Self-monitoring and self-administered overcorrection: The modification of nervous tics in children. *Behavior Modification, 5,* 75–84.

Ollendick, T. H. (1995). Cognitive behavioral treatment of panic disorder with agoraphobia in adolescents: A multiple baseline design analysis. *Behavior Therapy, 26,* 517–531.

Ollendick, T. H., & Cerny, J. A. (1981). *Clinical behavior therapy with children.* New York: Plenum Press.

Ollendick, T. H., & King, N. J. (2004). Empirically supported treatments for children and adolescents: Advances towards evidence-based practice. In P. M. Barrett & T. H. Ollendick (Eds.), *Handbook of interventions that work with children and adolescents: Prevention and treatment* (pp. 3–25). New York: Wiley.

Ollendick, T. H., King, N. J., & Chorpita, B. F. (2006). Empirically supported treatments for children and adolescents. In P. C. Kendall (Ed.), *Child and adolescent therapy: Cognitive-behavioral procedures* (3rd ed., pp. 482–520). New York: Guilford Press.

Ollendick, T. H., Öst, L., Reuterskiöld, L., Costa, N., Cederlund, R., Sirbu, C., . . . Jarrett, M. A. (2009). One-session treatment of specific phobias in youth: A randomized clinical trial in the United States and Sweden. *Journal of Consulting and Clinical Psychology, 77,* 504–516.

O'Shea, G., Spence, S. H., & Donovan, C. L. (2015). Group versus individual interpersonal psychotherapy for depressed adolescents. *Behavioural and Cognitive Psychotherapy, 43,* 19.

Öst, L. G., Svensson, L., Hellström, K., & Lindwall, R. (2001). One-session treatment of specific phobias in youths: A randomized clinical trial. *Journal of Consulting and Clinical Psychology, 69,* 814–824.

Ott, M. J. (1996). Imagine the possibilities!: Guided imagery with toddlers and preschoolers. *Pediatric Nursing, 22,* 34–39.

Overholser, J. C. (1998). Cognitive-behavioral treatment of depression, part x: Reducing the risk of relapse. *Journal of Contemporary Psychotherapy, 28,* 381–396.

Parron, D. L. (1997). The fusion of cultural horizons: Cultural influences on the assessment of psychopathology on children. *Applied Developmental Science, 1,* 156–159.

Pavlov, I. P. (1927). *Conditioned reflexes: An investigation of the physiological activity of the cerebral cortex.* Oxford, UK: Oxford University Press.

Pediatric OCD Treatment Study Team (2004). Cognitive-behavioral therapy, sertraline, and their combination for children and adolescents with obsessive–compulsive disorder: The Pediatric OCD Treatment Study (POTS) randomized controlled trial. *Journal of the American Medical Association, 292,* 1969–1976.

Pentz, M. A., & Kazdin, A. E. (1982). Assertion modeling and stimuli effects on assertive behavior and self-efficacy in adolescents. *Behaviour Research and Therapy, 20,* 365–371.

Peris, T. S., Compton, S. N., Kendall, P. C., Birmaher, B., Sherrill, J., March, J., . . . Piacentini, J. (2015). Trajectories of change in youth anxiety during cognitive-behavior therapy. *Journal of Consulting and Clinical Psychology, 83,* 239–252.

Peterson, L., Schultheis, K., Ridley-Johnson, R., Miller, D. J., & Tracy, K. (1984). Comparison of three modeling procedures for the presurgical and postsurgical reactions of children. *Behavior Therapy, 15,* 197–203.

Peterson, L., & Shigetomi, C. (1981). The use of coping techniques to minimize anxiety in hospitalized children. *Behavior Therapy, 12,* 1–14.

Phillips, D., Fischer, S. C., & Singh, R. (1977). A children's reinforcement survey schedule. *Journal of Behavior Therapy and Experimental Psychiatry, 8*, 131–134.

Piacentini, J., & Langley, A. K. (2004). Cognitive-behavioral therapy for children who have obsessive–compulsive disorder. *Journal of Clinical Psychology, 60*, 1181–1194.

Piacentini, J., Langley, A., & Roblek, T. (2007). *Cognitive-behavioral treatment of childhood OCD: It's only a false alarm, therapist guide*. New York: Oxford University Press.

Piaget, J. (1972). Intellectual evolution from adolescence to adulthood. *Human Development, 15*, 1–12.

Pina, A. A., & Silverman, W. K. (2004). Clinical phenomenology, somatic symptoms, and distress in Hispanic/Latino and European American youths with anxiety disorders. *Journal of Clinical Child and Adolescent Psychology, 33*, 227–236.

Pina, A. A., Silverman, W. K., Fuentes, R. M., Kurtines, W. M., & Weems, C. F. (2003). Exposure-based cognitive-behavioral treatment for phobic and anxiety disorders: Treatment effects and maintenance for Hispanic/Latino relative to European-American youths. *Journal of the American Academy of Child and Adolescent Psychiatry, 42*, 1179–1187.

Pincus, D. (2000). *I can relax!: CD for children*. Boston: Child Anxiety Network.

Plienis, A. J., Hansen, D. J., Ford, F., Smith, S., Stark, L. J., & Kelly, J. A. (1987). Behavioral small group training to improve the social skills of emotionally-disordered adolescents. *Behavior Therapy, 18*, 17–32.

Premack, D. (1965). Reinforcement theory. In D. Levine (Ed.), *Nebraska Symposium on Motivation* (pp. 123–180). Lincoln: University of Nebraska Press.

Prien, R. F., Carpenter, L. L., & Kupfer, D. J. (2005). The definition and operational criteria for treatment outcome of major depressive disorder: A review of the current research literature. *Archives of General Psychiatry, 48*, 796–800.

Prins, P. J., & Ollendick, T. H. (2003). Cognitive change and enhanced coping: Missing mediational links in cognitive behavior therapy with anxiety-disordered children. *Clinical Child and Family Psychology Review, 6*, 87–105.

Rapee, R. M., Abbott, M. J., & Lyneham, H. J. (2006). Bibliotherapy for children with anxiety disorders using written materials for parents: A randomized controlled trial. *Journal of Consulting and Clinical Psychology, 74*, 436–444.

Rapee, R. M., & Spence, S. H. (2004). The etiology of social phobia: Empirical evidence and an initial model. *Clinical Psychology Review, 24*, 737–767.

Reaven, J. (2011). The treatment of anxiety symptoms in youth with high-functioning autism spectrum disorders: Developmental considerations for parents. *Brain Research, 1380*, 255–263.

Rehm, L. P. (1977). A self-control model of depression. *Behavior Therapy, 8*, 787–804.

Reinecke, M., DuBois, D., & Schultz, T. (2001). Social problem solving, mood, and suicidality among inpatient adolescents. *Cognitive Therapy and Research, 25*, 743–756.

Reynolds, W. M., & Coats, K. I. (1986). A comparison of cognitive-behavioral therapy and relaxation training for the treatment of depression in adolescents. *Journal of Consulting and Clinical Psychology, 54*, 653–660.

Reynolds, W. M., & Stark, K. D. (1985). *Procedures for the development of Pleasant Activity Schedules for Children*. Unpublished manuscript.

Reynolds, W. M., & Stark, K. D. (1987). School-based intervention strategies for the treatment of depression in children and adolescents. *Special Services in the Schools, 3,* 69–88.

Ritter, B. (1968). The group desensitization of children's snake phobias using vicarious and contact desensitization procedures. *Behaviour Research and Therapy, 65,* 1–6.

Robin, A., Schneider, M., & Dolnick, M. (1976). The turtle technique: An extended case study of self-control in the classroom. *Psychology in the Schools, 13,* 449–453.

Rogers, C. R. (1951). *Client-centered therapy.* Boston: Houghton Mifflin.

Rogers, C. R. (1961). *On becoming a person.* Boston: Houghton Mifflin.

Rohde, P., Clarke, G. N., Mace, D. E., Jorgensen, J. S., & Seeley, J. R. (2004). An efficacy/effectiveness study of cognitive-behavioral treatment for adolescents with comorbid major depression and conduct disorder. *Journal of the American Academy of Child and Adolescent Psychiatry, 43,* 660–668.

Rohde, P., Lewinsohn, P. M., & Seeley, J. R. (1994). Response of depressed adolescents to cognitive-behavioral treatment: Do differences in initial severity clarify the comparison of treatments? *Journal of Consulting and Clinical Psychology, 62,* 851–854.

Ronan, K. R., Kendall, P. C., & Rowe, M. (1994). Negative affectivity in children: Development and validation of a self-statement questionnaire. *Cognitive Therapy and Research, 18,* 509–528.

Ropovik, I. (2014). Do executive functions predict the ability to learn problem-solving principles? *Intelligence, 44,* 64–74.

Rose, D. T., & Abramson, L. Y. (1992). Developmental predictors of depressive cognitive style: Research and theory. In D. Cicchetti & S. L. Toth (Eds.), *Developmental perspectives on depression* (pp. 323–350). Rochester, NY: University of Rochester Press.

Rosenthal, T. L., & Bandura, A. (1978). Psychological modeling: Theory and practice. In S. L. Garfield & A. E. Bergin (Eds.), *Handbook of psychotherapy and behavior change: An empirical analysis* (2nd ed., pp. 621–658). New York: Wiley.

Rosselló, J., & Bernal, G. (1996). Adapting cognitive-behavioral and interpersonal treatments for depressed Puerto Rican adolescents. In E. D. Hibbs & P. S. Jensen (Eds.), *Psychosocial treatments for child and adolescent disorders: Empirically based strategies for clinical practice* (pp. 157–185). Washington, DC: American Psychological Association.

Rosselló, J., & Bernal, G. (1999). The efficacy of cognitive-behavioral and interpersonal treatments for depression in Puerto Rican adolescents. *Journal of Consulting and Clinical Psychology, 67,* 734–745.

Rosselló, J., & Bernal, G. (2005). New developments in the cognitive-behavioral and interpersonal treatments for depressed Puerto Rican adolescents. In E. D. Hibbs & P. Jensen (Eds.), *Psychosocial treatments for child and adolescent disorders* (pp. 157–187). Washington, DC: American Psychological Association.

Rosselló, J., Bernal, G., & Rivera-Medina, C. (2008). Individual and group CBT and IPT for Puerto Rican adolescents with depressive symptoms. *Cultural Diversity and Ethnic Minority Psychology, 14,* 234–245.

Rosselló, J., Bernal, G., & Rivera-Medina, C. (2012). Individual and group CBT and IPT for Puerto Rican adolescents with depressive symptoms. *Journal of Latina/o Psychology, 1*(Suppl.), 36–51.

Roth, A. D., & Pilling, S. (2008). Using an evidence-based methodology to identify the competences required to deliver effective cognitive and behavioural therapy for depression and anxiety disorders. *Behavioural and Cognitive Psychotherapy, 36,* 129–147.

Rotter, J. (1954). *Social learning and clinical psychology.* Englewood Cliffs, NJ: Prentice-Hall.

Ruggiero, K. J., Morris, T. L., Hopko, D. R., & Lejeuz, C. W. (2007). Application of behavioral activation treatment for depression to an adolescent with a history of child maltreatment. *Clinical Case Studies, 6,* 64–78.

Rush, A. J., Kraemer, H. C., Sackeim, H. A., Fava, M., Trivedi, M. H., Frank, E., . . . Schatzberg, A. F. (2006). Report by the ACNP Task Force on response and remission in major depressive disorder. *Neuropsychopharmacology, 31,* 1841–1853.

Rutner, I. T., & Bugle, C. (1969). An experimental procedure for modification of psychotic behavior. *Journal of Consulting and Clinical Psychology, 33,* 651–653.

Ryff, C. D., & Singer, B. (1996). Psychological well-being: Meaning, measurement, and implications for psychotherapy research. *Psychotherapy and Psychosomatics, 65,* 12–23.

Sacco, W. P., & Graves, D. J. (1984). Childhood depression, interpersonal problem-solving, and self-ratings of performance. *Journal of Clinical Child Psychology, 13,* 10–15.

Safran, J. D., & Greenberg, L. S. (1991). *Emotion, psychotherapy, and change.* New York: Guilford Press.

Salter, A. (1949). *Conditioned reflex therapy.* New York: Capricorn.

Samuel, G. (2008). *The origins of yoga and tantra: Indic religions to the thirteenth century.* New York: Cambridge University Press.

Sanchez-Barker, T. N. (2003). Coping with depression: Adapted for use with incarcerated Hispanic youth. *Dissertation Abstracts International: Section B. Sciences and Engineering, 64*(5–B), 2403.

Santrock, J. W. (2010). *Children* (11th ed.). New York: McGraw-Hill.

Sarver, N. W., Beidel, D. C., & Spitalnick, J. S. (2014). The feasibility and acceptability of virtual environments in the treatment of childhood social anxiety disorder. *Journal of Clinical Child & Adolescent Psychology, 43,* 63–73.

Schachter, S., & Singer, J. E. (1962). Cognitive, social, and physiological determinants of emotional state. *Psychological Review, 69,* 379–399.

Schneider, B. H. (1992). Didactic methods for enhancing children's peer relations: A quantitative review. *Clinical Psychology Review, 12,* 363–382.

Schneider, M. (1974). Turtle technique in the classroom. *Teaching Exceptional Children, 7,* 21–24.

Schunk, D. H., & Pajares, F. (2005). Competence perceptions and academic functioning. In A. J. Elliot & C. S. Dweck (Eds.), *Handbook of competence and motivation* (pp. 85–104). New York: Guilford Press.

Schwoeri, L. D., & Sholevar, G. P. (2003). Psychoeducational family intervention. In G. P. Sholevar & L. D. Schwoeri (Eds.), *Textbook of family and couples therapy* (pp. 173–192). Washington, DC: American Psychiatric Publishing.

Scott, T. J. L., & Feeny, N. C. (2006). Relapse prevention techniques in the treatment of childhood anxiety disorders: A case example. *Journal of Contemporary Psychotherapy, 36,* 151–157.

Segrin, C. (2000) Social skills deficits associated with depression. *Clinical Psychology Review, 20,* 379–403.

Seligman, L. D., & Ollendick, T. H. (2011). Cognitive behavioral therapy for anxiety disorders in youth. *Child and Adolescent Psychiatric Clinics of North America, 20,* 217–238.

Selye, H. (1956). *The stress of life.* New York: McGraw-Hill.

Selye, H. (1993). History and present status of the stress concept. In L. Goldberg & S. Breznitz (Eds.), *Handbook of stress: Theoretical and clinical aspects* (2nd ed., pp. 7–17). New York: Free Press.

Shapiro, E. S., & Cole, C. L. (1999). Self-monitoring in assessing children's problems. *Psychological Assessment, 11,* 448–457.

Sharf, R. S. (2012). *Theories of psychotherapy and counseling: Concepts and cases* (5th ed.). Belmont, CA: Brooks/Cole.

Shirk, S. R., Crisostomo, P. S., Jungbluth, N., & Gudmundsen, G. R. (2013). Cognitive mechanisms of change in CBT for adolescent depression: Associations among client involvement, cognitive distortions, and treatment outcome. *International Journal of Cognitive Therapy, 6,* 311–324.

Shirk, S. R., & Karver, M. (2003). Prediction of treatment outcome from relationship variables in child and adolescent therapy: A meta-analytic review. *Journal of Consulting and Clinical Psychology, 71,* 452–464.

Shirk, S. R., & Saiz, C. (1992). Clinical, empirical, and developmental perspectives on the therapeutic relationship in child psychotherapy. *Development and Psychopathology, 4,* 713–728.

Shure, M., & Spivack, G. (1980). Interpersonal problem solving as a mediator of behavioral adjustment in preschool and kindergarten children. *Journal of Applied Developmental Psychology, 1,* 29–44.

Shure, M. B., Spivack, G., & Gordon, R. (1972). Problem-solving thinking: A preventive mental health program for preschool children. *Reading World, 11,* 259–273.

Shure, M. B., Spivack, G., & Jaeger, M. (1971). Problem-solving thinking and adjustment among disadvantaged preschool children. *Child Development, 42,* 1791–1803.

Siegler, R. S. (1998). *Children's thinking* (3rd ed.). Upper Saddle River, NJ: Prentice-Hall.

Silverman, W. K., Ginsburg, G. S., & Kurtines, W. M. (1995). Clinical issues in treating children with anxiety and phobic disorders. *Cognitive and Behavioral Practice, 21,* 93–117.

Silverman, W. K., Kurtines, W. M., Ginsburg, G. S., Weems, C. F., Lumpkin, P. W., & Carmichael, D. H. (1999). Treating anxiety disorders in children with group cognitive-behavioral therapy: A randomized clinical trial. *Journal of Consulting and Clinical Psychology, 67,* 995–1003.

Silverman, W. K., Ortiz, C. D., Viswesvaran, C., Burns, B. J., Kolko, D. J., Putnam, F. W., & Amaya-Jackson, L. (2008). Evidence-based psychosocial treatments for child and adolescent exposed to traumatic events: A review and meta-analysis. *Journal of Clinical Child and Adolescent Psychology, 37,* 156–183.

Silverman, W. K., Pina, A. A., & Viswesvaran, C. (2008). Evidence-based psychosocial treatments for phobic and anxiety disorders in children and adolescents. *Journal of Clinical Child and Adolescent Psychology, 37,* 105–130.

Simons, A. D., Marti, N. C., Rohde, P., Lewis, C. C., Curry, J., & March, J. (2012). Does homework "matter" in cognitive behavioral therapy for adolescent depression? *Journal of Cognitive Psychotherapy, 26,* 390–404.

Skinner, B. F. (1953a). *Science and human behavior.* New York: Macmillan.

Skinner, B. F. (1953b). Some contributions of an experimental analysis of behavior to psychology as a whole. *American Psychologist, 8,* 69–78.

Skinner, B. F. (1969). *Contingencies of reinforcement: A theoretical analysis.* New York: Appleton.

Smith, A. J., Jordan, J. A., Flood, M. F., & Hansen, D. J. (2010). Social skills interventions. In D. W. Nangle, D. J. Hansen, C. A. Erdley, & P. J. Norton (Eds.), *Practitioner's guide to empirically based measures of social skills* (pp. 99–115). New York: Springer.

Solomon, P., Gordon, B., & Davis, J. M. (1984). Assessing the service needs of the discharged psychiatric patient. *Social Work in Health Care, 10,* 61–69.

Southam-Gerow, M., & Chorpita, B. F. (2006). Fears and anxieties. In E. J. Mash & R. A. Barkley (Eds.), *Treatment of childhood disorders* (3rd ed., pp. 271–335). New York: Guilford Press.

Southam-Gerow, M. A., Kendall, P. C., & Weersing, V. (2001). Examining outcome variability: Correlates of treatment response in a child and adolescent anxiety clinic. *Journal of Clinical Child Psychology, 30,* 422–436.

Spence, S. H. (2003). Social skills training with children and young people: Theory, evidence, and practice. *Child and Adolescent Mental Health, 8,* 84–96.

Spiegler, M. D. (2016). *Contemporary behavior therapy* (6th ed.). Boston: Cengage.

Spivack, G., Platt, J. J., & Shure, M. B. (1976). *The problem-solving approach to adjustment.* San Francisco: Jossey-Bass.

Stark, K. D. (1990). *Childhood depression: School-based intervention.* New York: Guilford Press.

Stark, K. D., Brookman, C. S., & Frazier, R. (1990). A comprehensive school-based treatment program for depressed children. *School Psychology Quarterly, 5,* 111–140.

Stark, K. D., Hargrave, J., Hersh, B., Greenberg, M., Herren, J., & Fisher, M. (2008). Treatment of childhood depression: The ACTION treatment program. In J. R. Z. Abela & B. L. Hankin (Eds.), *Handbook of depression in children and adolescents* (pp. 224–229). New York: Guilford Press.

Stark, K. D., Hargrave, J., Sander, J., Custer, G., Schnoebelen, S., Simpson, J., & Molnar, J. (2006). Treatment of childhood depression: The ACTION treatment program. In P. C. Kendall (Ed.), *Child and adolescent therapy: Cognitive-behavioral procedures* (3rd ed., pp. 169–216). New York: Guilford Press.

Stark, K. D., Hoke, J., Ballatore, M., Valdez, C., Scammaca, N., & Griffin, J. (2005). Treatment of child and adolescent depressive disorders. In E. D. Hibbs & P. S. Jensen (Eds.), *Psychosocial treatments for child and adolescent disorders: Empirically based practices for clinical practice* (2nd ed., pp. 239–265). Washington, DC: American Psychological Association.

Stark, K. D., & Kendall, P. C. (1996). *Treating depressed children: Therapist manual for "Taking Action."* Ardmore, PA: Workbook.

Stark, K. D., Kendall, P. C., McCarthy, M., Stafford, M., Barron, R., & Thomeer, M. (1996). *ACTION: A workbook for overcoming depression.* Ardmore, PA: Workbook.

Stark, K. D., Reynolds, W. M., & Kaslow, N. J. (1987). A comparison of the relative efficacy of self-control therapy and a behavioral problem-solving therapy for depression in children. *Journal of Abnormal Child Psychology, 15,* 91–113.

Stark, K. D., Sander, J., Hauser, M., Simpson, J., Schnoebelen, S., Glenn, R., & Molnar, J. (2006). Depressive disorders during childhood and adolescence. In E. J.

Mash & R. A. Barkley (Eds.), *Treatment of childhood disorders* (3rd ed., pp. 336–407). New York: Guilford Press.

Stark, K. D., Simpson, J., Schnoebelen, S., Hargrave, J., Molnar, J., & Glen, R. (2007). *Treating depressed youth: Therapist manual for "ACTION."* Ardmore, PA: Workbook.

Stark, K. D., Streusand, W., Krumholz, L. S., & Patel, P. (2010). Cognitive-behavioral therapy for depression. In J. R. Weisz & A. E. Kazdin (Eds.), *Evidence-based psychotherapies for children and adolescents* (2nd ed., pp. 295–311). New York: Guilford Press.

Stark, K. D., Swearer, S., Kurowski, C., Sommer, D., & Bowen, B. (1996). Targeting the child and the family: A holistic approach to treating child and adolescent depressive disorders. In E. D. Hibbs & P. S. Jensen (Eds.), *Psychosocial treatments of child and adolescent disorders: Empirically based strategies for clinical practice* (pp. 207–238). Washington, DC: American Psychological Association.

Steinberg, L. (2013). *Adolescence* (10th ed.). New York: McGraw-Hill.

Steinberg, L., & Avenevoli, S. (2000). The role of context in the development of psychopathology: A conceptual framework and some speculative propositions. *Child Development, 71,* 66–74.

Stokes, T. F., & Baer, D. M. (1977). An implicit technology of generalization. *Journal of Applied Behavior Analysis, 10,* 349–367.

Stokes, T. F., & Baer, D. M., & Jackson, R. L. (1974). Programming the generalization of a greeting response in four retarded children. *Journal of Applied Behavior Analysis, 7,* 599–610.

Stokes, T. F., & Osnes, P. G. (1989). An operant pursuit of generalization. *Behavior Therapy, 20,* 337–355.

Sue, S. (1988). Psychotherapeutic services for ethnic minorities: Two decades of research findings. *American Psychologist, 43,* 301–308.

Suveg, C., Comer, J. S., Furr, J. M., & Kendall, P. C. (2006). Adapting manualized CBT for a cognitively delayed child with multiple anxiety disorders. *Clinical Case Studies, 5,* 488–510.

Suveg, C., Hoffman, B., Zeman, J. L., & Thomassin, K. (2009). Common and specific emotion-related predictors of anxious and depressive symptoms in youth. *Child Psychiatry and Human Development, 40,* 223–239.

Suveg, C., Payne, M., Thomassin, K., & Jacob, M. L. (2010). Electronic diaries: A feasible method of assessing emotional experiences in youth? *Journal of Psychopathology and Behavioral Assessment, 32,* 57–67.

Suveg, C., Roblek, T. L., Robin, J., Krain, A., Aschenbrand, S., & Ginsburg, G. S. (2006). Parental involvement when conducting cognitive-behavioral therapy for children with anxiety disorders. *Journal of Cognitive Psychotherapy, 20,* 287–299.

Suveg, C., Sood, E., Comer, J. S., & Kendall, P. C. (2009). Changes in emotion regulation following cognitive-behavioral therapy for anxious youth. *Journal of Clinical Child & Adolescent Psychology, 38,* 390–401.

Suveg, C., & Zeman, J. (2004). Emotion regulation in children with anxiety disorders. *Journal of Clinical Child and Adolescent Psychology, 33,* 750–759.

Sweeney, P. D., Anderson, K., & Bailey, S. (1986). Attributional style in depression: A meta-analytic review. *Journal of Personality and Social Psychology, 50,* 974–991.

Task Force on Promotion and Dissemination of Psychological Procedures. (1995). Training in and dissemination of empirically-validated psychological treatments: Report and recommendations. *Clinical Psychologist, 48,* 3–23.

Thakker, J., Ward, T., & Strongman, K. T. (1999). Psychopathology and cross-cultural psychology: A constructivist perspective. *Clinical Psychology Review, 19,* 843–874.

Thomas, E. J., Abrams, K. S., & Johnson, J. B. (1971). Self-monitoring and reciprocal inhibition in the modification of multiple tics of Gilles de la Tourette's syndrome. *Journal of Behavior Therapy and Experimental Psychiatry, 2,* 159–171.

Thomassin, K., Morelen, D., & Suveg, C. (2012). Emotion reporting using electronic diaries reduces anxiety symptoms in girls with emotion dysregulation. *Journal of Contemporary Psychotherapy, 42,* 207–213.

Thorndike, E. L. (1911). *Animal intelligence.* New York: Macmillan.

Thorndike, E. L. (1913). *Educational psychology: Vol. 2. The psychology of learning.* New York: Teachers College.

Thorndike, E. L. (1935). *The psychology of wants, interests and attitudes.* Oxford, UK: Appleton-Century.

Timberlake, W., & Allison, J. (1974). Response deprivation: An empirical approach to instrumental performance. *Psychological Review, 81,* 146–164.

Titlebaum, H. (1988). Relaxation. In R. P. Zahourek (Ed.), *Relaxation and imagery: Tools for therapeutic communication and intervention* (pp. 28–52). Philadelphia: Saunders.

Tiwari, S., Kendall, P. C., Hoff, A. L., Harrison, J. P., & Fizur, P. (2013). Characteristics of exposure sessions as predictors of treatment response in anxious youth. *Journal of Clinical Child & Adolescent Psychology, 42,* 34–43.

Tolman, E. C. (1938). The determiners of behavior at a choice point. *Psychological Review, 45,* 1–41.

Tolman, E. C. (1948). Cognitive maps in rats and men. *Psychological Review, 55,* 189–208.

Torp, N. C., Dahl, K. Skarphedinsson, G., Thomsen, P. H., Valderhaug, R., Weidle, B., . . . Ivarsson, T. (2015). Effectiveness of cognitive behavior treatment for pediatric obsessive–compulsive disorder: Acute outcomes from the Nordic Long-Term OCD Treatment Study (NordLOTS). *Behaviour Research and Therapy, 64,* 15–23.

Torrey, E. F. (1997). *Out of the shadows: Confronting America's mental illness crisis.* Oxford, UK: Wiley.

Treadwell, K. R. H., Flannery-Schroeder, E. C., & Kendall, P. C. (1995). Ethnicity and gender in relation to adaptive functioning, diagnostic status, and treatment outcome in children from an anxiety clinic. *Journal of Anxiety Disorders, 9,* 373–384.

Treatment for Adolescents with Depression Study (TADS) Team. (2003). Treatment for Adolescents with Depression Study (TADS): Rationale, design, and methods. *Journal of the American Academic of Child and Adolescent Psychiatry, 42,* 531–542.

Treatment for Adolescents with Depression Study (TADS) Team. (2004). Fluoxetine, cognitive-behavioral therapy, and their combination for adolescents with depression: Treatment for Adolescents with Depression Study (TADS) randomized controlled trial. *Journal of the American Medical Association, 292,* 807–820.

Treatment for Adolescents with Depression Study (TADS) Team. (2005). Treatment for Adolescents with Depression Study (TADS): Demographic and clinical characteristics. *Journal of the American Academic of Child and Adolescent Psychiatry, 44,* 28–40.

Trower, P., Bryant, B., & Argyle, M. (1978). *Social skills and mental health*. London, UK: Methuen.

Ultee, C. A., Griffioen, D., & Schellekens, J. (1982). The reduction of anxiety in children: A comparison of the effects of "systematic desensitization in vitro" and "systematic desensitization in vivo." *Behaviour Research and Therapy, 20*, 61–67.

Umaña-Taylor, A., & Fine, M. A. (2001). Methodological implications of grouping Latino adolescents into one collective ethnic group. *Hispanic Journal of Behavioral Sciences, 23*, 347–362.

Van Hasselt, V. B., Hersen, M., Bellack, A. S., Rosenblum, N. D., & Lamparski, D. (1979). Tripartite assessment of the effects of systematic desensitization in a multi-phobic child: An experimental analysis. *Journal of Behavior Therapy and Experimental Psychiatry, 10*, 51–55.

Van Hasselt, V. B., Hersen, M., Whitehill, M. B., & Bellack, A. S. (1979). Social skills assessment and training for children: An evaluative review. *Behaviour Research and Therapy, 17*, 413–437.

Vande Voort, J. L., Svecova, J., Brown Jacobsen, A., & Whiteside, S. P. (2010). A retrospective examination of the similarity between clinical practice and manualized treatment for childhood anxiety disorders. *Cognitive and Behavioral Practice, 17*, 322–328.

Varela, R., Vernberg, E. M., Sanchez-Sosa, J. J., Riveros, A., Mitchell, M., & Mashunkashey, J. (2004). Anxiety reporting and culturally associated interpretation biases and cognitive schemas: A comparison of Mexican, American, and European American families. *Journal of Clinical Child and Adolescent Psychology, 33*, 237–247.

Vasey, M. W. (1993). Development and cognition in childhood anxiety: The example of worry. *Advances in Clinical Child Psychology, 15*, 1–39.

Vecchio, J., & Kearney, C. A. (2007). Assessment and treatment of a Hispanic youth with selective mutism. *Clinical Case Studies, 6*, 34–43.

Verdeli, H., Mufson, L., Lee, L., & Keith, J. A. (2006). Review of evidence-based psychotherapies for pediatric mood and anxiety disorders. *Current Psychiatry Reviews, 2*, 395–421.

Verduin, T. L., & Kendall, P. C. (2008). Peer perceptions and liking of children with anxiety disorders. *Journal of Abnormal Child Psychology, 36*, 459–469.

Walker, C. E. (1979). Treatment of children's disorders by relaxation training: The poor man's biofeedback. *Journal of Clinical Child Psychology, 8*, 22–25.

Walker, H. M., & Hops, H. (1973). The use of group and individual reinforcement contingencies in the modification of social withdrawal. In L. A. Hamerlynck, L. C. Hardy, & E. J. Mash (Eds.), *Behavior change: Methodology, concepts, and practice* (pp. 269–307). Champaign, IL: Research Press.

Walker, J. V., III, & Lampropoulos, G. K. (2014). A comparison of self-help (homework) activities for mood enhancement: Results from a brief randomized controlled trial. *Journal of Psychotherapy Integration, 24*, 46–64.

Walkup, J. T., Albano, A. M., Piancentini, J., Birmaher, B., Compton, S. N., Sherrill, J. T., . . . Kendall, P. C. (2008). Cognitive behavioral therapy, sertraline, or a combination in childhood anxiety. *New England Journal of Medicine, 359*, 2753–2766.

Watson, J. B. (1924). *Behaviorism*. Chicago: University of Chicago Press.

Weersing, V. R., Gonzalez, A., Campo, J. V., & Lucas, A. N. (2008). Brief behavioral therapy for anxiety and depression: Piloting an integrated treatment approach. *Cognitive and Behavioral Practice, 15*, 126–139.

Wei, C., & Kendall, P. C. (2014). Parental involvement: Contribution to childhood anxiety and its treatment. *Clinical Child and Family Psychology Review, 17*, 319–339.

Weinstein, S. M., Henry, D. B., Katz, A. C., Peters, A. T., & West, A. E. (2015). Treatment moderators of child- and family-focused cognitive-behavioral therapy for pediatric bipolar disorder. *Journal of the American Academy of Child and Adolescent Psychiatry, 54*, 116–125.

Weiss, B., Tram, J. M., Weisz, J. R., Rescorla, L., & Achenbach, T. M. (2009). Differential symptom expression and somatization in Thai versus U.S. children. *Journal of Consulting and Clinical Psychology, 77*, 987–992.

Weiss, B., & Weisz, J. R. (1995). Relative effectiveness of behavioral versus nonbehavioral child psychotherapy. *Journal of Consulting and Clinical Psychology, 63*, 317–320.

Weiss, M. G., Raguram, R., & Channabasavanna, S. M. (1995). Cultural dimensions of psychiatric illness: A comparison of the DSM-III-R and illness explanatory models in South India. *British Journal of Psychiatry, 166*, 353–359.

Weisz, J. R., Chorpita, B. F., Palinkas, L. A., Schoenwald, S. K., Miranda, J., Bearman, S. K., . . . Gibbons, R. D. (2012). Testing standard and modular designs for psychotherapy treating depression, anxiety, and conduct problems in youth: A randomized effectiveness trial. *Archives of General Psychiatry, 69*, 274–282.

Weisz, J. R., & Kazdin, A. E. (Eds.). (2010). *Evidence-based psychotherapies for children and adolescents* (2nd ed.). New York: Guilford Press.

Weisz, J. R., Weiss, B. Alicke, M. D., & Klotz, M. L. (1987). Effectiveness of psychotherapy with children and adolescents: A meta-analysis for clinicians. *Journal of Consulting and Clinical Psychology, 55*, 542–549.

Weisz, J. R., Weiss, B., Han, S., Granger, D. A., & Morton, T. (1995). Effects of psychotherapy with children and adolescents revisited: A meta-analysis of treatment outcome studies. *Psychological Bulletin, 117*, 450–468.

Wells, A. (2004). A cognitive model of GAD: Metacognitions and pathological worry. In R. G. Heimberg, C. L. Turk, & D. S. Mennin (Eds.), *Generalized anxiety disorder: Advances in research and practice* (pp. 164–186). New York: Guilford Press.

West, A. E., Henry, D. B., & Pavuluri, M. N. (2007). Maintenance model of integrated psychosocial treatment in pediatric bipolar disorder: A pilot feasibility study. *Journal of the American Academy of Child and Adolescent Psychiatry, 46*, 205–212.

Westen, D., & Weinberger, J. (2005). In praise of clinical judgment: Meehl's forgotten legacy. *Journal of Clinical Psychology, 61*, 1257–1276.

Wierzbicki, M., & Sayler, M. K. (1991). Depression and engagement in pleasant and unpleasant activities in normal children. *Journal of Clinical Psychology, 47*, 499–505.

Wilson, C., & Hughes, C. (2011). Worry, beliefs about worry and problem solving in young children. *Behavioural and Cognitive Psychotherapy, 39*, 507–521.

Winer, J. I., Hilpert, P. L., Gesten, E. L., Cowen, E. L., & Schubin, W. E. (1982). The evaluation of a kindergarten social problem-solving program. *Journal of Primary Prevention, 2*, 205–216.

Wolpe, J. (1958). *Psychotherapy by reciprocal inhibition*. Stanford, CA: Stanford University Press.

Wolpe, J. (1958). *The practice of behavior therapy*. Elmsford, NY: Maxwell House.

Wolpe, J. (1969). *The practice of behavior therapy* (2nd ed.). New York: Pergamon Press.

Wood, D., Bruner, J. S., & Ross, G. (1976). The role of tutoring in problem solving. *Journal of Child Psychology and Psychiatry and Allied Disciplines, 17*(2), 89–100.

Wood, J. J., Chiu, A. W., Hwang, W. C., Jacobs, J., & Ifekwunigwe, M. (2008). Adapting cognitive-behavior therapy for Mexican American students with anxiety disorders: Recommendations for school psychologists. *School Psychology Quarterly, 23,* 515–532.

Wright, J. H., Basco, M. R., & Thase, M. E. (2006). *Learning cognitive behavioral therapy: An illustrated guide.* Washington, DC: American Psychiatric Publishing.

Wuthrich, V. M., Rapee, R. M., Cunningham, M. J., Lyneham, H. J., Hudson, J. L., & Schniering, C. A. (2012). A randomized controlled trial of the Cool Teens CD-ROM computerized program for adolescent anxiety. *Journal of the American Academy of Child and Adolescent Psychiatry, 51,* 261–270.

Yu, D., & Seligman, M. E. P. (2002). Preventing depressive symptoms in Chinese children. *Prevention and Treatment, 5,* Article 9.

Zelazo, P. D., & Müller, U. (2002). Executive function in typical and atypical development. In U. Goswami (Ed.), *Handbook of childhood cognitive development* (pp. 445–469). Oxford, UK: Blackwell.

Zigler, E., & Phillips, L. (1961). Social competence and outcome in psychiatric disorder. *Journal of Abnormal and Social Psychology, 63,* 264–271.

Zipkin, D. (1985). Relaxation techniques for handicapped children: A review of the literature. *Journal of Special Education, 19,* 283–289.

# Index

Note: *f* or *t* following a page number indicates a figure or table.